Antioxidant and Anti-Aging Action of Plant Polyphenols

Antioxidant and Anti-Aging Action of Plant Polyphenols

Special Issue Editor
Christophe Hano

MDPI • Basel • Beijing • Wuhan • Barcelona • Belgrade • Manchester • Tokyo • Cluj • Tianjin

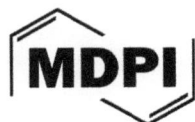

Special Issue Editor
Christophe Hano
University of Orleans
France

Editorial Office
MDPI
St. Alban-Anlage 66
4052 Basel, Switzerland

This is a reprint of articles from the Special Issue published online in the open access journal *Medicines* (ISSN 2305-6320) (available at: https://www.mdpi.com/journal/medicines/special_issues/plant_polyphenols).

For citation purposes, cite each article independently as indicated on the article page online and as indicated below:

LastName, A.A.; LastName, B.B.; LastName, C.C. Article Title. *Journal Name* **Year**, *Article Number*, Page Range.

ISBN 978-3-03936-507-4 (Hbk)
ISBN 978-3-03936-508-1 (PDF)

© 2020 by the authors. Articles in this book are Open Access and distributed under the Creative Commons Attribution (CC BY) license, which allows users to download, copy and build upon published articles, as long as the author and publisher are properly credited, which ensures maximum dissemination and a wider impact of our publications.

The book as a whole is distributed by MDPI under the terms and conditions of the Creative Commons license CC BY-NC-ND.

Contents

About the Special Issue Editor . . . . **vii**

Preface to "Antioxidant and Anti-aging Action of Plant Polyphenols" . . . . **ix**

Christophe Hano and Duangjai Tungmunnithum
Plant Polyphenols, More than Just Simple Natural Antioxidants: Oxidative Stress, Aging and Age-Related Diseases
Reprinted from: *Medicines* 2020, 7, 26, doi:10.3390/medicines7050026 . . . . **1**

Duangjai Tungmunnithum, Areeya Thongboonyou, Apinan Pholboon and Aujana Yangsabai
Flavonoids and Other Phenolic Compounds from Medicinal Plants for Pharmaceutical and Medical Aspects: An Overview
Reprinted from: *Medicines* 2018, 5, 93, doi:10.3390/medicines5030093 . . . . **11**

Aicha Hennia, Maria Graça Miguel and Said Nemmiche
Antioxidant Activity of *Myrtus communis* L. and *Myrtus nivellei* Batt. & Trab. Extracts: A Brief Review
Reprinted from: *Medicines* 2018, 5, 89, doi:10.3390/medicines5030089 . . . . **27**

Duangjai Tungmunnithum, Darawan Pinthong and Christophe Hano
Flavonoids from *Nelumbo nucifera* Gaertn., a Medicinal Plant: Uses in Traditional Medicine, Phytochemistry and Pharmacological Activities
Reprinted from: *Medicines* 2018, 5, 127, doi:10.3390/medicines5040127 . . . . **95**

Noémi Koczka, Éva Stefanovits-Bányai and Attila Ombódi
Total Polyphenol Content and Antioxidant Capacity of Rosehips of Some *Rosa* Species
Reprinted from: *Medicines* 2018, 5, 84, doi:10.3390/medicines5030084 . . . . **109**

Lucky Legbosi Nwidu, Philip Cheriose Nzien Alikwe, Ekramy Elmorsy and Wayne Grant Carter
An Investigation of Potential Sources of Nutraceuticals from the Niger Delta Areas, Nigeria for Attenuating Oxidative Stress
Reprinted from: *Medicines* 2019, 6, 15, doi:10.3390/medicines6010015 . . . . **119**

Moussa COMPAORE, Sahabi BAKASSO, Roland Nâg Tiero MEDA and Odile Germaine NACOULMA
Antioxidant and Anti-Inflammatory Activities of Fractions from *Bidens engleri* O.E. Schulz (Asteraceae) and *Boerhavia erecta* L. (Nyctaginaceae)
Reprinted from: *Medicines* 2018, 5, 53, doi:10.3390/medicines5020053 . . . . **135**

Masaaki Minami, Toru Konishi and Toshiaki Makino
Effect of Hochuekkito (Buzhongyiqitang) on Nasal Cavity Colonization of Methicillin-Resistant *Staphylococcus aureus* in Murine Model
Reprinted from: *Medicines* 2018, 5, 83, doi:10.3390/medicines5030083 . . . . **143**

Anh V. Le, Sophie E. Parks, Minh H. Nguyen and Paul D. Roach
Optimisation of the Microwave-Assisted Ethanol Extraction of Saponins from Gac (*Momordica cochinchinensis* Spreng.) Seeds
Reprinted from: *Medicines* 2018, 5, 70, doi:10.3390/medicines5030070 . . . . **155**

About the Special Issue Editor

Christophe Hano, who completed his Ph.D. in 2005 in Plant Physiology, Biochemistry, and Molecular Biology, is now an Assistant Professor at the University of Orleans at Research INRAE Lab LBLGC USC1328 and a member of the Cosm'ACTIFS Research Group (CNRS GDR3711). His research career has focused on applied plant metabolism and plant biotechnology. He has written more than 100 scientific papers, reviews, and book chapters in internationally renowned journals, and edited a variety of journal topical issues on plant secondary metabolism, including polyphenols. He is the Assistant Editor and an Editorial Board Member of several renowned Q1 Journals in Plant Biochemistry and Biotechnology. Currently, he is developing research projects aimed at studying plant secondary metabolism to lead to the development of natural products with interests in pharmacology or cosmetics. His research focuses on the elucidation of biosynthetic mechanisms of plant natural products and their exploitation by metabolic engineering approaches. He conducts research projects in cooperation with industrial companies and he coordinates the European Le Studium® Consortium Action on the bioproduction of bioactive extracts for cosmetic applications through plant cell in vitro cultures. In this context, he is exploring the potential of the Loire Valley Flora Area for cosmetic applications.

Preface to "Antioxidant and Anti-aging Action of Plant Polyphenols"

Polyphenols are plant non-nutrient natural products, or the plant secondary metabolites, found in fruits, vegetables, and seeds that we consume daily. Their intakes from fruit, vegetables, seeds, and nuts are associated with lower risks of chronic and age-related degenerative diseases. Aging is a dynamic and complex biological process involving multiple actors and is subject to a number of genetic and/or environmental influences. A variety of theories have been suggested to explain the aging process, including the famous free radical theory of aging proposed by Prof. Harman in 1956. According to this hypothesis, free radicals lead to oxidative damage, causing cellular dysfunctions and physiological decline, being responsible for aging, with the appearance of degenerative diseases and eventually death. From this hypothesis, antioxidant molecules are capable of slowing the aging process through the successful scavenging of radical oxygen and nitrogen species. Polyphenols have been shown to prolong the lifespan of different model species operating through a well-conserved antioxidant mechanism. This collection of research and review articles, "Antioxidant and Antiaging Action of Plant Polyphenols", covers the most recent advances in the use of plant polyphenols ranging from their biological properties and possible functions as medicines; the importance of traditional medicines as a source of inspiration; the rationalization of new uses of plant extracts, which has led to applications in modern medicine; the status of modern green-chemistry extraction methods; and some reflections on future prospects.

Christophe Hano
Special Issue Editor

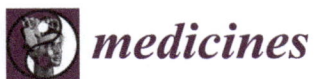

Editorial

Plant Polyphenols, More than Just Simple Natural Antioxidants: Oxidative Stress, Aging and Age-Related Diseases

Christophe Hano [1,2,*] and Duangjai Tungmunnithum [1,2,3]

1. Laboratoire de Biologie des Ligneux et des Grandes Cultures (LBLGC), INRAE USC1328, Université d'Orléans, 21 rue de Loigny la Bataille, F-28000 Chartres, France; duangjai.tun@mahidol.ac.th
2. Bioactifs et Cosmétiques, CNRS GDR3711, 45067 Orléans CEDEX 2, France
3. Department of Pharmaceutical Botany, Faculty of Pharmacy, Mahidol University, 447 Sri-Ayuthaya Road, Rajathevi, Bangkok 10400, Thailand
* Correspondence: hano@univ-orleans.fr; Tel.: +33-237-309-753; Fax: +33-237-910-863

Received: 6 May 2020; Accepted: 9 May 2020; Published: 9 May 2020

Abstract: The present editorial serves as an introduction to the Special Issue "Antioxidant and Anti-aging Action of Plant Polyphenols". It also provides a summary of the polyphenols, their biological properties and possible functions as medicines, the importance of traditional medicines as a source of inspiration, the rationalization of new uses of plant extracts which lead to applications in modern medicine, the status of modern green-chemistry extraction methods, and some reflections on future prospects. Here, the articles from this Special Issue, and the main aspects of the antioxidant and anti-aging effects of plant polyphenols are discussed in the form of seven questions.

Keywords: aging; age-related diseases; antioxidant; coumarins; flavonoids; lignans; phenolic acids; polyphenols; stilbenes

---

1. What Are These Polyphenols?

Polyphenols are plant non-nutrient natural products or the so-called plant secondary metabolites found in fruits, vegetables and seeds that we consume daily. Polyphenols are a large family of compounds derived from secondary metabolism that are widespread in the plant kingdom. Most of these are derived from l-phenylalanine through the phenylpropanoid pathway. Sensu stricto, polyphenols are characterized by the presence of at least two phenolic groups associated in more or less complex structures, generally of high molecular weight, but simple phenolics (aka phenolic acids), that could be polyphenol precursors, are also considered to belong to this group. The most commonly used definition is: "The term "polyphenol" should be used to define compounds exclusively derived from the shikimate/phenylpropanoid and/or the polyketide pathway, featuring more than one phenolic unit and deprived of nitrogen-based functions" [1]. Polyphenols, therefore, include, but are not limited to, phenolic acids, coumarins, flavonoids, stilbenes and lignans (Figure 1). Other polymerized forms, such as tannins and lignins, are also included. Some of them are responsible for the aroma, color, antioxidant properties of the fruit, vegetables, seeds and nuts that we consumed. Polyphenols are becoming increasingly important, in particular because of their beneficial effects on health. Indeed, their role as natural antioxidants is increasing in the prevention and treatment of cancer [2–4], inflammatory, cardiovascular and neurodegenerative diseases [1]. Their intakes from fruit, vegetables, seeds, and nuts have been associated with lower risks of chronic and age-related degenerative diseases [5,6]. They have a wide range of applications as food supplements, pharmaceutical and cosmetic additives [1–14].

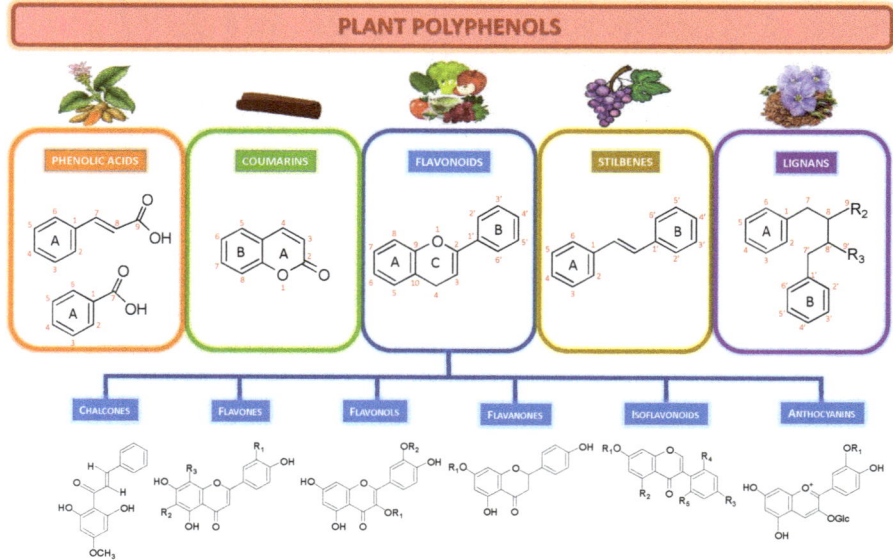

Figure 1. Polyphenol classification including phenolic acids, coumarins, flavonoids and their subgroups, stilbenes, and lignans.

The various main classes of natural polyphenols are shown in Figure 1.

Phenolic acids (or phenolcarboxylic acids) are types of compound aromatic acids that contain an organic carboxylic acid function and a phenolic ring. Hydroxybenzoic acids (C6–C1 backbone), and hydroxycinnamic acids (C6–C3 backbone) are two essential forms of naturally occurring phenolic acids. These groups include benzoic acid, p-coumaric acid, but also more complex phenolic acids, such as curcumin from turmeric.

Coumarins are benzopyrone (1,2-benzopyrones or 2H-1-benzopyran-2-ones) derivatives widely distributed in nature. Their name derives from the French word "coumarou" for the Tonka bean (*Dipteryx odorata*, Fabaceae), from which Vogel isolated coumarin in 1820. Chinese cinnamon is rich in coumarin derivatives.

Flavonoids are C6-C3-C6 phenylpropanoids consisting of two phenyl rings (rings A and B) and one heterocyclic ring (ring C). This group encompasses most antioxidants from fruits and vegetables, such as quercetin, kaempferol, isorhamnetin, fisetin, genistein. Flavonoids can be subdivided into different subgroups according to the carbon of the ring C connected to the ring B and the degree of unsaturation and oxidation of the ring C. Flavonoids in which the B ring is connected to position 3 of the C ring are called isoflavones. Those in which the B ring is associated in position 2 of the C ring can be further subdivided into several subgroups:

- Chalcones, characterized by the absence of ring C, therefore also called open-chain flavonoids.
- Flavones, with a double bond between positions 2 and 3 and a ketone on the ring C at position 4. Most of them have a hydroxy group in position 5 of the ring A, while hydroxylation in other positions, often in position 7 of the A ring or positions 3' and 4' of the B ring, are also commonly observed.
- Flavonols, the most common and the largest flavonoid subgroup, with a ketone and a hydroxyl group in position 3 of ring C. Flavonols exhibit various patterns of hydroxylation, methylation, and glycosylation. They can constitute the building blocks of proanthocyanin.

- Flavanones, with a fully saturated ring C. Unlike flavones, the double bond between positions 2 and 3 is saturated: this is the unique structural difference between these two subgroups.
- Anthocyanins, pigments responsible for the coloring of plants, flowers and fruits, which can vary depending on the methylation or acylation of the hydroxyl groups on the rings A and B but also the pH.

Stilbenes (aka stilbenoids) have a carbon backbone C6-C2-C6, namely the *trans*- ((E)-stilbenes) and *cis*-((Z)-stilbenes) 1,2-diphenylethylene structures. This group includes resveratrol from grape and wine.

Lignans are biphenolic compounds formed from the oxidative coupling of two monolignol (hydroxycinnamic alcohol) units. These same basic units are also used by plants to synthesize lignin, present in the walls of the conducting vessels. There are very many lignans, which differ in the type of bond between the two units and the changes that occur after dimerization. Secoisolariciresinol is one of the most common dietary lignans found in high amounts in flaxseeds.

2. How Can Simple Antioxidant Polyphenols Counteract Aging and Age-Related Diseases?

Aging is a dynamic and complex biological process involving multiple actors and subject to a number of genetic and/or environmental influences [15]. A variety of theories were suggested to explain the aging process, including the free radical theory of aging proposed by Prof. Harman in 1956 [16]. Undoubtedly, this theory was the most widely studied and continues to be revised, and so far, it remains a sound theory [17]. The theory explains that aging can be caused by excessive oxidative stress (Figure 2) [17].

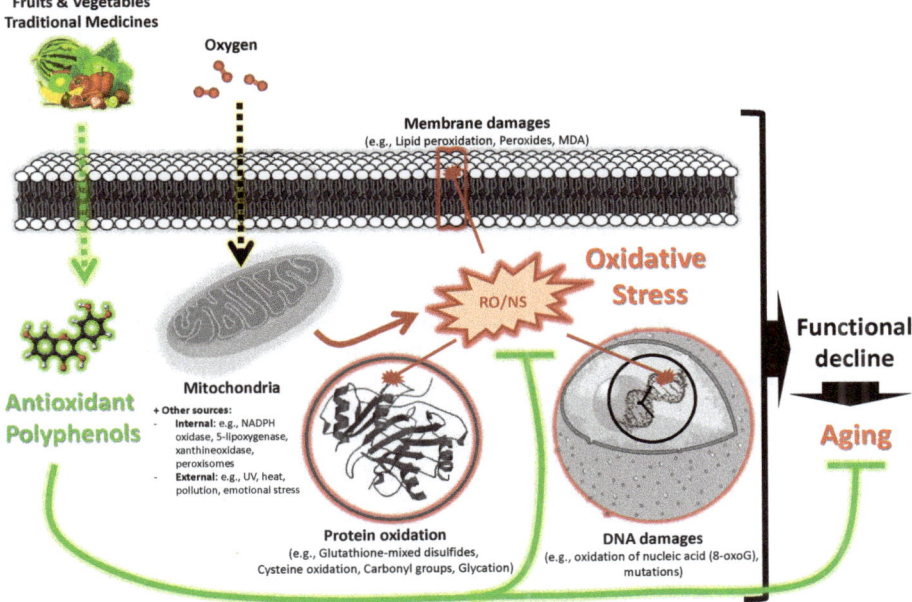

Figure 2. Schematic view of the premise behind the free radical theory of aging [16,17]. Mitochondria and other internal or external sources produced excessive oxidative stress (ROS/RNS) leading to oxidative damage to various cell macromolecules (membrane lipids, proteins and DNA) resulting in functional declines, aging and ultimately death.

During oxidative phosphorylation, reactive oxygen and nitrogen species (ROS/RNS) are mainly formed within mitochondria, although these are generated by additional endogenous and exogenous factors. A network of endogenous and exogenous antioxidants neutralizes ROS/RNS, although some ROS/RNS still bypass these defensive systems. These escaped ROS/RNS subsequently cause oxidative damage to cellular components, including lipids, proteins, nucleic acids, etc. While mechanisms exist for repairing oxidatively damaged biomolecules, some damage remains. From this observation, the free radical aging theory assumes that ROS/RNS induce oxidative damage, causing cell dysfunction and physiological decline, leading to aging, with the appearance of degenerative diseases, and eventually death. This hypothesis therefore indicates that antioxidants which were successful in scavenging ROS/RNS are capable of slowing down the aging process. In line with this, studies have shown that different plant-derived antioxidants, in particular polyphenols, may have a therapeutic potential for aging and age-related diseases [18–21].

Evidence that polyphenols such as resveratrol and quercetin have prolonged the lifespan of different species, operating through a well-conserved mechanism, was first described in yeast and then confirmed in many other model species such as *Caenorhabditis elegans*, *Drosophila melanogaster* and mice [18,19,22]. Yeast cells prove to be an excellent model for evaluating the in vivo antioxidant capacity of polyphenols in the context of cellular oxidative stress [10,23–28]. It is also an attractive and stable eukaryotic model, whose mechanisms of defense and adaptation to oxidative stress are well established and can be extrapolated to human cells [23–25].

3. What Are the Polyphenols Used to Promote Human Health?

Beyond the simple antioxidant activity, the question of the health promotion action of polyphenols is a vast one. This point has been discussed in several papers in this Special Issue. In particular, in their review "Flavonoids and Other Phenolic Compounds from Medicinal Plants for Pharmaceutical and Medical Aspects: An Overview", Tungmunnithum et al. [6] provide a comprehensive and synthetic description of the biological activities of plant polyphenols (flavonoids and phenolic compounds) in relation to their applied or potential pharmaceutical and medicinal potential. The authors present the effects of plant flavonoids and other phenolic substances on the promotion of human health, curing and prevention of diseases, including their antioxidant, antibacterial, anti-cancer, cardioprotective, immune system promoting, anti-inflammatory and skin protective actions. The natural plant phenolics and flavonoids with an interest in menopausal and postmenopausal women are also presented. Interestingly, the work of profiling and surveying flavonoids and other phenolics from medicinal plants is critically discussed, in particular, on the significant impact on the phytochemical quantity and composition of genetic (e.g., various ecotypes) and environmental factors, which represent a major challenge for the rationalization of traditional uses of medicinal plants, but also for their future use in modern medicine. Future perspectives and interesting directions for future research are also presented.

It is now recognized that the health-promoting effects of polyphenols are broader than their "basic" antioxidant function. The control of aging and degenerative diseases by polyphenols has also been linked to their ability to inhibit some enzymes such as cyclooxygenases and lipoxygenase 15 involved in inflammation [29] or acetylcholinesterase [30], associated with some neurodegenerative diseases in which oxidative stress and cholinergic deficiency create favorable conditions for Alzheimer's disease or Parkinson's disease. Minami et al. [31] describe an interesting action with Hochuekkito, a polyphenol-rich formula composed of 10 herbal medicines in traditional Kampo medicine, for the treatment of methicillin-resistant *Staphylococcus aureus* nasal colonization in the murine model, thus suggesting it as a serious therapeutic candidate for successful therapy in humans. Oxidative stress cross-talk between the host and *S. aureus* has been described as essential for nasal colonization [32,33]. It is therefore not excluded that polyphenols may interfere with this oxidative cross-talk.

4. To What Extent Can Traditional Medicines Be a Source of Inspiration?

The medical use of plants to treat, diagnose and prevent disease or maintain health is an important part of traditional medicine. Traditional medicines are an important source of inspiration for so-called modern medicine, which can contribute to the (re)discovery of lead remedies, as demonstrated by the success of antimalaria artemisinin and the Nobel Prize for the work of Prof. Tu Youyou. Beyond this well-deserved individual award, which comes to reward outstanding work, this award also highlights traditional medicines. We need to keep in mind that this is not an isolated case. Many plants have been used as an essential ingredient for various traditional medicines, such as traditional Chinese, Indian, Japanese, Thai, Korean, African, American or European medicines, and many new or unknown bioactive compounds have been discovered thanks to this ancient knowledge. In order to exemplify this traditional knowledge and how it continues to influence modern medicine through this special topic, a focus is placed on several plant species grown in various regions across the world, and used in various traditional medicines around the globe.

Some papers focused on a single plant species, such as *Nelumbo nucifera*, widely used as an active component of traditional Chinese, Indian, Japanese, Thai and Korean medicines, and many others for a number of medicinal purposes, as shown in the review by Tungmunnithum et al. [34]. Le et al. [35] propose a green extraction of bioactive compounds from the fruits of Gac or *Momordica cochinchinensis* (Lour.) Spreng., a medicinally essential plant from northeastern Australia but also found in southern China, Thailand, Laos, Myanmar, Cambodia and Vietnam.

Other papers pointed to the interest of several species of the same genus, allowing interesting cross-species comparisons, as reported by Koczka et al. [36] with *Rosa* species cultivated since ancient times, with a particular focus on *R. spinosissima, R. canina, R. rugosa, R. gallica* present throughout Europe, temperate Asia and North America, which have been used for their medicinal benefits for thousands of years. This is also the case with the work presented by Hennia et al. [37] on two *Myrtus* species, from the Mediterranean region (*M. communis* L., myrtle) and the Central Saharan Mountains (*M. nivellei* Batt. and Trab, Saharan myrtle)) used in folk medicines at the crossroads of different forms of traditional knowledge from both sides of the Mediterranean Basin.

Also considered were different plant species from the same regions. Campaore et al. [29] presented work on two plant species from the Gampela region, located in the middle east of Kadiogo (central region, Burkina Faso), *Bidens engleri* (O.E. Schulz, Asteraceae) and the erect spiderling *Boerhavia erecta* (L., Nyctaginaceae), two well-known medicinal plants traditionally used in Burkina Faso and Cote d'Ivoire. Nwidu et al. [30] present a comprehensive ethnobotanical survey of plants from Niger Delta region (Nigeria) showing in particular the interest in *Musa paradisiaca, Dennettia tripetala, Moringa oleifera, Tetrapleura tetraptera, Terminalia catappa* and *Mangifera indica*.

Traditional medicine often used complex mixtures of various plant species in which the beneficial action resulted from synergies. As a result, the rationalization of the biological activity involved very challenging research in this situation. Minami et al. [31] present very interesting results on the biological evaluation (*in vitro* and animal model) of Hochuekkito, a formula composed 10 herbal medicines from traditional Kampo medicine. Minami et al. [31], in particular, show that if a single crude extract from *Astragali radix, Bupleuri radix, Zingiberis rhizoma*, and *Cimicifugae rhizome* is excluded from the Hochuekkito formula, the biological activity of the resulting new formula is significantly weakened.

5. How Can the Biological Activity of Conventional Plant Uses Be Rationalized Scientifically?

Scientific validation of the traditional uses of a medicinal plant is a crucial step before it becomes a lead drug, there are many applicants and few are chosen to consider the success of artemisinin as exceptional. Most of the traditional uses of medicinal plant species extracts need more research investigations before contributing to the discovery and large-scale production of potent drugs. Without being exhaustive, this Special Issue sheds light on a number of important considerations concerning the scientific rationalization of the biological activity of traditional medicinal plants. There may be several local names for the same plant, depending on the region and country, for the use of traditional medicines, and there may also be a similar name for another plant. Consequently, the authentication of a plant species is a critical issue to consider [34,37], and must be carried out before the biological evaluation or its use for medical and pharmaceutical applications. Authentication is a first step but several genetic and/or environmental factors may influence the phytochemical profile of a plant extract, and hence its biological activity [34,36]. The same observation can be made for extraction, and the conditions of extraction, in particular the selection of the extract solvent, can have a significant effect on the phytochemical composition of the extract and therefore on its activity [29,36]. The more complete phytochemical characterization of the extract is essential for achieving reproducible results, but our understanding of this composition is affected by the choice of the analytical method (UV-visible absorption, HPLC or GC coupled or not with mass spectrometry) and its resolution [34,37]. Identifying the bioactive compound(s) may be relevant, but sometimes the observed activity may be the result of complex synergism between different compounds from different plant extracts making it difficult to identify them [31]. Biological evaluation may be carried out in vitro as a first high-throughput screening, allowing the simultaneous evaluation of several extracts from different plants/conditions, prior to their evaluation *in cellulo* and/or with animal models, and prior to a more comprehensive toxicity assessment, clinical trials or epidemiological studies [29–31,34–37].

6. What Position Do the Modern Green-Chemistry Extraction Methods Have?

A number of methods for extracting natural antioxidants from various natural matrices have been developed. Conventional methods are based on maceration, infusion, and decoction but these are time-consuming processes. The use of plants is intended to return to more naturalness; hence the use of environmentally friendly extraction methods makes sense. More recently it has been shown that green extraction methods, including microwave-assisted extraction or ultrasound-assisted extraction, are especially successful. Le et al. [35] described the development of a green microwave-assisted extraction of bioactive compounds from *M. cochinchinensis* fruit. Such extraction methods have been shown to promote the increased solubility of compounds and the yields of extraction, as well as the reduction in extraction time and solvent consumption. When developing an extraction process, a key parameter to decide is solvent selection. Various solvents, including methanol, ethanol (EtOH), water or acetone, are used routinely for extraction of plant polyphenols but they are not all consistent with a green extraction process. Interestingly, water and ethanol, two of the most readily available solvents, are considered green solvents [36] and can be used in the development of green extraction methods [35]. Indeed, EtOH is one of the least toxic solvents for humans and more environmentally friendly than other organic solvents, such as methanol. In addition, the extraction capacity of EtOH can be easily modulated by adding water, making it an ideal solvent for the extraction of a wide variety of compounds with variable polarity [35]. These green extraction technologies have attracted a great deal of interest in industrial applications and are now considered to be one of the most efficient energy-saving processes in terms of length, selectivity and reproducibility.

7. Future Prospects: Does the Use of Plants in Modern Medicine Still Have A Future Today?

Most of the time, plants are readily available, cheap and relatively rich in polyphenols, which is why they were in the spotlight for traditional and alternative medicines as well as for research on health-promoting compounds. However, it must be borne in mind that this is a long way off. Complete knowledge of the phytochemical composition of a bioactive extract and its biological activity is important but not sufficient. Plant identification/authentication, harvesting and post-harvest treatment are important issues to consider. Genetics and/or the environment can have a significant impact on the phytochemical profile of the extract, affecting both its biological activity and its safety for the consumer. The rational identification of the bioactive compounds from the raw extract as well as the molecular targets of the compounds responsible for the activity are also important steps. The source plant, which does not necessarily produce a compound in sufficient quantities for industrial use, may be rare or endangered species. It is therefore sometimes necessary to design alternative methods of production.

In addition to renewable sources, growing attention is being given to environmentally sustainable and consumer-friendly methods of extraction based on the principles of green chemistry. "Plant extract" or "natural product" does not inherently mean 'safer' than synthetic products in particular, as we still see so much in the minds of the general audience or the mass press, so toxicity and/or potential side effects need to be investigated. Targeted compounds should be used in biomedical and pharmaceutical research, ranging from in vitro to in vivo and clinical studies, to assess the safety, efficacy and side effects both short and long term of the candidate compounds tested. Despite all these obstacles before the discovery of an active molecule that will become a lead compound, polyphenols remain, and will certainly continue to be, serious potential candidates in the pharmaceutical and medical sectors to promote human health, prevent and cure various diseases. If we consider that only 15 per cent of the approximately 300,000 described terrestrial plant species have been systematically studied for their biological activities and/or phytochemical profiles, sometimes using ancient methods or not systematically and comprehensively, a vast field of exploration still appears to be open for the research on health-promoting polyphenols.

Author Contributions: C.H. and D.T. conceived, designed, and wrote the editorial. All authors have read and agreed to the published version of the manuscript.

Funding: This research was supported by Cosmetosciences, a global training and research program dedicated to the cosmetic industry. Located in the heart of the Cosmetic Valley, this program led by University of Orléans is funded by the Region Centre-Val de Loire. This research was supported by Ligue contre le Cancer, Comité d'Eure et Loir.

Acknowledgments: D.T. gratefully acknowledges the support of French government via the French Embassy in Thailand in the form of Junior Research Fellowship Program. C.H. and D.T. gratefully acknowledges the support of Campus France through the PHC SIAM (PNPIA, Project 44926WK) C.H. and D.T. would like to thank Medicines for offering us the opportunity to make this special issue a reality, and in particular Bonnie Yang for her availability, professionalism, help, constant support and kindness.

Conflicts of Interest: The authors declare no conflict of interest.

References

1. Quideau, S.; Deffieux, D.; Douat-Casassus, C.; Pouységu, L. Plant polyphenols: Chemical properties, biological activities, and synthesis. *Angew. Chem. Int. Ed.* **2011**, *50*, 586–621. [CrossRef] [PubMed]
2. Chen, D.; Daniel, K.G.; Kuhn, D.J.; Kazi, A.; Bhuiyan, M.; Li, L.; Dou, Q.P. Green tea and tea polyphenols in cancer prevention. *Front. Biosci.* **2004**, *9*, 2618. [CrossRef] [PubMed]
3. Lainé, E.; Hano, C.; Lamblin, F.F. *Phytoestrogens: Lignans*; Knasmüller, S., DeMarini, D.M., Johnson, I., Gerhäuser, C., Eds.; WILEY-VCH: Weinheim, Germany, 2009; ISBN 9783527320585.
4. Younas, M.; Hano, C.; Giglioli-Guivarc'h, N.; Abbasi, B.H. Mechanistic evaluation of phytochemicals in breast cancer remedy: Current understanding and future perspectives. *RSC Adv.* **2018**, *8*, 29714–29744. [CrossRef]
5. Nayak, B.; Liu, R.H.; Tang, J. Effect of Processing on Phenolic Antioxidants of Fruits, Vegetables, and Grains—A Review. *Crit. Rev. Food Sci. Nutr.* **2015**, *55*, 887–919. [CrossRef] [PubMed]
6. Tungmunnithum, D.; Thongboonyou, A.; Pholboon, A.; Yangsabai, A. Flavonoids and Other Phenolic Compounds from Medicinal Plants for Pharmaceutical and Medical Aspects: An Overview. *Medicines* **2018**, *5*, 93. [CrossRef]
7. Hano, C.; Renouard, S.; Molinié, R.; Corbin, C.; Barakzoy, E.; Doussot, J.; Lamblin, F.; Lainé, E. Flaxseed (*Linum usitatissimum* L.) extract as well as (+)-secoisolariciresinol diglucoside and its mammalian derivatives are potent inhibitors of α-amylase activity. *Bioorg. Med. Chem. Lett.* **2013**, *23*, 3007–3012. [CrossRef]
8. Hano, C.; Corbin, C.; Drouet, S.; Quéro, A.; Rombaut, N.; Savoire, R.; Molinié, R.; Thomasset, B.; Mesnard, F.; Lainé, E. The lignan (+)-secoisolariciresinol extracted from flax hulls is an effective protectant of linseed oil and its emulsion against oxidative damage. *Eur. J. Lipid Sci. Technol.* **2017**, *119*, 1600219. [CrossRef]
9. Tungmunnithum, D.; Garros, L.; Drouet, S.; Renouard, S.; Lainé, E.; Hano, C. Green Ultrasound Assisted Extraction of *trans* Rosmarinic Acid from *Plectranthus scutellarioides* (L.) R.Br. Leaves. *Plants* **2019**, *8*, 50. [CrossRef]

10. Nazir, M.; Tungmunnithum, D.; Bose, S.; Drouet, S.; Garros, L.; Giglioli-Guivarc'h, N.; Abbasi, B.H.; Hano, C. Differential Production of Phenylpropanoid Metabolites in Callus Cultures of Ocimum basilicum L. With Distinct In Vitro Antioxidant Activities and In Vivo Protective Effects against UV stress. *J. Agric. Food Chem.* **2019**, *67*, 1847–1859. [CrossRef]
11. Drouet, S.; Abbasi, B.H.; Falguières, A.; Ahmad, W.S.; Ferroud, C.; Doussot, J.; Vanier, J.R.; Lainé, E.; Hano, C. Single Laboratory Validation of a Quantitative Core Shell-Based LC Separation for the Evaluation of Silymarin Variability and Associated Antioxidant Activity of Pakistani Ecotypes of Milk Thistle (*Silybum Marianum* L.). *Molecules* **2018**, *23*, 904.
12. Drouet, S.; Doussot, J.; Garros, L.; Mathiron, D.; Bassard, S.; Favre-Réguillon, A.; Molinié, R.; Lainé, É.; Hano, C. Selective Synthesis of 3-O-Palmitoyl-Silybin, a New-to-Nature Flavonolignan with Increased Protective Action against Oxidative Damages in Lipophilic Media. *Molecules* **2018**, *23*, 2594. [CrossRef] [PubMed]
13. Drouet, S.; Leclerc, E.A.; Garros, L.; Tungmunnithum, D.; Kabra, A.; Abbasi, B.H.; Lainé, É.; Hano, C. A Green Ultrasound-Assisted Extraction Optimization of the Natural Antioxidant and Anti-Aging Flavonolignans from Milk Thistle Silybum marianum (L.) Gaertn. Fruits for Cosmetic Applications. *Antioxidants* **2019**, *8*, 304. [CrossRef] [PubMed]
14. Tungmunnithum, D.; Elamrani, A.; Abid, M.; Drouet, S.; Kiani, R.; Garros, L.; Kabra, A.; Addi, M.; Hano, C. A Quick, Green and Simple Ultrasound-Assisted Extraction for the Valorization of Antioxidant Phenolic Acids from Moroccan Almond (Prunus dulcis (Mill.) DA Webb) Cold-Pressed Oil Residues. *Preprints* **2020**. [CrossRef]
15. Pomatto, L.C.D.; Davies, K.J.A. Adaptive homeostasis and the free radical theory of ageing. *Free Radic. Biol. Med.* **2018**, *124*, 420–430. [CrossRef] [PubMed]
16. Harman, D. Aging: A theory based on free radical and radical chemistry. *J. Gerontol.* **1956**, *11*, 298–305. [CrossRef]
17. Harman, D. The free radical theory of aging. *Antioxid. Redox Signal.* **2003**, *5*, 557–561. [CrossRef]
18. Howitz, K.T.; Bitterman, K.J.; Cohen, H.Y.; Lamming, D.W.; Lavu, S.; Wood, J.G.; Zipkin, R.E.; Chung, P.; Kisielewski, A.; Zhang, L.-L. Small molecule activators of sirtuins extend Saccharomyces cerevisiae lifespan. *Nature* **2003**, *425*, 191–196. [CrossRef]
19. Baur, J.A.; Sinclair, D.A. Therapeutic potential of resveratrol: The in vivo evidence. *Nat. Rev. Drug Discov.* **2006**, *5*, 493–506. [CrossRef]
20. Hubbard, B.P.; Sinclair, D.A. Small molecule SIRT1 activators for the treatment of aging and age-related diseases. *Trends Pharmacol. Sci.* **2014**, *35*, 146–154. [CrossRef]
21. Bonkowski, M.S.; Sinclair, D.A. Slowing ageing by design: The rise of NAD+ and sirtuin-activating compounds. *Nat. Rev. Mol. Cell Biol.* **2016**, *17*, 679. [CrossRef]
22. Wood, J.G.; Rogina, B.; Lavu, S.; Howitz, K.; Helfand, S.L.; Tatar, M.; Sinclair, D. Sirtuin activators mimic caloric restriction and delay ageing in metazoans. *Nature* **2004**, *430*, 686–689. [CrossRef] [PubMed]
23. Steels, E.L.; Learmonth, R.P.; Watson, K. Stress tolerance and membrane lipid unsaturation in *Saccharomyces cerevisiae* grown aerobically or anaerobically. *Microbiology* **1994**, *140*, 569–576. [CrossRef] [PubMed]
24. Wolak, N.; Kowalska, E.; Kozik, A.; Rapala-Kozik, M. Thiamine increases the resistance of baker's yeast Saccharomyces cerevisiae against oxidative, osmotic and thermal stress, through mechanisms partly independent of thiamine diphosphate-bound enzymes. *FEMS Yeast Res.* **2014**, *14*, 1249–1262. [CrossRef] [PubMed]
25. Bisquert, R.; Muñiz-Calvo, S.; Guillamón, J.M. Protective role of intracellular Melatonin against oxidative stress and UV radiation in Saccharomyces cerevisiae. *Front. Microbiol.* **2018**, *9*, 1–11. [CrossRef] [PubMed]
26. Garros, L.; Drouet, S.; Corbin, C.; Decourtil, C.; Fidel, T.; De Lacour, J.L.; Leclerc, E.A.; Renouard, S.; Tungmunnithum, D.; Doussot, J.; et al. Insight into the influence of cultivar type, cultivation year, and site on the lignans and related phenolic profiles, and the health-promoting antioxidant potential of flax (*Linum usitatissimum* L.) seeds. *Molecules* **2018**, *23*, 2636. [CrossRef]
27. Tungmunnithum, D.; Abid, M.; Elamrani, A.; Drouet, S.; Addi, M.; Hano, C. Almond Skin Extracts and Chlorogenic Acid Delay Replicative Aging by Enhanced Oxidative Stress Response Involving SIR2 and SOD2 in Yeast. *Preprints* **2020**, 2020040429. [CrossRef]
28. Reddy, V.P.; Aryal, P.; Robinson, S.; Rafiu, R.; Obrenovich, M.; Perry, G. Polyphenols in Alzheimer's Disease and in the Gut–Brain Axis. *Microorganisms* **2020**, *8*, 199. [CrossRef]

29. Compaore, M.; Bakasso, S.; Meda, R.N.T.; Nacoulma, O.G. Antioxidant and Anti-Inflammatory Activities of Fractions from *Bidens engleri* O.E. Schulz (Asteraceae) and *Boerhavia erecta* L. (Nyctaginaceae). *Medicines* **2018**, *5*, 53. [CrossRef]
30. Nwidu, L.L.; Alikwe, P.C.N.; Elmorsy, E.; Carter, W.G. An Investigation of Potential Sources of Nutraceuticals from the Niger Delta Areas, Nigeria for Attenuating Oxidative Stress. *Medicines* **2019**, *6*, 15. [CrossRef]
31. Minami, M.; Konishi, T.; Makino, T. Effect of Hochuekkito (Buzhongyiqitang) on Nasal Cavity Colonization of Methicillin-Resistant *Staphylococcus aureus* in Murine Model. *Medicines* **2018**, *5*, 83. [CrossRef]
32. Hampton, M.B.; Kettle, A.J.; Winterbourn, C.C. Involvement of superoxide and myeloperoxidase in oxygen-dependent killing of Staphylococcus aureus by neutrophils. *Infect. Immun.* **1996**, *64*, 3512–3517. [CrossRef] [PubMed]
33. Cosgrove, K.; Coutts, G.; Jonsson, M.; Tarkowski, A.; Kokai-Kun, J.F.; Mond, J.J.; Foster, S.J. Catalase (KatA) and alkyl hydroperoxide reductase (AhpC) have compensatory roles in peroxide stress resistance and are required for survival, persistence, and nasal colonization in *Staphylococcus aureus*. *J. Bacteriol.* **2007**, *189*, 1025–1035. [CrossRef] [PubMed]
34. Tungmunnithum, D.; Pinthong, D.; Hano, C. Flavonoids from *Nelumbo nucifera* Gaertn., a Medicinal Plant: Uses in Traditional Medicine, Phytochemistry and Pharmacological Activities. *Medicines* **2018**, *5*, 127. [CrossRef] [PubMed]
35. Le, A.V.; Parks, S.E.; Nguyen, M.H.; Roach, P.D. Optimisation of the Microwave-Assisted Ethanol Extraction of Saponins from Gac (*Momordica cochinchinensis* Spreng.) Seeds. *Medicines* **2018**, *5*, 70. [CrossRef] [PubMed]
36. Koczka, N.; Stefanovits-Bányai, É.; Ombódi, A. Total Polyphenol Content and Antioxidant Capacity of Rosehips of Some *Rosa* Species. *Medicines* **2018**, *5*, 84. [CrossRef] [PubMed]
37. Hennia, A.; Miguel, M.G.; Nemmiche, S. Antioxidant Activity of *Myrtus communis* L. and *Myrtus nivellei* Batt. & Trab. Extracts: A Brief Review. *Medicines* **2018**, *5*, 89.

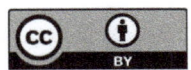

© 2020 by the authors. Licensee MDPI, Basel, Switzerland. This article is an open access article distributed under the terms and conditions of the Creative Commons Attribution (CC BY) license (http://creativecommons.org/licenses/by/4.0/).

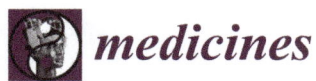

Review

Flavonoids and Other Phenolic Compounds from Medicinal Plants for Pharmaceutical and Medical Aspects: An Overview

Duangjai Tungmunnithum [1,2,*], Areeya Thongboonyou [1], Apinan Pholboon [1] and Aujana Yangsabai [1]

- [1] Department of Pharmaceutical Botany, Faculty of Pharmacy, Mahidol University, Bangkok 10400, Thailand; areeya.tho@hotmail.com (A.T.); smart.lady.angel@gmail.com (A.P.); Por.aujana@gmail.com (A.Y.)
- [2] Department of Botany, Tsukuba Botanical Garden, National Museum of Nature and Science, 4-1-1 Amakubo, Tsukuba 305-0005, Japan
- * Correspondence: duangjai.tun@mahidol.ac.th; Tel.: +66-264-486-96

Received: 17 July 2018; Accepted: 22 August 2018; Published: 25 August 2018

Abstract: Phenolic compounds as well as flavonoids are well-known as antioxidant and many other important bioactive agents that have long been interested due to their benefits for human health, curing and preventing many diseases. This review attempts to demonstrate an overview of flavonoids and other phenolic compounds as the interesting alternative sources for pharmaceutical and medicinal applications. The examples of these phytochemicals from several medicinal plants are also illustrated, and their potential applications in pharmaceutical and medical aspects, especially for health promoting e.g., antioxidant effects, antibacterial effect, anti-cancer effect, cardioprotective effects, immune system promoting and anti-inflammatory effects, skin protective effect from UV radiation and so forth are highlighted.

Keywords: flavonoid; medicinal and pharmaceutical applications; medicinal plants; phenolics

1. Introduction

Flavonoids and the other phenolic compounds are commonly known as plant secondary metabolites that hold an aromatic ring bearing at least one hydroxyl groups. More than 8000 phenolic compounds as naturally occurring substances from plants have been reported [1,2]. It is very interesting to note that half of these phenolic compounds are flavonoids presenting as aglycone, glycosides and methylated derivatives [1,2]. These phytochemical substances are presented in nutrients and herbal medicines, both flavonoids and many other phenolic components have been reported on their effective antioxidants, anticancer, antibacteria, cardioprotective agents, anti-inflammation, immune system promoting, skin protection from UV radiation, and interesting candidate for pharmaceutical and medical application [1,3–6]. Since a few decades ago, the research studies focusing on flavonoids and the other phenolic compounds from medicinal plant species have increased considerably, because of their versatile benefits for human health [1,2,7–11]. Most of the recent reviews focused on one precise aspect of flavonoids or phenolics action on human health.

This work aims to provide an overview of flavonoids and other phenolic phytochems as the potential sources of pharmaceutical and medical applications from the recent published studies as well as some interesting directions for future researches. The key word searches for flavonoids, phenolics, medicinal plant were performed on June, 2018 using Scopus, Google scholar and PubMed. The 351 resulted publications were found and carefully read, in order to find the more recent and non-redundant publications meeting the objective of this work with a few older publications to highlight some necessary points were also used. The 105 selected publications were employed in this review.

2. Effects of Plant Flavonoids and Other Phenolics on Human Health Promoting, Diseases Curing and Preventing

2.1. Antioxidant Effects

During the production of adenosine triphosphate (ATP) to generate energy for the cells by using oxygen, reactive oxygen species (ROS) and reactive nitrogen species (RNS) are produced as the by-products from these cellular redox reaction. At the balance level, ROS and RNS are beneficial compounds for cellular functions and immune responses, but the unbalance concentration of ROS and RNS will lead to oxidative stress which can cause chronic and degenerative disorders [12,13]. The naturally occurring antioxidant molecules have significantly increased in both usages and research studies; many natural antioxidant compounds have been employed in medical and pharmaceutical products as the substitute compounds for artificial antioxidant ones which have suspected to be one of the major causes for carcinogenesis [14]. Medicinal plants have long been reported as a prospective hub of natural antioxidant compounds, particularly plant secondary metabolites i.e., phenolic compounds and flavonoids which are generated by plant to defend itself or to promote the growth under unfavorable conditions. In addition, functional group arrangement, configuration, substitution, the number of hydroxyl groups were also influenced by antioxidant activity of flavonoids, for example radical scavenging activity and/or metal ion chelation ability [15]. Phenolics and flavonoids are commonly known as the largest phytochemical molecules with antioxidant properties from plants [5,9,10,16–19].

Oki and his team examined antioxidant activity of anthocyanins and other phenolic compounds from various cultivars of purple-fleshed sweet potato (*Ipomoea batatas* (L.) Lam.), an edible and economic medicinal species in Japan by diphenyl-2-picrylhydrazyl (DPPH) radical-scavenging activity; the obtained results showed the positive correlation between phenolic content and the activity of free-radical scavenging. In addition, chlorogenic acid was the phenolic compounds that acted as dominant DPPH radical-scavenger in "Miyanou-36" and "Bise" cultivars of *I. batatas*, whereas anthocyanins were the dominant DPPH radical-scavengers of "Ayamurasaki" and "Kyushu-132" cultivars [11]. *Bauhinia variegata* L., a medicinal plant that was used in traditional medicine in Pakistan, India and other Asian countries, was studied by Mishra and his group. The researchers found that leaf extracts of *B. variegate* contained flavonoid compounds, and presented antioxidant properties against oxidative damage by radical neutralization, iron binding and reducing power abilities [17]. The antioxidant activity and phytochemical characterization of young and adult cladodes, peel of the fruit and pulp of the fruits from six Spanish Mediterranean cultivars of *Opuntia ficus-indica* (L.) Mill. were analyzed by Andreu and his team. This research team discovered that the significant levels of total phenolic compounds in the best antioxidant cultivar played a significant role against oxidative stress [5]. The antioxidant property and bioactive compounds from the fruits of *Aesculus indica* (Wall. ex Cambess.) Hook, a medicinal plant from temperate regions of Asia i.e., Pakistan, Nepal, India and Afghanistan, were analyzed by the research group of Zahoor; their results indicated that 2-hydroxy-2-phenyle acetic acid (mandelic acid) and 2-(3,4-dihydroxy phenyl)-3,5,7-trihydroxy-4H-Chromen-4-one (quercetin) were the major bioactive molecules with significant antioxidant property to decrease oxidative stress caused by ROS [19]. Furthermore, the rhizomes extracts of *Polygonatum verticillatum* (L.) All., an Indian medicinal plant, were also exhibited antioxidant activity which is associated with the level of phenolic composition [20]. The research group of Meng evaluated the biological activity and phytochemical profiling from the leaves extract of *Camellia fangchengensis* S. Ye Liang and Y.C. Zhong, a wild tea species which local people have been used for green tea or black tea production, that is an endemic tea species in Guangxi province, Republic of China. The acquired results proved that flavan-3-ol oligomers and monomers were the potent antioxidant compounds and abundantly found in this species [6].

Besides the angiosperms or flowering plants, the antioxidant property of phenolic compounds was also reported in gymnosperms, the necked-seed plants. Ustun and his research group studied twig and needle extracts and essential oils of the 5 Turkish *Pinus* species such as *P. brutia* Tenore (Turkish pine), *P. pinea* L. (stone pine or umbrella pine), *P. halepensis* Miller (Aleppo pine), *P. sylvestris* L. (Scots pine) and *P. nigra* J.F. Arnold (European black pine), as well as pycnogenol which is the bark extract from *P. pinaster*, in order to investigate their phytochemical compounds and antioxidant activities by using DPPH and *N,N*-dimethyl-*p*-phenylendiamine (DMPD) radical scavenging, ferric-reducing antioxidant power (FRAP), and metal-chelating assays. Their results indicated that pycnogenol had the richest total phenol content, and revealed effective antioxidant effects [21]. Likewise, Apetrei and his collaborators conducted their study on phytochemical compounds and biological activity of *Pinus cembra* L., a native species of Central European Alps and the Carpathian mountains; they discovered that hydromethanolic extract from bark provided higher concentration of total phenolics and flavonoids than that of needle extract. Additionally, the bark extract showed better ability as free radical scavenger [22].

2.2. Antibacterial Effect

Interestingly, there are a large number of flavonoids and phenolics which exhibit antibacterial effect; such those compounds can be widely found in non-flowering medicinal plants to the flowering ones. The fern, *Aspleniumnidus nidus* L., contained gliricidin 7-*O*-hexoside and quercetin-7-O-rutinoside that can fight against the 3 pathogens e.g., *Proteus mirabilis* Hauser, *Proteus vulgaris* Hauser and *Pseudomonas aeruginosa* (Schroeter) Migula [23]. Moreover, flavonoid and phenolic compounds are synthesized by various plant groups including many medicinal plant species that are employed in traditional medicine or dietary consumption. An obvious example is nutmeg or *Myristica fragrans* Houtt.; this plant is mostly used traditionally as flavoring agent in Indonesia and other countries in South East Asia [24,25]. However, ethanolic extract of the nutmeg seed which contained 3′,4′,7-trihydroxyflavone showed effective potential against MDR gram-negative bacteria e.g., *Providencia stuartii* Ewing and *Escherichia coli* (Migula) Castellani and Chalmers. [25]. Similarly, *Pseudarthria hookeri* Wight and Arn which has been used as traditional herbal medicine in Africa [26,27] for the treatment of pneumonia, abdominal pains, cough and diarrhea. According to the antibacterial study of this medicinal species, Dzoyem and his team found that flavonoids from this plant showed the highest antibacterial effect against both gram-positive and gram-negative bacteria e.g., *E. coli*, *Klebsiella pneumonia* (Schroeter) Trevisan, *Pseudomonas aeruginosa* (Schroeter) Migula, *Enterococcus faecalis* (Andrew and Horder) Schleifer and Kilpper-Blazand, and *Staphylococcus aureus* Rosenbach; the highest antibacterial activities found in pseudarflavone A and 6-prenylpinocembrin [27]. In addition, Rajarathinam and his group found that *Pseudomonas aeruginosa* (Schroeter) Migula, an important resistant strain that caused many problems in medical treatment can be eliminated by 2-(3′,4′ dihydroxy-phenyl) 3,5,7-trihydroxy-chromen-4-one from the aerial part extract of *Trianthema decandra* L.; this phytochemical compound showed antibacterial activity against this pathogen comparing to chloremphenical, an antibiotic [28]. Flavonoids and other phenolics have also been reported as antibacterial agent against *P. acnes* which are the major cause of skin acne problems. Kaempferol that isolated from the *Impatiens balsamina* L. exhibited potential activity to inhibit the growth of *P. acnes*; its combination with clindamycin and quercetin combined with clindamycin were reported as a better synergic effects [29]. Moreover, flavones which were isolated from the root of *Scutellaria baicalensis* Georgi were proved as potential antibacterial agents against *P. acnes*-induced skin inflammation both in vitro and in vivo models [30]. The study of Hsieh and his team focused on strictinin, the main phenolic compound isolated from the leaves of *Camellia sinensis* var. *assamica* (J.W. Mast.) Kitam which is a raw plant material of Pu'er teas. They discovered that strictinin was a good candidate for antibacterial molecule against this bacteria [31]. Phenolics from kernel extract of *Mangifera indica* L. were also showed anti-acne property to inhibit the growth of *P. acnes* [32].

2.3. Anti-Cancer Effect

It is no denying that cancer is one of the major causes of death worldwide; the imbalance and high level of free radicals such as ROS and RNS can also become mutagenic or carcinogenic agents which lead to the cancer development. Chemotherapy is globally employed in cancer treatment, however a large number of drawbacks is its limitation. For example, sometimes the undesired side effects occur during chemotherapeutic treatment. Thus, it is interesting to seek for the alternative treatments for cancer that are no side effects and not so expensive cost. Flavopiridol, a flavonoid-derived drugs from *Dysoxylum binectariferum* (Roxb.) Hook.f. ex Bedd. [Currently the correct scientific name is *Dysoxylum gotadhora* (Buch.-Ham.) Mabb. (http://www.theplantlist.org/tpl1.1/record/kew-2607025)] is an example of anticancer drugs originated from phytochemical compound for lymphomas and leukemia treatments [33,34]. In addition, dietary supplements also play an important role in preventing and curing various kinds of cancer. Phenolic compounds especially flavonoids have long been reported as chemopreventive agents in cancer therapy [2,17,35,36].

Likewise, Danciu and colleagues researched on the phenolic compounds and biological activities of ethanolic extracts from rhizome of *Zingiber officinale* Roscoe and *Curcuma longa* L. which are the core representative species of Zingiberaceae family. This research team proposed the extract of *C. longa* rhizome as the promising source of natural active compounds to fight against malignant melanoma due to its potential anticancer property on B164A5 murine melanoma cell line. The authors also suggested that the increase in anticancer activity was correlated with the increase in amount of polyphenol compounds [37]. Moreover, the results from many biomedical research teams indicated that various kinds of flavonoids can promote apoptosis in various cancer cells [17,35,38]. Quercetin, a flavonol member, is reported as an interesting anticancer substance against prostate and breast cancers [1,38]. Gliricidin7-O-hexoside and Quercetin 7-O-rutinoside which were the flavonoids isolated from the medicine fern (*Asplenium nidus*) was also purposed as the potential chemopreventive against human hepatoma HepG2 and human carcinoma HeLa cells [23]. According to the intense studied of Hashemzaei and his research group on quercetin and apoptosis-inducing ability both in vitro and in vivo levels. For in vitro studies, they tested anticancer activity of quercetin in 9 cancer cell lines: prostate adenocarcinoma LNCaP cells, colon carcinoma CT-26 cells, pheocromocytoma PC12 cells, human prostate PC3 cells, acute lymphoblastic leukemia MOLT-4 T-cells, estrogen receptor-positive breast cancer MCF-7 cells, ovarian cancer CHO cells, human myeloma U266B1 cells and human lymphoid Raji cells; the obtained results proved that quercetin can significantly induce apoptosis of every tested cell lines at $p < 0.001$ comparing with control group [39]. The in vivo experiments conducted in mouse models i.e., mice bearing MCF-7 tumors and mice bearing CT-26 tumors; the quercetin-treated group exhibited a significant decrease in tumor size and volume at $p < 0.001$ compared to the control group. The survival period of the quercetin-tested animals were also prolonged [39]. Besides, the research team of Clifford conducted their research to evaluate anticancer benefits of quercetin on patient-derived pancreatic tissue and 3 established pancreatic cancer cell lines: primary pancreatic cancer cell line ASANPaCa, AsPC1 and PANC1 to go deeper on the cross talk between quercetin a polyphenol phytochemical compound, microRNAs and Notch signaling in the regulation of self-renewing cancer stem cell divisions [40]. Notch is known as an important gene for signaling receptor encoding, which leads to proper development, the decision of cell fate, cell proliferation and survival [41,42]; it is suggested as a good marker of oncogene and symmetric cell division [43]. Clifford team showed that quercetin can induced miR-200b-3p to regulate the mode of self-renewing divisions of the tested pancreatic cancer [40]. The intense reviewed on genistein and its molecular effects on prostate cancer by Adjakly and his group pointed out that a soy isoflavone genistein inhibited the activation of Nuclear factor kappa B (NF-κB) signaling pathway that is occupied the balance of cell survival and apoptosis, this soy isoflavone could also take its action to fight against cell growth, apoptotic and metastasis processes, including epigenetic modifications in prostate cancer [44]. Curcumin is one of natural phenolic compounds exhibiting anticancer effects towards skin cancers, this phenolic can influence the cell cycle by acting as a pro-apoptotic agent [4]. Abusnina and his team investigated the antiproliferative effect of curcumin on melanoma cancer in in vitro level using B16F10 murine melanoma cells. They showed that curcumin acted as non-selective cyclic nucleotide phosphodiesterases (PDE) inhibitor to inhibit melanoma cell proliferation which is related to epigenetic integrator UHRF1; these researchers also suggested that curcumin occurring in diets might be help to prevent this cancer and contribute in the gene expression via epigenetic control [45]. Interestingly, Hisamitsu group investigated prostate cancer therapeutic potential of curcumin on the inhibitory effect of intracrine androgen synthesis using both in vitro and in vivo models. Their in vitro experiments conducted on human prostate cancer cell lines such as LNCaP and 22Rv1 cells; curcumin decreased the expression of genes evolving in steroidogenic acute regulatory proteins, supporting the decline of testosterone synthesis. Curcumin inhibited proliferation of the selected cell lines in this experiment and induced apoptosis of the cancer cells with dose-dependent response. Their in vivo study on transgenic adenocarcinoma of the mouse prostate (TRAMP) model with 1-month oral administration of curcumin displayed that the phytochemical compound regulate the expression of steroidogenic enzyme, including AKR1C2, and suppressed the growth prostate cancer cells by decreasing testosterone levels in prostate tissues of TRAMP mice [46].

2.4. Cardioprotective Effects

The cardioprotective effects from various kinds of phenolics and/or flavonoids occurring in medicinal plants have been investigated from many researches since many decades ago [1,47–57]. The comprehensive review of Razavi-Azarkhiavi and his team illustrated cardioprotective role of various phenolic compounds against cardiotoxicity of doxorubicin which is the extensively used anticancer medicine for lymphomas, leukemia and breast cancers in clinical application that contains vulnerable side effect as cardiotoxicity such as pericarditis, arrhythmias, myocarditis, and acute heart failure [52]. They found that antioxidant phenolics have been recommended as a promising approach to reduce adverse effects of this anticancer drug; many phenolic and flavonoid compounds have been studied and reported their cardioprotective properties via various mechanisms including inhibition of ROS generation, mitochondrial dysfunction, apoptosis, NF-kB, p53, and DNA damage both in vitro, in vivo, and clinical studies. Razavi-Azarkhiavi team also found that many flavonoid and phenolics i.e., kaempferol, rutin, luteolin and resveratrol showed their efficacy against doxorubicin-induced cardiotoxicity, but do not affect on the antitumor activity of this medicine [58–60]. The most interesting reported compound was isorhamnetin. Because, it provided cardioprotective effect against cardiotoxicity of doxorubicin, and potentiated the anticancer efficacy of this drug [52,61]. Recently, there is the research on phenolic composition from methanolic extracts of the aerial parts of the two medicinal plants in Poland: *Centaurea borysthenica* Gruner and *C. daghestanica* (Lipsky) Wagenitz [At present, the corrected scientific name of this plant is *Centaurea transcaucasica* Sosn. ex Grossh. (http://www.theplantlist.org/tpl1.1/record/gcc-95497?ref=tpl1)] were analyzed together with their protective effects on cardiomyocytes treated with doxorubicin [53]. The obtained results from oxidative stress, cell viability, and mitochondrial membrane potential tests displayed their cardioprotective activity of both *C. borysthenica* and *C. daghestanica* extracts on rat cardiomyocytes treated with doxorubicin anticancer drug. According to this study, they found an attractive point that *C. daghestanica* methanolic extracts did not affect on efficacy of doxorubicin in this experiment [53].

In addition, the research group of Alhaider evaluated the cardioprotective potential of *Phoenix dactylifera* L. or date palm in English name or Nakl in Arabic name. The total flavonoid, total phenolic, in vitro antioxidant capacity and in vivo rodent myocardial infarction models with fruit extracts from 4 different varieties of date palm in eastern provision of Saudi Arabia were confirmed. The high concentrations of phenolics and flavonoids were detected in the fruit extracts that contributed the potential antioxidant activities and high cardioprotective effect against various induced factors in vivo myocardial infarction models by mobilizing the circulating progenitor cells from both bone marrow to the site of myocardial infraction, in order to promote tissue repairing from ischemic injury [56]. Syama and his colleagues evaluated the major phenolic acids and flavonoids from the different fractions of seeds extract from *Syzygium cumini* (L.) Skeels, and their cardioprotective potential in in vitro H9c2 cardiac cell lines such as tertiary butyl hydrogen peroxide induced oxidative stress, LDL oxidation, HMG-CoA reductase and angiotensin converting enzyme modulation. The major phytochemical compounds from the analyzed fractions were gellagic acid, syringic acid, gallic acid, ferulic acid, cinnamic acid and quercetin. These fractions attenuated oxidative stress in H9c2 cardiomyoblasts and molecular docking demonstrated the positive correlation between the major phytochemical compounds and key enzymes for preventing cardiovascular diseases i.e., angiotensin converting enzyme [57]. Moreover, the research group of Garjani investigated the potential of aerial parts extract from *Marrubium vulgare* L., a medicinal plant from Iran focusing on its cardioprotective effects against ischemia-reperfusion injury in vivo Wistar rat model. They determined total phenolic and flavonoids content of aqueous fraction of the extract, and their effect on ischemia-reperfusion injury of the rat hearts using Langendroff method; the obtained result proved that aqueous fraction from *M. vulgare* consisting of cardioprotective potential against this cardiac injury [48]. Aspalathin and phenylpyruvic acid-2-O-β-D-glucoside, the two of the major compounds from *Aspalathus linearis* (Burm.f.) R. Dahlgren were demonstrated as potential protective compounds to protect myocardial infarction caused by chronic hyperglycemia [49]. Likewise, puerarin is a potential isoflavones that was reported as an interesting candidate for cardioprotection by protecting myocardium from ischemia and reperfusion damage by means of opening the Ca^{2+}-activated K^+ channel and activating the protein kinase C [51]; this research team conducted their study using in vivo Sprague–Dawley rats model. Tian and his group compared the cardioprotective effects between polyphenolic extracts from apple peel and apple flesh in in vivo mice model with cardiovascular risk factors; they found that the extracts of apple peels exhibited better cardioprotective ability than that of apple flesh in mice model [54]. This may probably due to the higher amount of both total phenolics and total flavonoids consisting in polyphenolic extracts from apple peel.

2.5. Immune System Promoting and Anti-Inflammatory Effects

Medicinal and pharmacological agents, nutrients, pollutants and other environmental factors play a necessary role in the human immune system. A large number of flavonoids and other phenolics have been proved their noteworthy effects on immune system function and inflammatory processes [62,63]. Quercetin, apigenin, hesperidin and luteolin were reported as flavonoids containing potential anti-inflammatory effects [1]. The research group of Rupasinghe examined the anti-inflammatory properties of Canadian medicinal plant extracts, *Lonicera caerulea* L. or haskap berry in various cultivars focusing on pro-inflammatory cytokines using in vitro human monocytic cell line THP-1 derived macrophages which stimulated by lipopolysaccharide. Borealis cultivar of Haskap berry presented the highest phenolic, flavonoid and anthocyanin content ($p < 0.05$), and exhibited comparable anti-inflammatory effects to diclofenac which is a COX inhibitory medicine [64]. In addition, the synergistic effects on immune and health promoting properties of bioactive compounds and probiotic bacteria are also currently interested by the scientists. For example, the study of Sisto's group to investigate effect of *Lactobacillus paracasei* culture filtrates and *Cynara scolymus* L. or artichoke phenolic extract from edible part of its fresh buds on cytokine producing by dendritic cells. The experimental result pointed out the interesting anti-inflammatory effect of a culture filtrate obtained after probiotic *L. paracasei* strain growing in the media supplemented with artichoke phenolic extract [65]. Moreover, the anti-inflammatory activity of polyphenolic compounds in *Gaillardia grandiflora* Hort. ex Van Houte and *Gaillardia pulchella* Foug from Egypt were reported with nontoxicity test in in vivo mice model; the newly reported compound, 8-hydroxyapigenin 6-O-β-D-apiofuranosyl-($1'''\rightarrow 6''$)-C-β-D-$^4C_1$-glucopyranoside, from *G. grandiflora* and other known compound i.e., luteolin 6-C-β-D-$^4C_1$-glucopyranoside 8-methyl ether, schaftoside, isoorientin, apigenin 6-C-β-D-$^4C_1$- glucopyranoside 8-methyl ether, 6-methoxyluteolin isovitexin and hispidulin were also isolated and tested in this research [66]. The inflammatory inhibition ability both tumor necrosis factor- (TNF-) and interleukin-6 (IL-6) of polyphenol fractions from sixteen cultivars of Chinese blueberries including 14 commercialized ones such as Bluecrop, Bluesource, Berkeley, Brigitta, Duke, Darrow, Misty, Northblue, Northland, Northcountry, O'Neal, Patriot, Reka and Southgood from China were employed in the study of Ma and his team. Their anti-inflammatory effect of these blueberry samples were tested using lipopolysaccharide induced RAW 264.7 macrophages; anti-inflammatory potential of the polyphenol fractions were in the same trend of their phenolic acid contents [67]. Likewise, anti-inflammatory activities of two medicinal plant species: *Bidens engleri* O.E. Schulz from Asteraceae family as well as *Boerhavia erecta* L. from Nyctaginaceae family were tested in various fractions and evaluated their total phenolic and total flavonoid contents [68]. This research team found that dichloromethane was the highest potential solvent to extract flavonoid compounds in both species and this fraction also exhibited anti-inflammatory effect via COX-2 and LOX-15 inhibition. Macrophages play an important role in controlling the switches of immune system by means of maintaining the balance of pro-inflammatory and anti-inflammatory activities. Dugo and his team proved that polyphenol extract from roasted cocoa beans (*Theobroma cacao* L.) significantly lowered pro-inflammatory cytokines secretion in in vitro THP-1 cells, as well as suppressed inflammation by promoting oxidative pathways, which lead to the increase in oxygen consumption by mitochondria and ATP production via oxidative phosphorylation [69]. Additionally, Lopes and his team characterized phenolic composition of *Lavandula pedunculata* (Mill.) Cav. samples from various different geographical origins in Portugal, and compared their bioactive activities in aqueous and hydroethanolic extracts. The obtained results pointed out that the *L. pedunculata* hydroethanolic extract from Alentejo area exhibited highest anti-inflammatory activity in rat RAW 264.7 macrophages by inhibiting nitric oxide production [70].

It is known that COX-2 syntheses prostaglandin E2 is an endogenous pain-producing substance, while COX-1 is a house-keeping enzyme. According to the molecular mechanism of some anti-inflammatory medicines which inhibit both cyclooxygenase-2 (COX-2) and COX-1 enzymes. Consequently, the medicines that inhibits both COX-1 and COX-2 concurrently can cause adverse side effects i.e., renal dysfunction or gastrointestinal bleeding. Therefore, the researchers have challenged to seek for the better candidate for drug development; some phenolics have been reported as the selective inhibiting compounds toward COX-2 expression. An interesting example is the study Ma and his team which aimed to validate the potential and mechanisms of polyphenols from inner bark of *Tabebuia avellanedae* Lorentz ex Griseb [Currently, the corrected species name of this plant is *Handroanthus impetiginosus* (Mart. ex DC.) Mattos; http://www.theplantlist.org/tpl1.1/record/kew-317146], a medicinal plant with extensively use as folk medicine in Central and South America, as an anti-inflammation agent without undesirable side effects from COX-1 inhibition. This work was conducted using in vitro free fatty acid-stimulated macrophage cell lines and combined molecular docking to investigate the interactions between the phenolic compounds and COX-2; the obtained results illustrated anti-inflammatory effects of phenolics from this medicinal plant to regulate macrophages by targeting COX-2 activity inhibition without any action on COX-1 activity [71]. Furthermore, phenolics and flavonoids from bark of *Vitex peduncularis* Wall. ex Schauer, a herbal drug, were characterization together with their anti-inflammatory activity by the research group of Ferreres. They found high content of apigenin, C-rhamnosyl flavones and luteolin derivatives in this methanolic bark extract which reduced nitric oxide levels in macrophages and significantly inhibited the activity of phospholipase A2, a mediate enzyme in inflammatory processes [72]. Additionally, Lu and his research group optimized the ethanolic rhizome extract of astilbin, a dihydroflavonol, from *Smilax glabra* Roxb and evaluated its anti-inflammatory effects in in vitro lipopolysaccharide-induced RAW264.7 macrophages. Their results pointed out that astilbin significantly suppressed nitric oxide production, tumor necrosis factor-α (TNF-α), mRNA expression of inducible nitric oxide synthase and TNF-α in the tested cells [73]. Recently, the isolated astilbin flavonoid from rhizome of *S. glabra* in China and its anti-inflammatory potential was also investigated by Dong and his group in in vivo complete Freund's adjuvant-induced adjuvant arthritis rats (AA rats) model. Their results showed noteworthy inhibitory properties of astilbin on TNF-α, IL-1β as well as IL-6 mRNA expression; serum cytokine levels of TNF-α, IL-1β, and IL-6 were also decreased in treated AA rats. They also proved that oral treatment of astilbin daily at 5.3 mg/kg can reduce joint damage in hind paw of the animal model; this therapeutic properties of astilbin flavonoid on the inhibition of cytokines production and reduction of inflammatory response in in vivo AA rats model were effective as equal as leflunomide, the frequently used antirheumatic drug [74]. Moreover, the double-blind, randomized, placebo-controlled clinical trial on inflammation of ferulic acid, an abundant phenolic compound from various plant including edible medicinal plant and cereal grains, were evaluated in hyperlipidemic subjects by the research team of Bumrungpert. They randomly divided hyperlipidemia subjects into 2 groups i.e., treatment group (n = 24) with ferulic acid 1000 mg daily and the control group (n = 24) with a placebo for six weeks; ferulic acid supplementation significantly decreased in the inflammatory markers with statistic different comparing with the control group [75].

2.6. Skin Protective Effect from UV Radiation

Overexposure to ultraviolet (UV) radiation can harm to skin. It induces extensive production of reactive oxygen species (ROS) and eventually causes skin damages [76]. However, there are several strategies applicable for skin protection. Phytochemical compound, especially phenolics and flavonoids is one of the most interesting choices that exhibits beneficial effects on UV-irradiated skin [77–79]. Flavonoids have photoprotective effects that are antioxidant properties by their capacity to chelate iron which can damage lipid and protein on cell membrane, and modulate several signaling pathways, for example, inhibit xanthine oxidase which is considered as a source of ROS that contributes to oxidative stress [80,81]. Several phenolic compounds are reported as potential antioxidant molecules for treatment of various skin disorders including diseases which caused by UV radiation [4,78].

Apigenin is a major flavones with skin protective effect from UV light; this flavone can be found in many edible medicinal plants or plants-derived beverages e.g., red wine, beer and chamomile tea [82,83]. Quercetin is a flavonols which can be found in onion skin, apple peel and *Hypericum perforatum* L. leaves [84]. Topical application with quercitin effectively inhibited UVB-induced skin damage in hairless mice [85]. In addition, *Ginkgo biloba* L. extract (EGb 761) that contains a lot of quercetin derivatives had an ability to decrease sunburn symptoms UVB-induced skin in in vivo study using UVB irradiated-skin mice model; the results indicated that oral intake of EGb 761 may act as a protective and therapeutic agent [86]. Silymarin, a standardized extract of flavonolignans from the milk thistle (*Silybum marianum* (L.) Gaernt.) fruits contains silybin, a major active component [87]. The topical treatment with silymarin stimulated the repair of UVB-induced DNA damage that leads to the prevention of apoptosis in UVB-exposed human epidermal keratinocytes as well as fibroblasts in in vitro study [88]. Genistein is a soybean isoflavone that was also reported as photoprotective molecule against photocarcinogenesis by inhibiting UV-induced DNA damage in human skin equivalent in vitro model [89]. Moreover, Wang and his team examined effect of genistein in human dermal fibroblasts on UVB-induced senescence via the mechanism of oxidative pathway; they found that genistein was able to maintain activities of antioxidant enzymes and modulate mitochondrial oxidative stress [90]. Equol is known as an isoflavonoid metabolite from isoflavone daidzein or genistein producing by gut microflora [91,92]. An in vivo study in hairless mice reported that topical application with equol prior to UV-irradiation can prevent UV-induced erythema-associated edema, immunosuppression and skin cancer by acting as a sunscreen and inhibiting DNA photodamage [92]. Additionally, the study of Choi and his group to evaluate skin protective effects of spent coffee ground on ultraviolet UVB-induced photo aging in in vivo hairless mice model showed that topical application of spent coffee ground extracts consisting of flavonoids and caffeine which were able to protect mouse skin by down-regulating of matrix metalloproteinases [93]. Interestingly, the research team of Kano investigated protective effect of isoflavones from fermented soymilk products on photodamage in the skin of ovariectomized hairless by oral administration for 28 days. The results indicated the increases of isoflavone concentration on mice skin and in their blood can effectively scavenge reactive oxygen species generating by UV irradiation, and also exerting estrogenic activity, resulting in photoprotective effect on skin of the animal model [94].

3. Naturally Occurring Plant Phenolics and Flavonoids for Menopausal and Post-Menopausal Women

There is pros and cons between using synthetic chemical compounds and phytochemical substances in pharmacy and medicine. Synthetic substances or medicines are easy and quickly to produce in large scale of drug development process and modify as many forms of consumption for patients. Conversely, many non-natural (or synthetic chemical compounds) cause several undesirable side effects, particularly long-term treatments [95]. Some synthetic medicines were not accept for clinical treatments because of their harmful side effects. An obvious example is synthetic estrogen which was commonly used in menopause women for hormone replacement therapy a few decades ago. This synthetic chemical compounds could work well to reduce menopause symptoms, long before there were a number of researches discovered its unwanted side effects i.e., an increase in the risk of breast, uterus and ovarian cancers [95–97].

Estrogen is a sex hormone mainly responsible for reproductive functions and the menstrual cycle of women. In postmenopausal women, estrogen is depleted due to the failure of the response of ovary to pituitary. When the level of estrogen decreases, it leads to many postmenopausal symptoms including cardiovascular disease. In particular, postmenopausal woman who also has metabolic syndrome (MetS) will increase in the risk of cardiovascular disease [98]. The research study of Squadrito and his group showed that flavonoid supplementation can also improve cardiovascular function in postmenopausal woman with metabolic syndrome [99]. Genistein is an obvious example of interesting choice of flavonoid phytoestrogen for improving endothelial functions in postmenopausal women with MetS [100]. Gregorio and his research team investigated the effects of genistein supplement on cardiac function of postmenopausal women with MetS; postmenopausal women patients with type-2 Diabetes mellitus and free from previous cardiovascular disease 120 subjects were employed in this study [98]. The patients were equally divided into 2 groups: Genistein supplementation group and control group who have got placebo by using a computer-generated double-blind randomization. The result indicated that genistein can improve the cardiac function in postmenopausal women with MetS [98].

The decrease of estrogen leads to postmenopausal bone loss or osteoporosis. Morabito research team found that genistein can be used as hormone-replacement therapy (HRT) for preventing osteoporosis in postmenopausal women [101]. This research team aims to compare the effect of genistein phytoestrogen with HRT (estrogen and its derivatives). The study conducted on 90 healthy women between 47–57 years who had bone mineral density at femoral neck of <0.795 g/cm^2. The 90 participant subjects were randomly and equally divided into three groups: Genistein, HRT and control group treating with placebo continuously for 1 year. The result indicated that using genistein in postmenopausal bone loss is more effective than HRT, because the undesirable side effects were not found in genistein group. Kruger and his team investigated the effects of bone turnover and the change in microflora between the groups of healthy New Zealand post-menopausal women who received daily isoflavone supplementation (daidzein and genistein) alone and those who consumed green kiwifruit combined with isoflavones for 4 months; their results indicated that the second group of post-menopausal women significantly improved bone health [102]. Nevertheless, the minimum and optimum dose are the essential point to concern. The concreted example can be seen in the study of Kaczmarczyk-Sedlak and his research group; their results indicated that moderate dose of isoflavane glabridin from root of *Glycyrrhiza glabra* L. or licorice plant showed no effect on bone loss in ovariectomized rats, an in vivo model of osteoporosis from estrogen deficiency in postmenopausal women [103]. The secondary metabolites discovered in medicinal plants such as flavonoids and other phenolics may avoid the negative side effect of synthetic medicines, because they must accumulate within the cells and tissues of living organisms [71,95,96]. Moreover, many medicinal herbs contain novel or valuable secondary metabolites with different biological properties, and a huge numbers of them are waiting for discovery.

4. Profiling Works and the Survey of Flavonoids and Other Phenolics from Medicinal Plants

For over four million years, flavonoids and other phenolic substances from medicinal herbs have been used or consumed by humans so as to live healthy and fight against undesirable diseases [1,22,51]. As a plant secondary metabolites, flavonoids and the other phenolics are found in several plant species, type and amount of the chemical components are vary depending on species and affecting by environmental factors i.e., mineral at the growth locality and geographic origin [70]. Nowadays, there is a significant increase in the number of research on potential of medicinal plant species for pharmaceutical and medical purposes focusing on natural phenolic compounds and flavonoids [1,4,9,16,18,51,63,71,73,104].

Though many flavonoids and other phenolic compounds were examined from medicinal plant species, a large amount of native or endemic medicinal herbs are still waiting for being survey and observing their novel compounds from profiling works. These processes are an indispensable step to promote the progression in drug discovery and development using phytochemical compounds. Asian region is well-known as one of the greatest hotspot of plant biodiversity including medicinal species, especially Japan, China, Thailand and related areas in tropical and sub-tropical regions [6,54,67,74,104,105]. However, a comprehensive profiling of many medicinal plants and functional evaluation of their chemical compound has not been completely conducted. According to our intense review in more than one hundred scientific publications, it is clear that the different parts of medicinal species such as floral parts, leaves, stems, root or rhizome consisting of different types and amount of phenolics and flavonoids. Furthermore, the harvesting season, cultivar and variety of the targeted plant species should be accounted and compared in phytochemical profiling works.

5. Future Perspectives and Interesting Directions for Future Researches

(1) The low cost of medicines and many other medical products is very important to allow all people to access to the drug. Consequently, the flavonoid and phenolic compounds which are abundant found in a large number of plant may possible be an interesting choice of molecules for drug and medical product development.

(2) In the same species of medicinal plants, the different cultivars may provide different amount of flavonoid and phenolic compounds as well as the biological activities. Thus, the cultivars of medicinal plant should be taken into account for the future medical and pharmaceutical research studies.

(3) The geographic areas of raw plant material should also be analyzed and compared in the future research. Since the environmental factors e.g., nutrients and mineral in soil are also effect on the quality and quantity of phytochemical compounds in some species of medicinal plant as discussed in this work.

(4) Not only local medicinal plant species but also the wild or endemic species are interesting for the future studies, in order to discover the novel phytochemical compounds to increase the alternative sources of raw material for medical and pharmaceutical applications.

(5) The molecular mechanism and signaling pathway of many known flavonoid and phenolic compounds are need to be done in the future, so as to apply this knowledge to the drug development processes.

(6) The need of purified compounds to confirm data obtained with the plant extracts.

(7) Epidemiological and in vitro studies are sometimes contradictory. In part because of the calculation of the intake based on general table estimated content without taking into account genetic variation among cultivars, geographic variations and so on. Also because of the possible need of metabolization by gut microflora for activation. Those of gut microflora are not taken into account, and quantification of the active circulating forms was not evaluated most of the time.

6. Conclusions

To recapitulate, the use of phenolic compounds and flavonoids are the potential candidate of bioactive agents in pharmaceutical and medicinal sectors to promote human health, prevent and cure various diseases. In order to discover and progress these alternative choice of using phytochemical compounds, the survey of medicinal plants together with intense profiling research needs to be done. The targeted compounds should be employed in biomedical and pharmaceutical research ranging from in vitro, in vivo, and clinical trial step to evaluate the safety, efficacy and also the side effects of the tested candidate compounds.

Author Contributions: D.T. conceived, designed, proved and edited the whole review manuscript. A.P. wrote the topic of "Antibacterial effect", A.T. wrote the topic of "Skin protective effect from UV radiation", A.Y. wrote a second half part of the topic "Naturally occurring plant phenolics and flavonoids for menopause and post-menopausal women", and D.T. wrote the remaining topics of the review.

Funding: This research received no external funding.

Acknowledgments: Duangjai Tungmunnithum would like to express her sincere thanks to the Development and the Promotion of Science and Technology Talent Project (DPST) from the Royal Thai Government for financial support for her collaborative research in Japan. Nonetheless, the funders had no role in the design of the study; in the collection, analyses, or interpretation of data; in the writing of the manuscript, and in the decision to publish the results. She also thanks to Tsukasa Iwashina, the director of Tsukuba Botanical Garden, and head of Department of Botany, National Museum of Nature and Science, Japan for broadening her horizons in phytochemistry of medicinal plants during the fruitful period of her post-doctoral research in Japan.

Conflicts of Interest: The authors declare no conflict of interest.

References

1. Kumar, S.; Pandey, A.K. Chemistry and biological activities of flavonoids: An overview. *Sci. World J.* **2013**, *2013*, 162750. [CrossRef] [PubMed]
2. Ahmed, S.I.; Hayat, M.Q.; Tahir, M.; Mansoor, Q.; Ismail, M.; Keck, K.; Bates, R.B. Pharmacologically active flavonoids from the anticancer, antioxidant and antimicrobial extracts of *Cassia angustifolia* Vahl. *BMC Complement. Altern. Med.* **2016**, *16*, 460. [CrossRef] [PubMed]
3. Chen, X.; Dang, T.T.T.; Facchini, P.J. Noscapine comes of age. *Phytochemistry* **2015**, *111*, 7–13. [CrossRef] [PubMed]
4. Działo, M.; Mierziak, J.; Korzun, U.; Preisner, M.; Szopa, J.; Kulma, A. The potential of plant phenolics in prevention and therapy of skin disorders. *Int. J. Mol. Sci.* **2016**, *17*, 160. [CrossRef] [PubMed]
5. Andreu, L.; Nuncio-Jáuregui, N.; Carbonell-Barrachina, Á.A.; Legua, P.; Hernández, F. Antioxidant properties and chemical characterization of Spanish *Opuntia ficus-indica* Mill. cladodes and fruits. *J. Sci. Food Agric.* **2018**, *98*, 1566–1573. [CrossRef] [PubMed]
6. Meng, X.H.; Liu, C.; Fan, R.; Zhu, L.F.; Yang, S.X.; Zhu, H.T.; Wang, D.; Yang, C.R.; Zhang, Y.J. Antioxidative flavan-3-ol dimers from the leaves of *Camellia fangchengensis*. *J. Agric. Food Chem.* **2018**, *66*, 247–254. [CrossRef] [PubMed]
7. Zhishen, J.; Mengcheng, T.; Jianming, W. The determination of flavonoid contents in mulberry and their scavenging effects on superoxide radicals. *Food Chem.* **1999**, *64*, 555–559. [CrossRef]
8. Wink, M. Modes of action of herbal medicines and plant secondary metabolites. *Medicines* **2015**, *2*, 251–286. [CrossRef] [PubMed]
9. Wang, J.; Cao, X.; Ferchaud, V.; Qi, Y.; Jiang, H.; Tang, F.; Yue, Y.; Chin, K.L. Variations in chemical fingerprints and major flavonoid contents from the leaves of thirty-one accessions of *Hibiscus sabdariffa* L. *Biomed. Chromatogr.* **2016**, *30*, 880–887. [CrossRef] [PubMed]
10. Okpuzor, J.; Ogbunugafor, H.; Kareem, G.K.; Igwo-Ezikpe, M.N. In vitro investigation of antioxidant phenolic compounds in extracts of *Senna alata*. *Res. J. Phytochem.* **2009**, *3*, 68–76. [CrossRef]
11. Oki, T.; Masuda, M.; Furuta, S.; Nishiba, Y.; Terahara, N.; Suda, A.I. Involvement of anthocyanins and other phenolic compounds in radical scavenging activity of purple-fleshed sweet potato cultivars. *J. Food Sci.* **2002**, *67*, 1752–1756. [CrossRef]
12. Valko, M.; Rhodes, C.J.; Moncol, J.; Izakovic, M.; Mazur, M. Free radicals, metals and antioxidants in oxidative stress-induced cancer. *Chem. Biol. Interact.* **2006**, *160*, 1–40. [CrossRef] [PubMed]

13. Pham-Huy, L.A.; He, H.; Pham-Huy, C. Free radicals, antioxidants in disease and health. *Int. J. Biomed. Sci.* **2008**, *4*, 89–96. [PubMed]
14. Carocho, M.; Barreiro, M.F.; Morales, P.; Ferreira, I.C.F.R. Adding molecules to food, pros and cons: A review on synthetic and natural food additives. *Compr. Rev. Food Sci. Food Saf.* **2014**, *13*, 377–399. [CrossRef]
15. Heim, K.E.; Tagliaferro, A.R.; Bobilya, D.J. Flavonoid antioxidants: Chemistry, metabolism and structure-activity relationships. *J. Nutr. Biochem.* **2002**, *13*, 572–584. [CrossRef]
16. Ryu, S.W.; Jin, C.-W.; Lee, H.-S.; Lee, J.-Y.; Sapkota, K.; Lee, B.-G.; Yu, C.-Y.; Lee, M.-K.; Kim, M.-J.; Cho, D.-H. Changes in total polyphenol, total flavonoid contents and antioxidant activities of *Hibiscus cannabinus* L. *Korean J. Med. Crop Sci.* **2006**, *14*, 307–310.
17. Mishra, A.; Sharma, A.K.; Kumar, S.; Saxena, A.K.; Pandey, A.K. *Bauhinia variegata* leaf extracts exhibit considerable antibacterial, antioxidant, and anticancer activities. *Biomed. Res. Int.* **2013**, *2013*, 915436. [CrossRef] [PubMed]
18. Wang, L.; Tian, X.; Wei, W.; Chen, G.; Wu, Z. Fingerprint analysis and quality consistency evaluation of flavonoid compounds for fermented *Guava* leaf by combining high-performance liquid chromatography time-of-flight electrospray ionization mass spectrometry and chemometric methods. *J. Sep. Sci.* **2016**, *39*, 3906–3916. [CrossRef] [PubMed]
19. Zahoor, M.; Shafiq, S.; Ullah, H.; Sadiq, A.; Ullah, F. Isolation of quercetin and mandelic acid from *Aesculus indica* fruit and their biological activities. *BMC Biochem.* **2018**, *19*, 5. [CrossRef] [PubMed]
20. Kumar Singh, S.; Patra, A. Evaluation of phenolic composition, antioxidant, anti-inflammatory and anticancer activities of *Polygonatum verticillatum* (L.). *J. Integr. Med.* **2018**, *16*, 273–282. [CrossRef] [PubMed]
21. Ustun, O.; Senol, F.S.; Kurkcuoglu, M.; Orhan, I.E.; Kartal, M.; Baser, K.H.C. Investigation on chemical composition, anticholinesterase and antioxidant activities of extracts and essential oils of *Turkish Pinus* species and pycnogenol. *Ind. Crops Prod.* **2012**, *38*, 115–123. [CrossRef]
22. Apetrei, C.L.; Tuchilus, C.; Aprotosoaie, A.C.; Oprea, A.; Malterud, K.E.; Miron, A. Chemical, antioxidant and antimicrobial investigations of *Pinus cembra* L. bark and needles. *Molecules* **2011**, *16*, 7773–7788. [CrossRef] [PubMed]
23. Jarial, R.; Thakur, S.; Sakinah, M.; Zularisam, A.W.; Sharad, A.; Kanwar, S.S.; Singh, L. Potent anticancer, antioxidant and antibacterial activities of isolated flavonoids from Asplenium nidus. *J. King Saud Univ.-Sci.* **2018**, *30*, 185–192. [CrossRef]
24. Nagja, T.; Vimal, K.; Sanjeev, A. Myristica Fragrans: A comprehensive review. *Int. J. Pharm. Pharm. Sci.* **2016**, *8*, 27–30.
25. Dzotam, J.K.; Simo, I.K.; Bitchagno, G.; Celik, I.; Sandjo, L.P.; Tane, P.; Kuete, V. In vitro antibacterial and antibiotic modifying activity of crude extract, fractions and 3′,4′,7-trihydroxyflavone from *Myristica fragrans* Houtt against MDR Gram-negative enteric bacteria. *BMC Complement. Altern. Med.* **2018**, *18*, 15. [CrossRef] [PubMed]
26. Tchamgoue, J.; Hafizur, R.M.; Tchouankeu, J.C.; Kouam, S.F.; Adhikari, A.; Hameed, A.; Green, I.R.; Choudhary, M.I. Flavonoids and other constituents with insulin secretion activity from *Pseudarthria hookeri*. *Phytochem. Lett.* **2016**, *17*, 181–186. [CrossRef]
27. Dzoyem, J.P.; Tchamgoue, J.; Tchouankeu, J.C.; Kouam, S.F.; Choudhary, M.I.; Bakowsky, U. Antibacterial activity and cytotoxicity of flavonoids compounds isolated from *Pseudarthria hookeri* Wight & Arn. (Fabaceae). *S. Afr. J. Bot.* **2018**, *114*, 100–103. [CrossRef]
28. Geethalakshmi, R.; Sundaramurthi, J.C.; Sarada, D.V.L. Antibacterial activity of flavonoid isolated from *Trianthema decandra* against *Pseudomonas aeruginosa* and molecular docking study of FabZ. *Microb. Pathog.* **2018**, *121*, 87–92. [CrossRef] [PubMed]
29. Lim, Y.-H.; Kim, I.-H.; Seo, J.-J. In vitro activity of kaempferol isolated from the *Impatiens balsamina* alone and in combination with erythromycin or clindamycin against *Propionibacterium acnes*. *J. Microbiol.* **2007**, *45*, 473–477. [PubMed]
30. Tsai, P.J.; Huang, W.C.; Hsieh, M.C.; Sung, P.J.; Kuo, Y.H.; Wu, W.H. Flavones isolated from *Scutellariae radix* suppress *Propionibacterium acnes*-induced cytokine production in vitro and in vivo. *Molecules* **2016**, *21*, 15. [CrossRef] [PubMed]
31. Hsieh, S.K.; Xu, J.R.; Lin, N.H.; Li, Y.C.; Chen, G.H.; Kuo, P.C.; Chen, W.Y.; Tzen, J.T.C. Antibacterial and laxative activities of strictinin isolated from Pu'er tea (*Camellia sinensis*). *J. Food Drug Anal.* **2016**, *24*, 722–729. [CrossRef] [PubMed]

32. Poomanee, W.; Chaiyana, W.; Mueller, M.; Viernstein, H.; Khunkitti, W.; Leelapornpisid, P. In-vitro investigation of anti-acne properties of *Mangifera indica* L. kernel extract and its mechanism of action against *Propionibacterium acnes*. *Anaerobe* **2018**, *52*, 64–74. [CrossRef] [PubMed]
33. Cragg, G.M.; Newman, D.J. Plants as a source of anti-cancer agents. *J. Ethnopharmacol.* **2005**, *100*, 72–79. [CrossRef] [PubMed]
34. Shah, U.; Shah, R.; Acharya, S.; Acharya, N. Novel anticancer agents from plant sources. *Chin. J. Nat. Med.* **2013**, *11*, 16–23. [CrossRef]
35. Brusselmans, K.; De Schrijver, E.; Heyns, W.; Verhoeven, G.; Swinnen, J.V. Epigallocatechin-3-gallate is a potent natural inhibitor of fatty acid synthase in intact cells and selectively induces apoptosis in prostate cancer cells. *Int. J. Cancer* **2003**, *106*, 856–862. [CrossRef] [PubMed]
36. Block, V.; Patterson, B.; Subar, A. Fruit, vegetables, and cancer prevention: A review of the epidemiological evidence. *Nutr. Cancer* **1992**, *18*, 1–29. [CrossRef] [PubMed]
37. Danciu, C.; Vlaia, L.; Fetea, F.; Hancianu, M.; Coricovac, D.E.; Ciurlea, S.A.; Şoica, C.M.; Marincu, I.; Vlaia, V.; Dehelean, C.A.; et al. Evaluation of phenolic profile, antioxidant and anticancer potential of two main representants of Zingiberaceae family against B164A5 murine melanoma cells. *Biol. Res.* **2015**, *48*, 1. [CrossRef] [PubMed]
38. Brusselmans, K.; Vrolix, R.; Verhoeven, G.; Swinnen, J.V. Induction of cancer cell apoptosis by flavonoids is associated with their ability to inhibit fatty acid synthase activity. *J. Biol. Chem.* **2005**, *280*, 5636–5645. [CrossRef] [PubMed]
39. Hashemzaei, M.; Far, A.D.; Yari, A.; Heravi, R.E.; Tabrizian, K.; Taghdisi, S.M.; Sadegh, S.E.; Tsarouhas, K.; Kouretas, D.; Tzanakakis, G.; et al. Anticancer and apoptosis-inducing effects of quercetin in vitro and in vivo. *Oncol. Rep.* **2017**, *38*, 819–828. [CrossRef] [PubMed]
40. Nwaeburu, C.C.; Abukiwan, A.; Zhao, Z.; Herr, I. Quercetin-induced miR-200b-3p regulates the mode of self-renewing divisions in pancreatic cancer. *Mol. Cancer* **2017**, *16*, 23. [CrossRef] [PubMed]
41. Yuan, X.; Wu, H.; Xu, H.; Xiong, H.; Chu, Q.; Yu, S.; Wu, G.S.; Wu, K. Notch signaling: An emerging therapeutic target for cancer treatment. *Cancer Lett.* **2015**, *369*, 20–27. [CrossRef] [PubMed]
42. Capaccione, K.M.; Pine, S.R. The Notch signaling pathway as a mediator of tumor survival. *Carcinogenesis* **2013**, *34*, 1420–1430. [CrossRef] [PubMed]
43. Ellisen, L.W.; Bird, J.; West, D.C.; Soreng, A.L.; Reynolds, T.C.; Smith, S.D.; Sklar, J. TAN-1, the human homolog of the Drosophila *Notch* gene, is broken by chromosomal translocations in T lymphoblastic neoplasms. *Cell* **1991**, *66*, 649–661. [CrossRef]
44. Adjakly, M.; Ngollo, M.; Boiteux, J.P.; Bignon, Y.J.; Guy, L.; Bernard-Gallon, D. Genistein and daidzein: Different molecular effects on prostate cancer. *Anticancer Res.* **2013**, *33*, 39–44. [PubMed]
45. Abusnina, A.; Keravis, T.; Yougbaré, I.; Bronner, C.; Lugnier, C. Anti-proliferative effect of curcumin on melanoma cells is mediated by PDE1A inhibition that regulates the epigenetic integrator UHRF1. *Mol. Nutr. Food Res.* **2011**, *55*, 1677–1689. [CrossRef] [PubMed]
46. Ide, H.; Lu, Y.; Noguchi, T.; Muto, S.; Okada, H.; Kawato, S.; Horie, S. Modulation of AKR1C2 by curcumin decreases testosterone production in prostate cancer. *Cancer Sci.* **2018**, *109*, 1230–1238. [CrossRef] [PubMed]
47. Craig, W.J. Health-promoting properties of common herbs. *Am. J. Clin. Nutr.* **1999**, *70*, 491S–499S. [CrossRef] [PubMed]
48. Garjani, A.; Tila, D.; Hamedeyazdan, S.; Vaez, H.; Rameshrad, M.; Pashaii, M.; Fathiazad, F. An investigation on cardioprotective potential of *Marrubium vulgare* aqueous fraction against ischaemia-reperfusion injury in isolated rat heart. *Folia Morphol.* **2017**, *76*, 361–371. [CrossRef] [PubMed]
49. Dludla, P.V.; Joubert, E.; Muller, C.J.F.; Louw, J.; Johnson, R. Hyperglycemia-induced oxidative stress and heart disease-cardioprotective effects of rooibos flavonoids and phenylpyruvic acid-2-O-β-D-glucoside. *Nutr. Metab.* **2017**, *14*, 45. [CrossRef] [PubMed]
50. Cook, N.C.; Samman, S. Flavonoids—Chemistry, metabolism, cardioprotective effects, and dietary sources. *J. Nutr. Biochem.* **1996**, *7*, 66–76. [CrossRef]
51. Gao, Q.; Yang, B.; Ye, Z.-G.; Wang, J.; Bruce, I.C.; Xia, Q. Opening the calcium-activated potassium channel participates in the cardioprotective effect of puerarin. *Eur. J. Pharmacol.* **2007**, *574*, 179–184. [CrossRef] [PubMed]

52. Razavi-Azarkhiavi, K.; Iranshahy, M.; Sahebkar, A.; Shirani, K.; Karimi, G. The protective role of phenolic compounds against doxorubicin-induced cardiotoxicity: A comprehensive review. *Nutr. Cancer* **2016**, *68*, 892–917. [CrossRef] [PubMed]
53. Korga, A.; Józefczyk, A.; Zgórka, G.; Homa, M.; Ostrowska, M.; Burdan, F.; Dudka, J. Evaluation of the phytochemical composition and protective activities of methanolic extracts of *Centaurea borysthenica* and *Centaurea daghestanica* (Lipsky) Wagenitz on cardiomyocytes treated with doxorubicin. *Food Nutr. Res.* **2017**, *61*, 1344077. [CrossRef] [PubMed]
54. Tian, J.; Wu, X.; Zhang, M.; Zhou, Z.; Liu, Y. Comparative study on the effects of apple peel polyphenols and apple flesh polyphenols on cardiovascular risk factors in mice. *Clin. Exp. Hypertens.* **2018**, *40*, 65–72. [CrossRef] [PubMed]
55. Olas, B. The multifunctionality of berries toward blood platelets and the role of berry phenolics in cardiovascular disorders. *Platelets* **2017**, *28*, 540–549. [CrossRef] [PubMed]
56. Alhaider, I.A.; Mohamed, M.E.; Ahmed, K.K.M.; Kumar, A.H.S. Date palm (*Phoenix dactylifera*) fruits as a potential cardioprotective agent: The role of circulating progenitor cells. *Front. Pharmacol.* **2017**, *8*, 592. [CrossRef] [PubMed]
57. Syama, H.P.; Arya, A.D.; Dhanya, R.; Nisha, P.; Sundaresan, A.; Jacob, E.; Jayamurthy, P. Quantification of phenolics in *Syzygium cumini* seed and their modulatory role on tertiary butyl-hydrogen peroxide-induced oxidative stress in H9c2 cell lines and key enzymes in cardioprotection. *J. Food Sci. Technol.* **2017**, *54*, 2115–2125. [CrossRef] [PubMed]
58. Repo-Carrasco-Valencia, R.; Hellström, J.K.; Pihlava, J.M.; Mattila, P.H. Flavonoids and other phenolic compounds in Andean indigenous grains: Quinoa (*Chenopodium quinoa*), kañiwa (*Chenopodium pallidicaule*) and kiwicha (*Amaranthus caudatus*). *Food Chem.* **2010**, *120*, 128–133. [CrossRef]
59. Morrison, D.K. MAP kinase pathways. *Cold Spring Harb. Perspect. Biol.* **2012**, *4*, a011254. [CrossRef] [PubMed]
60. Han, X.; Gao, S.; Cheng, Y.; Sun, Y.; Liu, W.; Tang, L.; Ren, D. Protective effect of naringenin-7-O-glucoside against oxidative stress induced by doxorubicin in H9c2 cardiomyocytes. *Biosci. Trends* **2012**, *6*, 19–25. [CrossRef] [PubMed]
61. Sun, J.; Sun, G.; Meng, X.; Wang, H.; Luo, Y.; Qin, M.; Ma, B.; Wang, M.; Cai, D.; Guo, P.; et al. Isorhamnetin protects against doxorubicin-induced cardiotoxicity in vivo and in vitro. *PLoS ONE* **2013**, *8*, e64526. [CrossRef] [PubMed]
62. Middleton, E.; Kandaswami, C. Effects of flavonoids on immune and inflammatory cell functions. *Biochem. Pharmacol.* **1992**, *43*, 1167–1179. [CrossRef]
63. Locatelli, M.; Macchione, N.; Ferrante, C.; Chiavaroli, A.; Recinella, L.; Carradori, S.; Zengin, G.; Cesa, S.; Leporini, L.; Leone, S.; et al. Graminex pollen: Phenolic pattern, colorimetric analysis and protective effects in immortalized prostate cells (PC3) and rat prostate challenged with LPS. *Molecules* **2018**, *23*, 1145. [CrossRef] [PubMed]
64. Vasantha Rupasinghe, H.P.; Boehm, M.M.A.; Sekhon-Loodu, S.; Parmar, I.; Bors, B.; Jamieson, A.R. Anti-inflammatory activity of haskap cultivars is polyphenols-dependent. *Biomolecules* **2015**, *5*, 1079–1098. [CrossRef] [PubMed]
65. Sisto, A.; Luongo, D.; Treppiccione, L.; De Bellis, P.; Di Venere, D.; Lavermicocca, P.; Rossi, M. Effect of *Lactobacillus paracasei* culture filtrates and artichoke polyphenols on cytokine production by dendritic cells. *Nutrients* **2016**, *8*, 635. [CrossRef] [PubMed]
66. Moharram, F.A.; El Dib, R.A.E.M.; Marzouk, M.S.; El-Shenawy, S.M.; Ibrahim, H.A. New apigenin glycoside, polyphenolic constituents, anti-inflammatory and hepatoprotective Activities of *Gaillardia grandiflora* and *Gaillardia pulchella* aerial parts. *Pharmacogn. Mag.* **2017**, *13*, S244–S249. [CrossRef] [PubMed]
67. Su, X.; Zhang, J.; Wang, H.; Xu, J.; He, J.; Liu, L.; Zhang, T.; Chen, R.; Kang, J. Phenolic acid profiling, antioxidant, and anti-inflammatory activities, and miRNA regulation in the polyphenols of 16 blueberry samples from China. *Molecules* **2017**, *22*, 312. [CrossRef] [PubMed]
68. Compaore, M.; Bakasso, S.; Meda, R.; Nacoulma, O. Antioxidant and anti-inflammatory activities of fractions from *Bidens engleri* O.E. Schulz (Asteraceae) and *Boerhavia erecta* L. (Nyctaginaceae). *Medicines* **2018**, *5*, 53. [CrossRef] [PubMed]

69. Dugo, L.; Belluomo, M.G.; Fanali, C.; Russo, M.; Cacciola, F.; MacCarrone, M.; Sardanelli, A.M. Effect of cocoa polyphenolic extract on macrophage polarization from proinflammatory M1 to anti-inflammatory M2 state. *Oxid. Med. Cell. Longev.* **2017**, *2017*, 6293740. [CrossRef] [PubMed]
70. Lopes, C.L.; Pereira, E.; Soković, M.; Carvalho, A.M.; Barata, A.M.; Lopes, V.; Rocha, F.; Calhelha, R.C.; Barros, L.; Ferreira, I.C.F.R. Phenolic composition and bioactivity of *Lavandula pedunculata* (Mill.) Cav. samples from different geographical origin. *Molecules* **2018**, *23*, 1037. [CrossRef] [PubMed]
71. Ma, S.; Yada, K.; Lee, H.; Fukuda, Y.; Iida, A.; Suzuki, K. Taheebo polyphenols attenuate free fatty acid-induced inflammation in murine and human macrophage cell lines as inhibitor of cyclooxygenase-2. *Front. Nutr.* **2017**, *4*, 63. [CrossRef] [PubMed]
72. Ferreres, F.; Duangsrisai, S.; Gomes, N.G.M.; Suksungworn, R.; Pereira, D.M.; Gil-Izquierdo, A.; Valentão, P.; Choowongkomon, K.; Andrade, P.B. Anti-inflammatory properties of the stem bark from the herbal drug *Vitex peduncularis* Wall. ex Schauer and characterization of its polyphenolic profile. *Food Chem. Toxicol.* **2017**, *106*, 8–16. [CrossRef] [PubMed]
73. Lu, C.L.; Zhu, Y.F.; Hu, M.M.; Wang, D.M.; Xu, X.J.; Lu, C.J.; Zhu, W. Optimization of astilbin extraction from the rhizome of *Smilax glabra*, and evaluation of its anti-inflammatory effect and probable underlying mechanism in lipopolysaccharide-induced RAW264.7 macrophages. *Molecules* **2015**, *20*, 625–644. [CrossRef] [PubMed]
74. Dong, L.; Zhu, J.; Du, H.; Nong, H.; He, X.; Chen, X. Astilbin from *Smilax glabra* Roxb. Attenuates inflammatory responses in complete Freund's adjuvant-induced arthritis rats. *Evid. Based Complement. Alternat. Med.* **2017**, *2017*, 8246420. [CrossRef] [PubMed]
75. Bumrungpert, A.; Lilitchan, S.; Tuntipopipat, S.; Tirawanchai, N.; Komindr, S. Ferulic acid supplementation improves lipid profiles, oxidative stress, and inflammatory status in hyperlipidemic subjects: A randomized, double-blind, placebo-controlled clinical trial. *Nutrients* **2018**, *10*, 713. [CrossRef] [PubMed]
76. Ichihashi, M.; Ueda, M.; Budiyanto, A.; Bito, T.; Oka, M.; Fukunaga, M.; Tsuru, K.; Horikawa, T. UV-induced skin damage. *Toxicology* **2003**, *189*, 21–39. [CrossRef]
77. Svobodová, A.; Psotová, J.; Walterová, D. Natural phenolics in the prevention of UV-induced skin damage. A review. *Biomed. Pap.* **2003**, *147*, 137–145. [CrossRef]
78. Korać, R.; Khambholja, K. Potential of herbs in skin protection from ultraviolet radiation. *Pharmacogn. Rev.* **2011**, *5*, 164–173. [CrossRef] [PubMed]
79. Saewan, N.; Jimtaisong, A. Photoprotection of natural flavonoids. *J. Appl. Pharm. Sci.* **2013**, *3*, 129–141. [CrossRef]
80. Ferrali, M.; Signorini, C.; Caciotti, B.; Sugherini, L.; Ciccoli, L.; Giachetti, D.; Comporti, M. Protection against oxidative damage of erythrocyte membrane by the flavonoid quercetin and its relation to iron chelating activity. *FEBS Lett.* **1997**, *416*, 123–129. [CrossRef]
81. Cos, P.; Ying, L.; Calomme, M.; Hu, J.P.; Cimanga, K.; Van Poel, B.; Pieters, L.; Vlietinck, A.J.; Vanden Berghe, D. Structure-activity relationship and classification of flavonoids as inhibitors of xanthine oxidase and superoxide scavengers. *J. Nat. Prod.* **1998**, *61*, 71–76. [CrossRef] [PubMed]
82. McKay, D.L.; Blumberg, J.B. A review of the bioactivity and potential health benefits of chamomile tea (*Matricaria recutita* L.). *Phyther. Res.* **2006**, *20*, 519–530. [CrossRef] [PubMed]
83. Gerhäuser, C. Beer constituents as potential cancer chemopreventive agents. *Eur. J. Cancer* **2005**, *41*, 1941–1954. [CrossRef] [PubMed]
84. Wach, A.; Pyrzyńska, K.; Biesaga, M. Quercetin content in some food and herbal samples. *Food Chem.* **2007**, *100*, 699–704. [CrossRef]
85. Casagrande, R.; Georgetti, S.R.; Verri, W.A.; Dorta, D.J.; dos Santos, A.C.; Fonseca, M.J.V. Protective effect of topical formulations containing quercetin against UVB-induced oxidative stress in hairless mice. *J. Photochem. Photobiol. B Biol.* **2006**, *84*, 21–27. [CrossRef] [PubMed]
86. Ozkur, M.K.; Bozkurt, M.S.; Balabanli, B.; Aricioglu, A.; Ilter, N.; Gurer, M.A.; Inaloz, H.S. The effect of EGb 761 on lipid peroxide levels and superoxide dismutase activity in sunburn. *Photodermatol. Photoimmunol. Photomed.* **2002**, *18*, 117–120. [CrossRef] [PubMed]
87. Bijak, M. Silybin, a major bioactive component of milk thistle (*Silybum marianum* L. Gaernt.)—Chemistry, bioavailability, and metabolism. *Molecules* **2017**, *22*, 1942. [CrossRef] [PubMed]

88. Katiyar, S.K.; Mantena, S.K.; Meeran, S.M. Silymarin protects epidermal keratinocytes from ultraviolet radiation-induced apoptosis and DNA damage by nucleotide excision repair mechanism. *PLoS ONE* **2011**, *6*, e21410. [CrossRef] [PubMed]
89. Moore, J.O.; Wang, Y.; Stebbins, W.G.; Gao, D.; Zhou, X.; Phelps, R.; Lebwohl, M.; Wei, H. Photoprotective effect of isoflavone genistein on ultraviolet B-induced pyrimidine dimer formation and PCNA expression in human reconstituted skin and its implications in dermatology and prevention of cutaneous carcinogenesis. *Carcinogenesis* **2006**, *27*, 1627–1635. [CrossRef] [PubMed]
90. Wang, Y.N.; Wu, W.; Chen, H.C.; Fang, H. Genistein protects against UVB-induced senescence-like characteristics in human dermal fibroblast by p66Shc down-regulation. *J. Dermatol. Sci.* **2010**, *58*, 19–27. [CrossRef] [PubMed]
91. Setchell, K.D.R.; Clerici, C. Equol: History, chemistry, and formation. *J. Nutr.* **2010**, *140*, 1355S–1362S. [CrossRef] [PubMed]
92. Widyarini, S. Protective effect of the isoflavone equol against DNA damage induced by ultraviolet radiation to hairless mouse skin. *J. Vet. Sci.* **2006**, *7*, 217–223. [CrossRef] [PubMed]
93. Choi, H.S.; Park, E.D.; Park, Y.; Han, S.H.; Hong, K.B.; Suh, H.J. Topical application of spent coffee ground extracts protects skin from ultraviolet B-induced photoaging in hairless mice. *Photochem. Photobiol. Sci.* **2016**, *15*, 779–790. [CrossRef] [PubMed]
94. Kano, M.; Kubota, N.; Masuoka, N.; Hori, T.; Miyazaki, K.; Ishikawa, F. Oral administration of fermented soymilk products protects the skin of hairless mice against ultraviolet damage. *Nutrients* **2016**, *8*, 514. [CrossRef] [PubMed]
95. Lahlou, M. The success of natural products in drug discovery. *Pharmacol. Pharm.* **2013**, *4*, 17–31. [CrossRef]
96. Burton, J.L.; Wells, M. The effect of phytoestrogens on the female genital tract. *J. Clin Pathol* **2002**, *55*, 401–407. [CrossRef] [PubMed]
97. Rachoń, D. Endocrine disrupting chemicals (EDCs) and female cancer: Informing the patients. *Rev. Endocr. Metab. Disord.* **2015**, *16*, 359–364. [CrossRef] [PubMed]
98. De Gregorio, C.; Marini, H.; Alibrandi, A.; Di Benedetto, A.; Bitto, A.; Adamo, E.B.; Altavilla, D.; Irace, C.; Di Vieste, G.; Pancaldo, D.; et al. Genistein supplementation and cardiac function in postmenopausal women with metabolic syndrome: Results from a pilot strain-echo study. *Nutrients* **2017**, *9*, 584. [CrossRef] [PubMed]
99. Squadrito, F.; Marini, H.; Bitto, A.; Altavilla, D.; Polito, F.; Adamo, E.B.; D'Anna, R.; Arcoraci, V.; Burnett, B.P.; Minutoli, L.; et al. Genistein in the metabolic syndrome: Results of a randomized clinical trial. *J. Clin. Endocrinol. Metab.* **2013**, *98*, 3366–3374. [CrossRef] [PubMed]
100. Irace, C.; Marini, H.; Bitto, A.; Altavilla, D.; Polito, F.; Adamo, E.B.; Arcoraci, V.; Minutoli, L.; Di Benedetto, A.; Di Vieste, G.; et al. Genistein and endothelial function in postmenopausal women with metabolic syndrome. *Eur. J. Clin. Investig.* **2013**, *43*, 1025–1031. [CrossRef] [PubMed]
101. Morabito, N.; Crisafulli, A.; Vergara, C.; Gaudio, A.; Lasco, A.; Frisina, N.; D'Anna, R.; Corrado, F.; Pizzoleo, M.A.; Cincotta, M.; et al. Effects of genistein and hormone-replacement therapy on bone loss in early postmenopausal women: A randomized double-blind placebo-controlled study. *J. Bone Miner. Res.* **2002**, *17*, 1904–1912. [CrossRef] [PubMed]
102. Kruger, M.C.; Middlemiss, C.; Katsumata, S.; Tousen, Y.; Ishimi, Y. The effects of green kiwifruit combined with isoflavones on equol production, bone turnover and gut microflora in healthy postmenopausal women. *Asia Pac. J. Clin. Nutr.* **2018**, *27*, 347–358. [CrossRef] [PubMed]
103. Kaczmarczyk-Sedlak, I.; Klasik-Ciszewska, S.; Wojnar, W. Glabridin and glycyrrhizic acid show no beneficial effect on the chemical composition and mechanical properties of bones in ovariectomized rats, when administered in moderate dose. *Pharmacol. Rep.* **2016**, *68*, 1036–1041. [CrossRef] [PubMed]
104. Malaivijitnond, S.; Tungmunnithum, D.; Gittarasanee, S.; Kawin, K.; Limjunyawong, N. Puerarin exhibits weak estrogenic activity in female rats. *Fitoterapia* **2010**, *81*, 569–576. [CrossRef] [PubMed]
105. Drouet, S.; Garros, L.; Hano, C.; Tungmunnithum, D.; Renouard, S.; Hagège, D.; Maunit, B.; Lainé, É. A critical view of different botanical, molecular, and chemical techniques used in authentication of plant materials for cosmetic applications. *Cosmetics* **2018**, *5*, 30. [CrossRef]

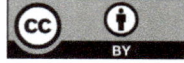

© 2018 by the authors. Licensee MDPI, Basel, Switzerland. This article is an open access article distributed under the terms and conditions of the Creative Commons Attribution (CC BY) license (http://creativecommons.org/licenses/by/4.0/).

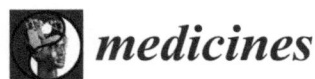

Review

Antioxidant Activity of *Myrtus communis* L. and *Myrtus nivellei* Batt. & Trab. Extracts: A Brief Review

Aicha Hennia [1], Maria Graça Miguel [2,*] and Said Nemmiche [3]

1. Department of Agronomy, Faculty of Nature and Life Sciences, University of Mostaganem, BP 188/227, Mostaganem 27000, Algeria; a.hennia@gmail.com
2. Departamento de Química e Farmácia, Faculdade de Ciências e Tecnologia, Universidade do Algarve, MeditBio, Campus de Gambelas, 8005-139 Faro, Portugal
3. Department of Biology, Faculty of Nature and Life Sciences, University of Mostaganem, BP 188/227, Mostaganem 27000, Algeria; snemiche@hotmail.com
* Correspondence: mgmiguel@ualg.pt; Tel.: +351-289-800-100

Received: 30 June 2018; Accepted: 8 August 2018; Published: 11 August 2018

Abstract: *Myrtus communis* L. (myrtle) and *Myrtus nivellei* Batt. & Trab. (Saharan myrtle) have been used in folk medicine for alleviating some ailments. *M. communis* is largely distributed in the Mediterranean Basin, whereas *M. nivellei* is confined in specific zones of the central Saharan mountains. The chemical composition and antioxidant activity of berry and leaf extracts isolated from myrtle are deeply documented, whereas those isolated from Saharan myrtle extracts are less studied. In both species, the major groups of constituents include gallic acid derivatives, flavonols, flavonol derivatives, and hydroxybenzoic acids. In coloured berries, anthocyanins are also present. In *M. nivellei* extracts are reported for some compounds not described in *M. communis* so far: 2-hydroxy-1,8-cineole-β-D-glucopyranoside, 2-hydroxy-1,8-cineole 2-O-α-L-arabinofuranosyl (1→6)-β-D-glucopyranoside, rugosin A, and rugosin B. Berries and leaves extracts of both species had antioxidant activity. Comparative studies of the antioxidant activity between leaf and berry myrtle extracts revealed that leaf extracts are best antioxidants, which can be assigned to the galloyl derivatives, flavonols, and flavonols derivatives, although the ratio of these groups of compounds might also have an important role in the antioxidant activity. The anthocyanins present in myrtle berries seem to possess weak antioxidant activity. The antioxidant activity of sample extracts depended on various factors: harvesting time, storage, extraction solvent, extraction type, and plant part used, among other factors. Leaf extracts of myrtle revealed to possess anti-inflammatory activity in several models used. This property has been attributed either to the flavonoids and/or hydrolysable tannins, nevertheless nonprenylated acylphloroglucinols (e.g., myrtucommulone and semimyrtucommulone) have also revealed a remarkable role in that activity. The biological activities of myrtle extracts found so far may direct its use towards for stabilizing complex lipid systems, as prebiotic in food formulations, and as novel therapeutic for the management of inflammation.

Keywords: Anti-inflammatory; berries; leaves; galloyl derivatives; flavonol derivatives; anthocyanins; myrtucommulone

---

1. Introduction

Myrtaceae is a family of woody flowering plants that encompasses around 5500 species, classified in 144 genera, and 17 tribes. Within Myrtaceae, the tribe Myrteae represents half of the family's biodiversity with 51 genera and about 2500 species mostly restricted to the Neotropics, though 15 genera and about 450 species are found in other continents, such as Southeast Asia, Northeast Australia, and the Pacific islands, including New Caledonia and New Zealand. The genus *Myrtus* is the sole found in European/Northern African, Asia, particularly in the Mediterranean region of southern Europe as far west as Macaronesia (Madeira and the Azores), the Saharan mountains and as far east as western Asia (Iran and Afghanistan) [1–3].

Two species can be found in the genus *Myrtus*: *Myrtus communis* L. and *Myrtus nivellei* Batt. & Trab. The latter is endemic to the central Saharan mountains growing in rocky and sandy wades and gorges, at high elevations, above 1400 m. The former can be found in the Mediterranean Basin, Macaronesia, Iran, and Afghanistan, particularly at elevations not exceeding c.a. 500 m a.s.l. [1]. Both species are shrubs with rough bark, opposite leaves, white flowers that are star-like (5–9 petals), and white, purple, blue, or even black berries. They differ in the following morphological characteristics: the leaves of *M. nivellei* are linear-lanceolate (4–5 cm in length) and narrower (6–8 mm) than the *M. communis* ones, which are ovate-lanceolate (2–5 cm long) and wider (10–20 mm); the fruits of *M. communis* are ellipsoid to subglobose, pyriform, elongated, or flat (7–9 mm length), whereas those of *M. nivellei* are globose and smaller (4–5 mm) [1,4–6]. *M. communis* grows to 0.5–3 m in height, while *M. nivelli* grows to 1–2 m in height [1].

Different parts (berries, branches, and leaves) of *M. communis* (myrtle) have been used in folk medicine for treating diarrhoea, peptic ulcers, haemorrhoids, inflammation, uterine bleeding, headache, palpitation, leucorrhoea, urethritis, epistaxis, conjunctivitis, excessive perspiration, and pulmonary and skin diseases [4,7]. Only few studies have reported a sedative effect of myrtle, as a anxiolytic and muscle relaxant without anticonvulsivant activity [8,9].

Myrtle leaves have been used for healing wounds or disorders of the digestive and urinary systems due to their astringent, tonic, and antiseptic properties [4,10]. From leaves is also possible to extract essential oils that have been used as anti-septic, anti-catarrhal, and to treat chest ailments, ulcers, and hemorrhoids [4,10–13].

Although the berries decoctions had been used to bathe newborns with reddened skin, and the decoctions of leaves and berries in sore washing, the most is used to produce the characteristic myrtle liqueur obtained by hydro-alcoholic infusion of the berries [4,14,15].

The biological properties assigned to diverse organs (leaves and berries) of myrtle can be due to diverse compounds such as volatile compounds or essential oils (terpenoids, particularly α-pinene, 1,8-cineole, geranyl acetate, and linalool), flavonoids (quercetin, catechin and myricetin derivatives, and anthocyanins), coumarins, oligomeric nonprenylated acylphloroglucinol compounds (myrtucommulone A and B and semimyrtucommulone), galloyl-glucosides, ellagitannins, galloyl-quinic acids, caffeic, gallic and ellagic acids, fatty acids (linoleic, palmitic, oleic, and stearic acids) in diverse organs [4]. Table 1 shows examples of biological properties assigned to *Myrtus communis*.

M. nivellei (Saharan myrtle) leaves in infusions are used against intestinal diseases (diarrhoea), fever, diabetes, and added to barley wafers is employed against blennorrhoea [16–18]. The crushed leaves added to oil or butter ointment has been used in the treatment of dermatosis and for hair and body care [16,17,19]. The decoction of leaves mixed with goat milk and heated on charcoal has been used for liver disorders by nomad Algerians of Tassili region [20]. The leaf infusion is used in this region as a common beverage, instead of green tea [20]. Berries are consumed either fresh or dried to treat mouth canker sores [19].

The chemical composition of Saharan myrtle is less studied than that of myrtle. The main constituents reported include volatile essential oils [16,21], phenols (flavonoids, anthocyanins, and tannins), norterpenoids [19–22].

The present review will focus on the antioxidant and anti-inflammatory activities of *M. communis* and *M. nivellei* in which the chemical composition is discriminated.

Table 1. Biological properties attributed to *Myrtus communis* (antioxidant and anti-inflammatory activities are not included).

Plant Part Used	Compounds	Biological Properties	References
		Antimicrobial	
Leaves	Not reported	Bacterial vaginosis	[23]
Leaves	Not reported	*Propionibacterium acnes*	[24]
Leaves and berries	Not reported	- Spoilage bacteria *Pseudomonas aeruginosa* IH, *Pseudomonas aeruginosa* CECT 118, *Pseudomonas aeruginosa* CECT 110T, *Pseudomonas fluorescens* CECT 378 and *Bacillus subtilis* DCM 3366 - Food-borne pathogenic bacteria, namely *Escherchia coli* K12, *Listeria innocua* CECT 4030, *Listeria monocytogenes* CECT 4032, *Enteroccus faecium* CECT 410, *Staphylococcus aureus* MBLA, *Staphylococcus aureus* CECT 976, *Staphylococcus aureus* CECT 794 and *Proteus vulgaris* CECT 484	[25]
Leaves	Not reported	One hundred and twenty strains of *Escherichia coli* isolated from the urine culture	[26]
Leaves	Not reported	*Streptococcus pneumoniae*, *Streptococcus pyogenes*, *Streptococcus agalactiae*, *Listeria monocytogenes*, *Campylobacter jejuni*, *Staphylococcus aureus*, *Micrococcus luteus*, *Escherichia coli*, *Proteus vulgaris*, and *Pseudomonas aeruginosa*	[27]
Leaves	Not reported	*Aeromonas hydrophila* isolated from four hundred and fifty samples from the intestines of the infected *Cyprinus carpio* fish	[28]
Leaves	Not reported	Ninety-six *P. aeruginosa* strains isolated from 400 burn patients (men and women) in Iranian hospital	[29]
Leaves	*Galloylated nonprenylated phloroglucinol glucosides:* Gallomyrtucommulone A Gallomyrtucommulone B Gallomyrtucommulone C Gallomyrtucommulone D	*Staphylococcus aureus* strain ATCC 25923 gift of E. Udo (Kuwait University, Kuwait) *S. aureus* RN4220 containing plasmid pUL5054, which carries the gene encoding the MsrA macrolide efflux protein, provided by J. Cove *S. aureus* XU-212 which possesses the TetK tetracycline efflux protein, provided by E. Udo *S. aureus* SA-1199B, which overexpresses the *norA* gene encoding the NorA MDR efflux protein, provided by G. Kaatz *S. aureus* EMRSA-15 is an epidemic strain of MRSA gift of P. Stapleton, School of Pharmacy, University of London	[30]

Table 1. Cont.

Plant Part Used	Compounds	Biological Properties	References
Seeds	Not reported	*Escherichia coli* (PTCC No. 1330), *Pseudomonas aeruginosa* (PTCC No. 1074), *P. fluorescens* (PTCC No. 1181), *Klebsiella pneumoniae* (PTCC No. 1053), *Bordetella bronchiseptica* (PTCC No. 1025), *Staphylococcus aureus* (PTCC No. 1112), *S. epidermidis* (PTCC No. 1114), *Micrococcus luteus* (PTCC No. 1170), *Bacillus cereus* (PTCC No. 1015), and *B. pumilis* (PTCC No. 1319)	[31]
Berry seeds	Hydroxybenzoic acid hexose Delphinidin-3-O-galactoside Delphinidin-3-O-glucoside Quercetin hexoside Delphinidin-3-O-rhamnoside Delphinidin rutinoside Delphinidin-3-(6 coumaroyl)-glucoside Petunidin-3-O-glucoside Petunidin diglucoside Petunidin malonylglucoside Petunidin-3-O-rutinoside Isorhamnetin-O-rhamnoside Malvidin-O-galactoside Malvidin-O-glucoside Peonidin diglucoside Petunidin methyl pentose	*Escherichia coli* ATCC 8739, *Salmonella typhimurium* NCTC 6017, *Staphylococcus aureus* ATCC 29213, *Pseudomonas aeruginosa* ATCC 27853, *Aeromonas hydrophila* EI, and *Bacillus cereus* ATCC 1247	[32]
Leaves	Not reported	*Streptococcus mutans* (PTCC 1683)	[33]
Leaves	Not reported	Gram-positive (*Listeria monocytogenes* and *Bacillus cereus*) Gram-negative (*Escherichia coli* O157:H7) bacterial strains Fungal strain (*Candida albicans*)	[34]
Leaves and berries	Not reported	*Staphylococcus aureus* (ATCC 6538), *Bacillus subtilis* (ATCC 6059), *Micrococcus flavus* (SBUG 16), *Escherichia coli* (ATCC 11229), *Pseudomonas aeruginosa* (ATCC 27853), and three multi-resistant *Staphylococcus* strains (*Staphylococcus epidermidis* 847, *Staphylococcus haemolyticus* 535, *Staphylococcus aureus* north German epidemic strain) *Candida maltosa* (SBUG)	[35]

Table 1. Cont.

Plant Part Used	Compounds	Biological Properties	References
Leaves	Not reported	Staphylococcus aureus, Staphylococcus epidermidis, Escherichia coli, Bacillus subtilis and Serratia marcescens	[36]
Leaves	Myrtucommulones J-L Myrtucommulone A	Staphylococcus aureus (ATCC 25923)	[37]
Leaves	Not reported	Enterococcus faecalis (ATCC 29212)	[38]
Leaves	Not reported	Bacterial vaginosis	[39]
Leaves	Not reported	Pseudomonas aeruginosa	[40]
Leaves	Not reported	Microsporum canis ATCC 32903, M. gypseum ATCC 14683, and Trichophyton mentagrophytes ATCC 1481 (var. interdigitale) from Tehran University of Medical Sciences	[41]
Aerial parts	Not reported	Trichophyton mentagrophytes, T. interdigitale, Microsporum canis, and M. gypseum (10 strain of each)	[42]
Leaves	Not reported	Escherichia coli O157:H7, Yersinia enterocolitica O9, Proteus spp., and Klebsiella pneumoniae	[43]
Berries	Not reported	Helicobacter pylori (12 clinical isolates)	[44]
Leaves	Not reported	Staphylococcus aureus (489 samples) isolated either from healthy carriers (nose and throat) or clinical samples S. aureus used as reference strains for comparison: ATCC 25923, ATCC 9144, ATCC 29737, ATCC 12596, and Bristol A 9596	[45]
Leaves	5-Acetoxy-4-hydroxy-4-isobutyl-2,2,6,6-tetramethylcyclohexan-1,3-dione β-Sitosterol Isomyrtucommulone-B Endoperoxide-G-3-hormone Gallic acid Myricetin-3-O-α-L-rhamnoside Myricetin-3-O-β-D-glucoside Myrncetin-3-O-β-D-galactoslde-6''-O-gallate (8)	Propionibacterium acnes NRRL (B-4224)	[46]

Table 1. Cont.

Plant Part Used	Compounds	Biological Properties	References
Leaves	Myrtucommulone A	Bacillus subtilis, Staphylococcus aureus, Escherichia coli, Saccharomyces cerevisiae, Escherichia coli B, E. coli CW 3747, E. coli K-12, Klebsiella pneumoniae, Proteus mirabilis, Proteus morganii, Shigella dysenteriae, S. flexneri, Salmonella typhimurium, Pseudomonas fluorescens, Vibrio cholerae, Serratia, Staphylococcus aureus, S. albus, Bacillus subtilis W23, B. subtilis 16, B. pumilus, Streptococcus faecalis, Corynebacterium diphtheriae, and C. xerosis	[47]
Leaves	Not reported	Helicobacter pylori	[48]
Leaves	Myrtucomvalones A–C Callistiviminene J-N	Respiratory syncytial virus (RSV)	[49]
Aerial parts	Myrtucommulone B-E Usnone A Tectochrysine 2,5-Dihydroxy-4-methoxybenzophenone (cearoin) β-Sitosterol Sideroxylin Ursolic acid Corosolic acid Arjunolic acid Erythrodiol Oleanolic acid Betulin	Escherichia coli, Bacillus subtilis, Shigella flexneri, Staphylococcus aureus, Pseudomonas aeruginosa, and Salmonella typhi	[50]
Leaves	Semimyrtucommulone myrtucommulone A	Staphylococcus aureus strains RN4220 (Msr(A)), XU212 (Tet(K)), 1199-B (Nor(A)), and ATCC 25923	[51]
Leaves	Myrtucommunins A-D 6-Methyl-isomyrtucommulone B 4-Methyl myrtucommulone B 2-Isobutyryl-4-methylphloroglucinol 1-O-β-D-glucopyranoside Chromone derivative, undulatoside A 6′-O-gallate	Escherichia coli, Staphylococcus aureus (MRSA), Staphylococcus aureus (MSSA), and Bacillus subtilis	[52]

Table 1. Cont.

Plant Part Used	Compounds	Biological Properties	References
Leaves	Silver nanoparticles synthesized using *Myrtus communis* L. leaf extract	*Escherichia coli*, *Bacillus subtilis*, *Pseudomonas aeruginosa*, *Staphylococcus aureus* methicillin-resistant, *Staphylococcus aureus*, and *Enterococcus faecalis*	[53]
Leaves	Before and after encapsulation in liposomes	*Staphylococcus aureus* (ATCC25923), *Staphylococcus epidermidis* (ATCC 12228), *Staphylococcus mutans* (ATCC 31989) and *Staphylococcus viridans* (ATCC 19952), *Pseudomonas aeruginosa* (ATCC 27853), *Escherichia coli* (ATCC 25922), *Enterobacter cloacae* (ATCC 13047) and *Klebsiella pneumoniae* (ATCC13883), *Candida albicans* (ATCC 10231), *Candida tropicalis* (ATCC 13801) and *Candida glabrata* (ATCC 28838), and *Listeria monocytogenes*	[54]
		Other organisms	
Leaves	Not reported	Anti-*Leishmania tropica* on an *in vitro* model	[55]
Aerial parts	Not reported	*In vivo*, anti-*Plasmodium berghei* in female Swiss albino mice, weight 18–20 g *In vitro*, chloroquine-sensitive strain (3D7) of *P. falciparum*	[56]
Not reported (myrtle was obtained from a local grocery for herbal plants)	Not reported	Induced programmed cell death in hydatid cyst protoscolices	[57]
Aerial part	Not reported	*In vitro*, anti-chloroquine-resistant (K1) and chloroquine-sensitive (3D7) strains of *Plasmodium falciparum* *In vivo*, anti-*Plasmodium berghei* infection in adult male albino mice	[58]
		Cytotoxicity	
Leaves	Not reported	Cytotoxic activities against J774 cells (Mouse BALB/c monocyte macrophage)	[55]
Leaves and berries	Not reported	Cytotoxic activities against urinary bladder 5637 and human breast carcinoma MCF-7 cell lines	[35]
Leaves	Myrtucommulones J-L Myrtucommulone A	Cytotoxic activities against human haematological tumor cell line MT-4. Cytotoxic activities against solid tumor cell lines (HepG2 or human liver cancer, DU145 or human prostate cancer cell lines), and against "normal" human tissue cells (CRL7065)	[37]
Leaves	Myrtucommulone A	Cytotoxic activities against U-937 (human lung (lymphoblast), K-562 (human blood (chronic myelogenous leukemia), leukemic cell line KBM-5, and MEG-01 (human bone marrow) cell lines	[59]

Table 1. Cont.

Plant Part Used	Compounds	Biological Properties	References
Aerial part	Not reported	Cytotoxic activities against MCF7 (breast adenocarcinoma), HepG2 (hepatocellular carcinoma), WEHI (fibrosarcoma), and MDBK (normal kidney cells)	[58]
Not reported	Not reported	L20B (cell line a mouse cell-line genetically engineered to express human poliovirus receptor, CD155 cell lines), RD (rhabdomyosarcom), and Vero (African green monkey kidney)	[60]
Not reported	Myrtucommulone A	Mitochondrial lysates from leukemic HL-60 cells	[61]
Leaves	Myrtucommulone Semi-myrtucommulone	Jurkat-A3 cells, caspase-8-deficient Jurkat cells, FADD deficient Jurkat cells, PC-3 (androgen-independent prostate carcinoma), LNCaP (androgen-dependent prostate carcinoma), H9 (cutaneous T-cell lymphoma), DLD-1 (colorectal adenocarcinoma), HL-60 (acute promyelocytic leukaemia), Jurkat (acute T-cell leukaemia) and Jurkat DD3 (mutated in CD95), KFR (rhabdomyosarcoma) and UKF-NB-3 (neuroblastoma) cells, mono Mac 6 (MM6, acute monocytic leukaemia) cells, and human peripheral blood mononuclear cells (PBMC)	[62]
Not reported	Myrtucommulone	Mouse Breast cancer cell line 4T1, mouse embryonic fibroblasts, and human dermal fibroblasts (hDFs)	[63]
Leaves	Myrtucomvalones A–C Callistiviminene J-N	Human larynx epidermoid carcinoma cells (HEp-2) cells	[49]
Leaves	Myricetin-3-O-galactoside Myricetin-3-O-rhamnoside	Human chronic myelogenous leukemia cell line K562	[64]
Leaves	3,5-O-Di-galloylquinic acid	Human chronic myelogenous leukemia CML cell line K562	[65]
Genotoxicity/mutagenicity			
Leaves	Not reported	Protective effect against genotoxicity on the SOS reponse induced by Aflatoxin B1 (AFB1) and Nifuroxazide in *Escherichia coli* PQ37	[66]
Leaves	Not reported	Protective effect against the mutagenicity induced by aflatoxin B1 (AFB1) in *Salmonella typhimurium* TA100 and TA98 assay systems, and against the mutagenicity induced by sodium azide in TA100 and TA1535 assay system	[67]

Table 1. Cont.

Plant Part Used	Compounds	Biological Properties	References
Leaves	Not reported	Protective effect against on the mutagenicity induced by aflatoxin B1 in *Salmonella typhimurium* TA100 or TA98	[68]
Leaves	Myricetin-3-O-galactoside Myricetin-3-O-rhamnoside	Protective effect against the mutagenicity induced by aflatoxin B1 in *Escherichia coli* PQ37 strain	[64]
Leaves	3,5-O-Di-galloylquinic acid	Inhibitory effect against H_2O_2-induced genotoxicity, using the comet assay	[65]
Gastrointestinal system			
Berry seeds	Hydroxybenzoic acid hexose Delphinidin-3-O-galactoside Delphinidin-3-O-glucoside Quercetin hexoside Delphinidin-3-O-rhamnoside Delphinidin rutinoside Delphinidin-3-(6 coumaroyl)-glucoside Petunidin-3-O-glucoside Petunidin diglucoside Petunidin malonylglucoside Petunidin-3-O-rutinoside Isorhamnetin-O-rhamnoside Malvidin-O-galactoside Malvidin-O-glucoside Peonidin diglucoside Petunidin methyl pentose	Anti-diarrhoeal in adult male Wistar rats after castor oil administration	[32]
Leaves	Not reported	Anti-diarrhoeal in Swiss albino mice of either sex weighing 20–30 g and aged 6–8 weeks, after castor oil administration	[69]
Berries	Not reported	Protective effect on gastric ulcer against ethanol, indomethacin, and pyloric ligation induced models in albino rats of Wistar strain weighing 150–200 g	[70]
Stems and seeds	Not reported	Protective effect on oral ulcer recovery process in white Spraque–Dawley rats weighing 250–300 g after punch to create a wound in the hard palate in the oral cavity	[71]

Table 1. Cont.

Plant Part Used	Compounds	Biological Properties	References
Berry seeds	Palmitic acid Stearic acid Oleic acid Linoleic acid Linolelaidic (trans, trans-C18:2) Arachidic acid	Protective effect on peptic ulcer against ethanol induced in adult male Wistar rats (weighing 220–240 g)	[72]
Berry seeds	Hydroxybenzoic acid hexose Delphinidin-3-O-galactoside Delphinidin-3-O-glucoside Quercetin hexoside Delphinidin-3-O-rhamnoside Delphinidin rutinoside Delphinidin-3-(6 coumaroyl)-glucoside Petunidin-3-O-glucoside Petunidin diglucoside Petunidin malonylglucoside Petunidin-3-O-rutinoside Isorhamnetin-O-rhamnoside Malvidin-O-galactoside Malvidin-O-glucoside Peonidin diglucoside Petunidin methyl pentose	Protective effect on acetic acid-induced ulcerative colitis in adult male Wistar rats (weighing 220–240 g)	[73]
Leaves	Not reported	Protective effect on acetic acid-induced ulcerative colitis in Wistar albino rats (weighing 250–300 g)	[74]
Leaves	Not reported	Protective effect on liver injury and fibrosis occurring in Wistar albino rats (weighing 250–300 g) with biliary obstruction by double ligatures with suture silk	[75]
Berries	Not reported	Decrease of reflux and dyspeptic scores as compared with the baseline, in double-blind randomized controlled clinical trial in adult aged from 18 to 60 years	[76]
Berries	Not reported	Decrease of the recurrence of symptoms in reflux patients after the discontinuance of proton pump inhibitors, in outpatient, double-blind, randomized, parallel treatment groups study	[77]
Leaves	Not reported	Decrease of the recurrent aphthous stomatitis in randomized, double blind, controlled before–after clinical trial	[78]

Table 1. *Cont.*

Plant Part Used	Compounds	Biological Properties	References
Leaves	Not reported	Decrease of recurrent aphthous stomatitis in a single-blind, placebo-controlled clinical trial	[79]
Aerial parts	Not reported	Upregulation of appetite related gene (ghrelin) and food intake in zebrafish	[80]
Aerial parts	Not reported	Spasmolytic: complete relaxation of spontaneous and K+ (80 mM)-induced contractions in isolated rabbit jejunum	[81]
		Cardiovascular system	
Leaves	Not reported	Anti-hypercholesterolemia by inhibition of 3-hydroxy-3-methylglutaryl coenzyme A reductase	[82]
Leaves	5,8-Dihydroxy-6,7,4′-trimethoxyflavone Quercetin-3-O-neohesperidoside, Quercetin-3-O-galactoside *trans*-1′,5′-5-(5-Carboxymethyl-2-oxocyclopentyl)-3Z-pentenyl-(6-O-galloyl) glucopyranoside, 3-Methoxy myricetin 7-O-β-L-rhamnopyranoside	Antiobesity effect on high fat diet induced male wistar albino obese rats	[83]
Aerial parts	Not reported	Vasodilator: Relaxation of phenylephrine (1 µM)- and K+ (80 mM)-induced contractions in isolated rabbit aorta	[81]
		Anti-hyperglycaemic	
Leaves	Not reported	Streptozotocin-induced diabetic female Swiss albino mice	[84]
Leaves	Not reported	Streptozotocin-induced diabetic 6-week-old male Albino Wistar rats	[85]
Not reported	Not reported	Inhibition of α-glucosidase from for baker's yeast, rabbit liver, and rabbit small intestine	[86]

Table 1. Cont.

Plant Part Used	Compounds	Biological Properties	References
Aerial parts	Myrtucommulone B-E Usnone A Tectochrysine 2,5-Dihydroxy-4-methoxybenzophenone (cearoin) β-Sitosterol Sideroxylin Ursolic acid Corosolic acid Arjunolic acid Erythrodiol Oleanolic acid Betulin	Inhibition of α-glucosidase from *Saccharomyces* species	[50]
Aerial parts	Not reported	Streptozocin-induced type 1 diabetes mellitus in Sprague–Dawley male rats (weighing 225–250 g)	[87]
		Respiratory system	
Aerial parts	Not reported	Relaxant effect on carbachol- and K^+ (80 mM)-induced contractions in isolated rabbit tracheal preparations	[81]
Berries	Not reported	Treatment of chronic rhinosinusitis in double-blinded randomized placebo-controlled trial	[88]
Leaves	Not reported	Inhibition of inflammation and fibrosis of lung parenchyma in both preventive and therapeutic methods in male albino rats weighting 180–200 g	[89]
		Nervous system	
Leaves	Not reported	Anxiolytic and muscle relaxant effect without anticonvulsant activities, hypnotic effects without effect on seizure threshold: Male NMRI mice subjected to open field, righting reflex, grip strength, and pentylentetrazole-induced seizure tests. Male Wistar rats used to evaluate the alterations in rapid eye movement (REM) and non-REM (NREM) sleep	[9]
Aerial parts	Not reported	Inhibition of acetylcholinesterse and butyrylcholinesterase	[90]

Table 1. *Cont.*

Plant Part Used	Compounds	Biological Properties	References
Aerial parts	Not reported	Antinociceptive activity using male albino mice weighing 25–30 g and the following tests: assessed using the hot plate and Writhing tests	[91]
		Skin	
Leaves	Not reported	Case report: Two patients with common warts	[92]
Leaves	Not reported	Treatment of dandruff: A double blinded randomized clinical trial comprised patients with dandruff aged 18–60 years visiting the dermatology out-patient clinic	[93]
		Genito-urinary system	
Berries	Not reported	A randomized, double-blind, placebo-controlled pilot study conducted on 30 women suffering from abnormal uterine bleeding-menometrorrhagia	[94]
		Longevity	
Leaves	Not reported	*Caenorhabditis elegans* used a model organism for longevity research and age-related diseases	[95]

The microorganisms reported in the Table are those that were used by the authors, such does not mean that samples have activity against all of the microorganisms.

2. *Myrtus communis*: Berries

All works regarding the antioxidant activity of berry extracts reported their capacity for preventing lipid peroxidation or capacity for scavenging free radicals. In the majority of cases, the evaluation was done *in vitro* as can be read below. The presentation of results was diverse, hampering many times the comparison of the results. In addition, in those cases where the identification of compounds was done, very few works correlate the contribution of each phenol compound on the antioxidant activity. Factors such as type of extraction, solvents, maturation stage, storage conditions, variety, different parts of the fruit, different organs that could influence the chemical profile, and antioxidant activity of myrtle extracts were evaluated by diverse teams, as can be read below. Sanjust et al. [96] had previously reviewed the antioxidant activity of myrtle liqueur along with other Mediterranean shrubs *Arbutus unedo*, *A. andrachne*, *Capparis spinosa*, *Opuntia ficus-indica*, *Rosa canina*, *Rosmarinus officinalis*, and *Rubus fruticosus*.

2.1. Myrtle Liqueur

One of the most applications of berries is to produce the myrtle liqueur obtained by hydro-alcoholic infusion of the berries. For this reason, there are some works evaluating the antioxidant of myrtle liqueur as described beneath.

Previously, Alamanni and Cossu [97] not only reported the antioxidant activity measured to the ability for scavenging DPPH (2,2-diphenyl-1-picrylhydrazyl) free radicals, conductimetric method, and the linoleic acid test of liquors made from berries and leaves *Myrtus communis* L. (eight industrially-prepared and three laboratory-prepared samples), as also correlated with the amounts of phenols in samples, although not identifying such metabolites. Simultaneously, the authors compare the activities of samples with some red wines and synthetic antioxidant standards (Butylated hydroxytoluene (BHT) and butylated hydroxyanisole (BHA)) and a natural standard (catechin). The results showed that samples had capacity for scavenging free radicals and had also higher antioxidant index and induction time in the conductimetric test. In both tests, the authors found a correlation between the activities and the phenol concentration of samples. This correlation was low in the linoleic acid test. For the same concentration of phenols, berry liquors showed higher protection against fatty acid oxidation and red wines presented better protection than liquors [97]. Concerning the capacity for scavenging free radicals, both berry and leaf liquours had higher activity than red wines. The amounts of phenols ranged from 0.17 to 1.47 g/L.

The correlation between phenol and anthocyanins amounts and antioxidant activity was poorly significant in the results obtained by Vacca et al. [98] when studying the effect of type and time of storage of myrtle liqueur on the accumulation of phenols and anthocyanins as well as in the capacity for scavenging the DPPH free radicals. The antioxidant activity of myrtle liqueur decreased over the time, with a loss of about 20% by the end of storage in opened bottles, in contrast to the unopened bottles in which the activity practically remained constant, even after one year of storage. Either in open or unopened bottles, the free and combined anthocyanins decreased, nevertheless faster and more intensively in last ones [98]. Montoro et al. [15] showed that berry extracts of *M. communis* prepared for liqueur recipe were not stable during one year of storage, being flavonoids and, particularly, anthocyanins the most unstable compounds. Their results have even allowed to state that the use of extracts should not exceed three months. During this period, the antioxidant activity (scavenging 2,2'-azino-*bis*-3-ethylbenzthiazoline-6-sulphonic acid (ABTS) free radicals capacity) would be preserved. In addition, the authors also identified by high performance liquid chromatography (HPLC) coupled with electrospray mass spectrometry (ESMS) the flavonoids and anthocyanins (Table 2) present in the extract, along with their quantification by HPLC coupled with Ultraviolet/visible detection (UV/Vis), over the storage period. For obtaining a final product of myrtle liqueur with the traditional characteristics, the starting material should be fresh or lyophilised and the extraction should be only the maceration, excluding other procedures such as the ultrasonic extraction. The initial extract had capacity for scavenging the ABTS free radical that increased after 3 months of storage.

Such is coincident with the hydrolysis of the flavon glycosides, that is, higher accumulation of myricetin, which leads to an additional hydroxyl group able to participate in the redox reaction. However, after 8 months of storage the antioxidant activity was stable and similar to the fresh extract, despite significant decrease of anthocyanins but higher amounts of myricetin [15].

For myrtle liqueur production, berries must be processed immediately after harvest to prevent quality loss such as decay and development of off flavours. For this reason, liqueur industries immediately process the berries and store the hydro-alcoholic extracts. Nevertheless, some anthocyanins decreased over time and the extract loses the initial characteristics [15]. Another approach is to store berries in cold conditions during a defined period, or even freeze them, however, some studies have also concluded that these procedures are not free of undesirable effects, namely in the alteration of fruit composition and, therefore, in the liqueur quality [99]. According to Fadda et al. [14], oxygen-enriched atmospheres have been successfully used to retain the quality of stored fruit and vegetables. For this reason, they proposed to evaluate the effect of different high oxygen treatments on physicochemical quality of myrtle berries and their corresponding hydro-alcoholic extracts used for the preparation of the liqueur. Oxygen treatments induced an increase of total phenols in stored berries, for example, berries held at 80% O_2 had higher total phenols than 60% O_2 and control fruit after 10 and 20 days of storage, nevertheless practically without differences after 30 days. Anthocyanins' contents were also higher in those berries submitted to higher levels of O_2, particularly after 10–20 days of storage. The capacity for scavenging DPPH free radicals was also higher in those samples held at 80% O_2 after 20 days, and decreasing afterwards. Oxygen treatments did not influence the ability of samples for quenching ABTS free radicals. Such results allowed concluding that myrtle fruit held at oxygen concentration between 60% and 80%, for 20 days at 2 °C, preserve quality with higher phenolic and anthocyanin concentration [14].

For producing liqueur of myrtle berries, Zam et al. [100] studied the effect of different extracts from Syrian wild myrtle berries and their mixtures with cloves and cinnamon added as flavours on the phenolic fractions and antioxidant activity. Hydroalcoholic mixtures in the range of 50–80% and a maceration process for 5 months were used. Concerning the total polyphenols the authors observed that the extraction mixture with higher percentage of water extracted higher amount of phenols than the extraction mixture with higher percentage of ethanol. According to the authors, such may be attributed to several factors: high concentrations of ethanol will denature proteins which prevent the dissolution of phenols, and low levels of ethanol in the extraction will permit to access easily into cells and dissociate the complex phenolic compounds bound to proteins and polysaccharides into the cell walls [100]. Only the addition of clove originates higher amounts of polyphenols in the samples. During the maceration period there was an increase of the amounts of total polyphenols being also dependent on the concentrations of ethanol. The highest phenol concentration was observed in the hydroalcoholic extract (50:50) with cloves, and after 60 days of maceration (7.82 g/100 g, dry weight). The antioxidant activity was also measured through the ability of samples for scavenging the DPPH free radicals. All samples presented variable antioxidant activity depending on the type of extract, concentration of alcohol, and time of maceration. The sample extracted with the hydroalcoholic (50:50) solution and after 60 days of maceration in myrtle berries:cinnamon:clove and myrtle berries:clove mixtures had the best capacity for scavenging the DPPH free radicals (80.95% and 80.02%, respectively). The results indicate a positive correlation between the total content of polyphenols and the antioxidant activity. At the end, the authors [100] concluded that the extract obtained with the mix ethanol/water (50:50) with cloves was the most adequate for providing the better characteristics for liqueur preparation.

The extraction efficiency in the preparation of myrtle liqueur was also evaluated by Snoussi et al. [101]. In order to achieve the objective, the authors assayed different alcohol–water mixtures (50–90% ethanol), for 40 days. Flavonoids and anthocyanins were identified (Table 2) by HPLC/ESMS and quantified by HPLC/UV/Vis. The antioxidant activity was assayed using the method of DPPH. The results showed that higher amounts of total polyphenols were obtained in the extract with 80% ethanol, coinciding with the highest capacity for scavenging the DPPH free radicals (87.5%). The minimum activity was found in the extract with 60% ethanol (65.0%). The best phenol extraction with mixtures of solvents with higher proportions of alcohol contrasts with those reported by [100]. In addition, during the maceration period, a reduction in the concentrations of the identified compounds was observed. For example, the content of the major constituent of the extract, malvidin-3-*O*-glucoside, decreased with a loss of 30–40% after 40 days of storage. According to the authors [101], such loss can be attributed to the degradation, combination with other compounds providing more stable polymeric pigments. Differences in the antioxidant activity can be attributed not only to the amounts of phenols but also to their structures, according to the authors, nevertheless none study was performed by them to clarify this statement [101].

Tuberoso et al. [102] used three methods (capacity for scavenging the DPPH and ABTS free radicals, and ferric reducing antioxidant power (FRAP)) for evaluating the antioxidant activity of liqueurs obtained by cold maceration of myrtle berries and compared the results with other two typical food products from the Mediterranean area (red wines Cannonau and strawberry-tree honey). Simultaneously, the authors [102] proceeded in identifying the secondary metabolites by LC-MS/MS (liquid chromatography tandem mass spectrometry) and also dosing them by HPLC-DAD (High-Performance Liquid Chromatography with Diode-Array Detection). Cannonau wine and myrtle liqueur showed high levels of total polyphenols (1978 and 1741 mg gallic acid equivalent/L, respectively). A positive correlation between the results of FRAP, ABTS, and DPPH assays and total polyphenols were observed by the authors [102]. Despite this correlation, myrtle liqueur, wines Cannonau and strawberry-tree honey presented different antioxidant activities. The authors did not determine the antioxidant activity of each phenol compound identified in samples and, therefore, they were not able to attribute those activities to any compound, nevertheless they suggested that the different types of phenols could be responsible for the differences observed. Only some examples pointed out by the authors [102]: myrtle liqueur was characterized by myricetin-3-*O*-arabinoside (not detected in Cannonau wine), quercetin-3-*O*-glucuronide and kaempferol-3-*O*-glucoside were detected only in Cannonau wine; strawberry-tree honey showed homogentisic acid as the most prominent phenolic compound, which was absent in myrtle liqueur and Cannonau wine. The antioxidant activities of myrtle liqueur found by the authors were as follows: 26.7 mmol Fe^{2+}/L, 9.3 mmol TEAC/L, and 11.5 mmol TEAC/L for the FRAP, DPPH, and ABTS assays, respectively [102].

The antioxidant capacity of myrtle liqueur obtained from white myrtle berry was also determined by Serreli et al. [103]. The identification and quantification of the phenols were followed by LC-MS/MS and HPLC-DAD, respectively. The antioxidant activity was determined through ABTS, DPPH, FRAP, and CUPRAC (CUPric Reducing Antioxidant Capacity) assays. The constituents of the volatile fraction of liqueur samples were also identified by gas chromatography and mass spectrometry (GC-MS) and quantified by GC-FID (GC-flame ionization detector) after headspace solid-phase microextraction (HS-SPME) and liquid–liquid extraction (LLE). According to the results obtained, lower amounts of total polyphenols were found by the authors in the white myrtle berry liqueur (636.3 mg gallic acid equivalent/L), when they compared their results with those of other authors that used purple berries (1741 mg gallic acid equivalent/L) [102]. Despite this difference, white myrtle berry liqueur did not exhibit poorer antioxidant activity than purple myrtle berry liqueur [102]. The antioxidant activities of white myrtle liqueur found by the authors were as follows: 30.21 mmol Fe^{2+}/L, 3.72 mmol TEAC/L, and 11.66 mmol TEAC/L for the FRAP, DPPH, and ABTS assays, respectively [103]. The antioxidant activity measured through the CUPRAC method was 11.30 mmol Fe^{2+}/L. Once again, the contribution of each compound on the antioxidant activity was not made by the authors; however they attributed the similar or even better activity of their samples (liqueurs obtained from white myrtle berries) to the highest amounts of gallic acid and their derivatives (Table 2), although other groups of polyphenols are also present in the liqueur samples (Table 2). In the volatile fraction, terpenes predominated in white myrtle berry liqueurs, nevertheless other ones could also be detected such as 4-hydroxybenzyl alcohol, ethyl 4-hydroxybenzoate, 4-hydroxybenzoic acid, vanillic acid, and ethyl vanillate, all of them shikimic acid pathway derivatives, which could also contribute to the antioxidant activity [103].

2.2. Antioxidant Activity of Berry Extracts

The antioxidant activities of berry extracts were also performed in diverse works. For example, [104] reported that the methanolic extracts of eight accessions of Turkish myrtle fruits had capacity for scavenging DPPH free radicals as well as inhibiting linoleic acid oxidation measured through the method of β-carotene-bleaching test, although with different strenght. In the DPPH assay, the IC_{50} values found ranged from 2.34 µg/mL, not significantly different to that of the reference α-tocopherol, and 8.24 µg/mL. In what concerns, the ability for preventing linoleic acid oxidation, the percentages of inhibition were always above 80%, nevertheless lower than the percentage registered for reference (α-tocopherol); that was 96.31%. The effect of extracting solvents on the total phenolic content, antioxidant, and antiradical activity of extracts of myrtle berry, collected in different places of Turkey, was also studied by Polat et al. [105]. The antioxidant activity, evaluated through the phosphomolybdenum spectrophotometric method, revealed that methanolic extract presented the highest antioxidant value (241.533 mg ascorbic acid equivalents/g dry extract). Overall, the phenol content ranged from 39.933 to 207.4 mg gallic acid equivalent/g. The capacity for scavenging DPPH free radicals ranged between 6.73% and 65.6%.

The antioxidant activity of extracts obtained from white and dark blue Tunisian berries was evaluated by [106]. The chemical composition was also evaluated by the authors: essential oils, fatty acids, and anthocyanins. Dark blue fruits produced extracts with higher antioxidant activity, measured through the capacity of scavenging the DPPH free radicals and ferric reducing antioxidant power (IC_{50} = 2.1 mg/mL and 2.6 mmol Fe^{2+}/g, respectively) than white fruits (2.8 mg/mL and 2.1 mmol Fe^{2+}/g, respectively). These results are different to those previously reported [103], because these authors did not observe lower activity in liqueurs made with white berries. However, and as expected, in both cases the levels of anthocyanins in white berries is lower than in red or dark purple berries (Table 2). Total polyphenols, flavonoids, and flavonols were higher in coloured berries than in white ones. The authors attributed the antioxidant capacity variation between the two myrtle types to their different phenolic contents [106].

Other factors that can influence the phenol/anthocyanin content and antioxidant activity of myrtle extracts have been studied by diverse research teams: variety [107,108], part of the berry [107], maturation [109], method of extraction, and type of solvent [110–112].

The antioxidant activity of myrtle berry extracts prepared with solvents at diverse polarities (water, alcohol, and ethyl acetate) was evaluated by Tuberoso et al. [110] for the first time. The authors evaluated the capacity of those extracts for scavenging the DPPH free radicals and their capacity to protect biological molecules using the cholesterol and LDL (low density lipoproteins) oxidation assays. In the same work, the identification of phenolic compounds was assigned by HPLC-DAD and HPLC-MS/MS (Table 2). The ethyl acetate extract had the highest capacity for inhibiting the reduction of polyunsaturated fatty acids and cholesterol, and the increase of their oxidative products [110]. Moreover, higher amounts of phenols were found in the aqueous and ethyl acetate extracts which coincided with the highest antioxidant activity, meaning a high correlation between the concentration of phenols and the antioxidant activity. However, the contribution of each phenol compound on the antioxidant activity, independent on the method used, was not clarified. Besides the protective effect of myricetin-3-O-galactoside and myricetin-3-O-rhamnoside on cholesterol and human LDL oxidation, since they are generally considered excellent in inhibiting free radical and lipid peroxidation, other compounds might have contributed to the best activity of the ethyl acetate extract, such as gallic acid derivatives [110].

Methanolic extracts of whole fruit, seed and pericarp of *M. communis* var. *italica* were analysed in terms of total phenols, flavonoids, anthocyanins, and antioxidant activity (DPPH, β-carotene-linoleic acid bleaching and reducing power assays) [107]. The total phenol and tannins contents varied among different parts of myrtle fruit; seed extract had higher total phenol and tannin contents than whole fruit, while total flavonoid contents were higher in pericarp. The compounds identified by the authors are depicted in Table 2. Methanolic seed extracts showed higher scavenging ability on DPPH radicals (IC_{50} = 8 µg/mL) than whole fruit (IC_{50} = 136 µg/mL) and pericarp (IC_{50} = 196 µg/mL), which can be attributed to the highest levels of hydrolysable tannins [107]. Seed methanolic extract also showed a higher ability to prevent the bleaching of β-carotene (IC_{50} = 70 µg/mL) than whole fruit (IC_{50} = 78 µg/mL) and pericarp (IC_{50} = 150 µg/mL). The reducing power of seed methanolic extract was also better than the remaining myrtle fruit parts. According to these results, myrtle seed is the structure within the fruit that has the strongest activity, probably due to the presence of galloyl derivatives [107]. Later on, these authors [108] studied the chemical composition and antioxidant activity of oil and methanolic extract of seeds of other variety of myrtle, *M. communis* var. *baetica*. The total phenol (25.25 mg/g), tannins (20.33 mg/g), flavonoids (0.75 mg/g), and proanthocyanidins (0.75 mg/g) were determined in the methanolic extracts. The capacity of this extract for scavenging DPPH free radicals (IC_{50} = 0.01 mg/mL), preventing the bleaching of β-carotene (IC_{50} = 0.07 mg/mL), chelating activity (3 mg/mL), and reducing power (0.01 mg/mL) were determined by the authors. The IC_{50} values found in this extract [108] were not significantly different to those reported for the methanolic extract of *M. communis* var. *italica* [107].

Babou et al. [109] also studied the chemical composition, antioxidant activity (ability for scavenging DPPH, superoxide, and nitric oxide free radicals) and inhibition of acetylcholinesterase of different parts of myrtle fruits and leaves. Simultaneously, they studied the influence of extraction processes (sonication followed by maceration with methanol:water 1:1 and decoction using water) and maturation stage (collection of plant material in September and December) on the chemical composition. The phenolic composition is depicted in Table 2. The concentrations of polyphenols in the extracts were dependent on both plant organ and extraction procedure. Hydroxybenzoic acids predominated in both seed extracts, whereas anthocyanins were at higher concentration in the pericarps (December), independent on the type of extract. Leaf aqueous extract from samples of December had higher amounts of flavonol glycosides and flavonol aglycones than the remaining samples, however, these groups of compounds were higher in methanolic/aqueous extract of leaves collected in September and seeds collected in December, respectively. Aqueous extracts extracted more amounts of phenols than the methanolic/aqueous extract. The capacity for scavenging DPPH free radicals, there was no significant difference between leaves-September (IC_{50} = 8.29–8.45 µg/mL) and leaves-December (IC_{50} = 9.44–9.51 µg/mL), berries-September (IC_{50} = 8.42 µg/mL) and seeds-December (IC_{50} = 3.89–6.50 µg/mL) samples. Significant differences in the capacity for scavenging the superoxide anion radical were not observed by the authors in both extraction procedures (except for pericarps-December extracts). The most active extracts were those of leaves-September (IC_{50} = 29.70–31.69 µg/mL) and leaves-December (IC_{50} = 33.70–34.69 µg/mL), berries-September (IC_{50} = 28.55–31.49 µg/mL) and seeds-December (IC_{50} = 24.19–28.32 µg/mL). Aqueous extracts of leaves-September (IC_{50} = 17.81 µg/mL), leaves-December (13.69 µg/mL), berries-September (22.16 µg/mL), and seeds-December (20.00 µg/mL) had the highest capacity for scavenging nitric oxide radicals [109]. The contribution of each phenolic compound in the antiradicalar activity was not evaluated by the authors but a statistical treatment allowed them to observe that the compounds contributing most for the antioxidant activity were the hydroxybenzoic acids (gallic and ellagic acids) and the flavonols (quercetin, quercetin-3-O-galactoside, quercetin-3-O-rutinoside, myricetin-3-O-rhamnoside, myricetin, and kaempferol). Although the highest amounts of phenols in both extracts of seeds, the anticholinesterase activity was weak [109].

Generally, maceration is the most common procedure for extracting phenols from myrtle berries, with some exception as reported above, in which the authors assayed other methods to compare the efficiency of phenol extraction, such as sonication or decoction [109]. Sonication or ultrasound-assisted extraction was also assayed by Pereira et al. [112] and supercritical fluid extraction [111] for extracting phenols and for evaluating the antioxidant activity of such extracts obtained from leaves and berries of

Portuguese *M. communis* L. Flavonoids from the family of quercetin and myricetin were present in the myrtle leaf extracts obtained by ultrasound-assisted extraction, and anthocyanins, hydrolysable tannins, and quinic acid (Table 2) were the constituents found in berries obtained by the same extraction method [112]. The antioxidant activity determined through the methods of ABTS and ORAC (oxygen radical antioxidant capacity) that measures the ability of samples for scavenging peroxyl free radicals, correlated with the phenol content, although the authors had not determined the contribution of individual phenol for the ability of quenching the free radicals. The samples were analysed by HPLC–DAD–ESI–MS/MS. The leaf extracts had higher antioxidant activity (358 µmol Trolox/g and 624 µmol Trolox/g) than berries extracts (179 µmol Trolox/g and 366 µmol Trolox/g) for ABTS and ORAC methods, respectively, although the anthocyanin content is quite high. Such finding may indicate that the best activity comes from the compounds belonging to the flavonols and not from the anthocyanins [112].

Pereira et al. [111] evaluated two extraction procedures of secondary metabolites from Portuguese leaves and berries of *M. communis* (liquid phase extraction and supercritical fluid extraction) on the composition and concentration of phenols (HPLC-DAD-MS/MS methods), and antiradicalar activity (ability for scavenging ABTS and peroxyl free radicals), during three years. In the liquid phase extraction, the extracts were obtained from the water dearomatized by hydrodistillation that was extracted with diisopropyl ether, whereas in the supercritical fluid extraction, the extracts were obtained at 23 MPa, 45 °C and a CO_2 flow of 0.3 kg/h using ethanol as cosolvent with a flow rate of 0.09 kg/h. The compounds found by the authors are listed in Table 2, flavonoids and anthocyanins were found in those extracts obtained by supercritical fluid extraction, whereas phenolic acids were only observed in the extracts obtained by liquid phase extraction. Extracts obtained by supercritical fluid extraction exhibited higher concentration of phenols and higher antioxidant activity, correlating well with the concentration of flavonol glycosides, the myricetin-O-glycosides [111]. In addition, leaf extracts were more active as antioxidants than berries in line with that already observed by [112] when used ultrasound-assisted extraction. The antiradicalar activities found by the authors were: ABTS (Leaves): 55–130 µmol Trolox/g; ABTS (Berries): 25–80 µmol Trolox/g; ORAC (Leaves): 530–759 µmol Trolox/g; ORAC (Berries): 130–250 µmol Trolox/g. With the exception of ORAC (Leaves), the activities found by Pereira et al. [111] for the extracts obtained by supercritical fluid extraction were lower than those obtained by ultrasound-assisted extraction. Such results demonstrated the importance of the extraction method on the antioxidant activity. The differences found by the authors [111] in the phenol content and antioxidant activity of the samples collected at different years were attributed to climatic factors since polyphenol content is affected by temperature [111].

The best antioxidant activity (DPPH radical scavenging capacity assay, the reducing antioxidant power assay and β-carotene linoleic acid assay) of leaf extracts had been already reported [113] for the different extract solvents (methanolic, ethanolic, and aqueous) of Moroccan myrtle. The amounts of total phenols were also higher in leaf extracts, independent on the extract, than berry extracts. The total phenol content of myrtle extracts ranged between 9.0 and 35.6 mg gallic acid equivalent/g extract. In leaf extracts, the overall antioxidant strength was in the order methanol > water > ethanol, whereas in berry extracts the order was methanol > ethanol > water. A positive correlation between the phenolic content with the antioxidant activity was observed by the authors: DPPH assay showed the highest correlation (r^2 = 0.949), followed by the reducing power assay (r^2 = 0.914) and the lowest for the β-carotene linoleic acid assay (r^2 = 0.722).

Later on, Amensour et al. [114] evaluated the amounts of total phenols and flavonoids of extracts of Moroccan leaves and berries of *M. communis* extracted with methanol, ethanol, ethyl acetate, and water. At the same time, they determined the antiradicalar capacity of all of these extracts using the ABTS method. Once again, the authors found that leaf extracts, independent on the extraction solvent, had higher activity that the remaining extracts. This higher activity is also coincident with the highest concentration of flavonoids and total phenols. In leaf and berry extracts, the overall antioxidant strengths were in the order methanol > water > ethanol > ethyl acetate, which were coincident with the order of flavonoids' concentration. In leaf and berry extracts, the order of total phenols was: water > methanol > ethanol > ethyl acetate. In addition, the authors observed higher positive correlation between capacity for scavenging the ABTS free radicals and total phenols (r^2 = 0.9452) than capacity for scavenging the ABTS free radicals and total flavonoids (r^2 = 0.5978), whereby the authors suggested that apart from flavonoids, there might be other phenolic compounds such as phenolic acids, tannic acid, and others responsible for the antioxidant activity.

Beyond the antioxidant activity of berry extracts, Serio et al. [115] also evaluated the anti-listerial activity. The hydroalcoholic extracts of red berries of *M. communis* exhibited antilisterial activity (two type strains and four isolates) and antioxidant activity (capacity for scavenging the ABTS free radicals) [115]. The authors used Central Composite Design (CCD) for studying the combined effect of sub-lethal concentrations of myrtle extract, NaCl (0–2.0 g/100 mL) and pH (5–7) on the growth of the six *Listeria monocytogenes* strains. The highest myrtle extract concentrations (0.117–0.195 mL/100 mL) combined with the lowest pH values (5.0–6.0) inhibited the growth of *L. monocytogenes*. This extract also possessed antioxidant activity that was stable during 70 days of storage in refrigerated conditions. According to the authors [115], such will permit to use this type of extracts with a certain quality assurance. The polyphenol content of the same extract was 5315.20 mg gallic acid equivalent/kg, and malvidin-3-*O*-glucoside was the most abundant anthocyanin in the same extract.

2.3. Anti-Inflammatory Activity of Berry Extracts

The anti-inflammatory activity of four species (*Myrtus communis*, *Smilax aspera*, *Lavandula stoechas*, and *Calamintha nepeta*) was evaluated by Amira et al. [116]. At the same time, the authors sought a possible correlation of anti-inflammatory activity with the antioxidant activity. The anti-inflammatory activity was done through the method of the carrageenan-induced paw oedema and the antioxidant activity through the following methods (DPPH, ABTS, galvinoxyl, superoxide and peroxynitrite scavenging activities, reducing power, and human plasma lipid peroxidation). Myrtle extract had the highest inhibitory activity in the paw oedema induced by carrageenan (60% at 3 h), in contrast to lavender that had the lowest inhibitory property (38%). Myrtle extract was the best among the extracts studied for scavenging the DPPH (163 µg Trolox equivalent/mg), ABTS (726 µg Trolox equivalent/mg) free radicals as well as reducing power (1351 µg ascorbic acid equivalent/mg); nevertheless *C. nepeta* extract was the best for scavenging galvinoxyl and superoxide radicals and peroxynitrite anion. *M. communis* extract was even unable to scavenge this anion, at least at the higher concentration tested (100 µg/mL) [116]. The inhibition of human plasma lipid peroxidation, assayed through the thiobarbituric acid reactive substance method, was higher in *C. nepeta* and *L. stoechas* extracts (>80%), while the inhibition percentage observed for myrtle extract was <25%. Reactive oxygen species, such as superoxide anion, peroxynitrite anion, and hydroxyl radicals, produced by neutrophils, have a role in the inflammatory processes, therefore, compounds able to scavenge or inhibit the production of these radicals may have a positive role in the inflammation. Myrtle extract had lower concentration of total phenols (117 µg quercetin equivalent/mg) than *L. stoechas* or *C. nepeta*, nevertheless exhibited high ability to reduce the FRAP reagent or scavenge the DPPH and ABTS free radicals, and the best anti-inflammatory activity, whereby the activities found cannot be attributed to the total amount of phenols, but to the type of phenolics or other compounds not quantified [116]. In addition, the best anti-inflammatory activity of myrtle observed by the authors cannot be attributed to its ability for scavenging superoxide anion and peroxynitrite anion, since the activities were low or even null.

The antidiarrheal effects of myrtle berries seeds aqueous extracts from Tunisia and their antioxidant activity were determined by Jabri et al. [32] in adult male Wistar rats. According to the authors, castor oil induces intestinal hypersecretion and diarrhoea, which is accompanied by an oxidative stress. Myrtle berries seeds aqueous extracts were able to reduce the intestinal fluid accumulation protecting against diarrhoea, and decreasing the oxidative stress, particularly reducing hydrogen peroxide, and free iron levels in a dose-dependent manner. Acute castor oil also increases lipoperoxidation with higher accumulation of malondialdehyde and decreases the thiol groups in intestinal mucosa, which is reversed by administering myrtle berries seeds aqueous extracts [32]. Eighteen compounds belonging to three major groups (hydroxybenzoic acid derivatives, anthocyanins derivatives, and flavonols derivatives) were identified in the extracts (Table 2).

The gastroesophageal reflux disease occurs because there is a lower esophageal sphincter dysfunction, decreased esophageal clearance capacity, esophageal mucosal barrier dysfunction, esophageal visceral hypersensitivity, and increased gastric acid secretion [117]. The chronicity of this disease leads to erosions, stenosis, ulcer, or metaplastic epithelium of lower esophagus [117]. Inflammatory cytokines (interleukin-6, IL-6 and interleukin-8, IL-8), leukocytes, and oxidative stress seem to have an important role in the development of the gastroesophageal reflux disease [118]. For this reason, Jabri et al. [117] determined the protective effect of the myrtle berry seed aqueous extract against gastroesophageal reflux, not only evaluating its capacity for scavenging *in vitro* ABTS free radicals and hydrogen peroxide, but also evaluating the free radical scavenging activities of plasma using the DPPH radical method, the capacity for preventing esophageal lipid peroxidation measured through the malondialdehyde (MDA) determination, as well as the influence of the extract on the nonenzymatic antioxidant levels and antioxidant enzyme activities (superoxide dismutase, catalase, and glutathione peroxidase). According to the authors [117], the effective concentrations 50 (EC_{50}) for ABTS and hydrogen peroxide scavenging activities were 184.34 and 380.96 μg/mL, respectively, higher than the control gallic acid (73.34 and 324.31 μg/mL, respectively), therefore poorer than the control. The oxidative stress in the esophageal tissue was significantly decreased (lower MDA accumulation), and the plasma scavenging activities, the esophageal nonenzymatic antioxidant levels and the antioxidant enzyme activities increased in a dose-dependent manner when animals (male Wistar rats) were treated with the extract or the controls (gallic acid and famotidine). In addition, the authors [117] also observed that the extract restored the pH that decreased in the presence of gastroesophageal reflux disease. The authors attributed these beneficial properties to the high amounts of total polyphenols (147.56 mg gallic acid equivalent/g) and total anthocyanins (5.01 cyanidin 3-glucoside equivalent/g) in the aqueous extract of myrtle berry seeds, although no correlation had been made by them [117]. In ulcerative colitis there is also an oxidative stress with the production of reactive oxygen species. Jabri et al. [73], studying the effect of aqueous extracts of berry seeds of myrtle against acetic acid-induced colonic lesions in rats, found that they decreased the formation of malondialdehyde, therefore decreased the colonic lipoperoxidation, and increased the nonenzymatic antioxidant levels, thiol groups, and glutathione, and the activity of superoxide dismutase, catalase, and glutathione peroxidase. The aqueous extract was predominantly constituted by phenols (Table 2).

2.4. Antioxidant Activity of Berry Foods

The evaluation of antioxidant activities of myrtle berries was predominantly *in vitro*, as reported above, with some very few exceptions, as those described above in which *ex vivo* and *in vivo* assays were used. The application of myrtle berry extracts in foods is also limited, although some works could be found and reported below.

Beyond the application of myrtle berries in liqueurs, they can also be used for making jam. Rosa et al. [119] evaluated the antioxidant activity of methanol extracts of myrtle berries jam and compared their results with other extracts obtained from prickly pear fruit jam and cream, and orange and mandarin-orange marmalades. The chemical profile of methanol extracts was characterized by ^{1}H-NMR (proton-nuclear magnetic resonance) spectroscopy. The antioxidant activity was followed through the determination of capacity of samples for preventing lipid peroxidation using liposomes as lipid substrate and measuring the inhibition of malondialdehyde production and the capacity for scavenging reactive oxygen species using the 2′,7′-dichlorofluorescein diacetate (DCFH-DA) in Caco-2 cells. The results showed that the extract of myrtle jam exhibited antioxidant activity, nevertheless the authors considered two possible factors responsible for such property: amount of phenols (206.33 gallic acid equivalent/100 g) found in the sample and the products from nonenzymatic browning reactions resulting from the jam production [119]. Extracts from prickly pear cream and myrtle berries jam preserved liposomes from oxidation, and extracts from prickly pear cream and citrus marmalades significantly reduced the reactive oxygen species generation in Caco-2 cell culture. Using the ^{1}H-NMR, the authors did not identify phenolic compounds in the methanolic extract of myrtle berries jam [119].

In the ice cream formulation, sometimes prebiotics, such as dietary fibers or oligosaccharides, were added. The utilization of fruits as prebiotics in ice cream formulation is scarce. Öztürk et al. [120] used dark blue and white myrtle berries along with the probiotic *Lactobacillus casei* (*L. casei*) 431 in the ice cream formulation. The aim of the work was to study the performance of *L. casei* strain in ice cream during frozen storage in association with dark blue and white myrtle berries. The sensory acceptability of the new formulation was also evaluated. The results showed that *L. casei* 431 kept viable throughout the storage period and increased with the freezing process, and the addition of myrtle fruits lead to an increase of total phenols (5 and 8 mg gallic acid equivalent/g, in the presence of white and dark blue berries, respectively), although the antioxidant activity had not undergone any alteration during the same storage period. The addition of pulp fruits to the ice cream with *L. casei* 431 improved the antioxidant activity, showing a positive effect of fruits on the probiotic *L. casei* 431. Ice cream samples with *L. casei* 431 and dark blue berries of myrtle exhibited higher antioxidant activity (EC_{50} = 90.25 after 8 weeks of storage—85.48 mg/L, on day 1) than when white pulps were added (EC_{50} = 263 after 8 weeks of storage—323 mg/L, on day 1), which may be explained by the highest total phenol content found in the ice cream with *L. casei* 431 and dark blue berries (22.5–26.5 mg gallic acid equivalent/100 g). In ice-cream formulation with *L. casei* 431 and white berries, the amounts of total phenols ranged from 8 to 13.5 mg gallic acid equivalent/100 g. The sensory was improved with the addition of myrtle fruits, particularly white ones, because the formulation in which *L. casei* 431 and white myrtles were added, the acidic taste characteristic of a fermentation process, was eliminated. With these results the authors suggest that dark blue and white berries should be used together in new probiotic product formulations [120].

Curiel et al. [121] used a selected lactic acid bacterium (*Lactobacillus plantarum* C2, which was previously isolated from carrots, identified by partial sequencing of 16S rRNA) in myrtle berries with the objective to improve their antioxidant activity and, consequently, to enhance the functional properties of *M. communis*. The authors determined the antioxidant activity either *in vitro* (capacity for scavenging ABTS and DPPH free radicals and lipid peroxidation inhibitory activity) or *ex vivo* on murine fibroblasts Balb3T3 using the dichloro-dihydro-fluorescein diacetate (DCFH-DA) method, which measures the intracellular reactive oxygen species generation, after analysing the cytotoxicity of extracts through the MTT (3-(4,5-dimethyl-2-yl)-2,5-diphenyltetrazolium bromide) method. Myrtle berries with yeast extract (0.4%) and fermented with *L. plantarum* C2 had significantly higher antioxidant activity *in vitro* than the control constituted by acidified homogenate without bacterial inoculum and submitted to the same experimental conditions. The antiradicalar activity, measured through the DPPH method, increased by 30% and the capacity for inhibiting linoleic acid peroxidation increased twice when compared to the control. The phenols (gallic and ellagic acids), flavonoids (myricetin and quercetin), and anthocyanins' contents also enhanced in the fermented samples, about 5–10 times higher than those found for the nonfermented samples (Table 2). The highest increase of gallic and ellagic acids can be attributed to tannase or tannin acyl hydrolase of *L. plantarum* that catalyzes the hydrolysis of ester bonds present in hydrolysable tannins and gallic acid esters [121]. Other esterases may also be responsible for the increase of the aglycones myricetin and quercetin in the fermented homogenates. The antioxidant activity of fermented homogenates was confirmed ex vivo. The results show that the antioxidant activity of myrtle berries can be improved through lactic acid fermentation [121].

Table 2. Phenols, flavonoids and anthocyanins in berry myrtle liqueurs and berry myrtle extracts.

Origin	Type of Extract	Identification/Quantification	Compounds	Reference
Italy (Sardinia)	- Traditional recipe for the preparation of the liqueur: maceration of fresh berries in ethanol:water (70:30) 960 mL for 40 days. - Lyophilized berries extracted by macerating berries in ethanol:water (70:30) for 40 days. - Fresh berries extracted by sonication for 1 h followed by maceration in ethanol:water (70:30) for one night. For quantitative determination: HPLC-UV/VIS using the internal standards cyanidin-3-O-galactopyranoside for anthocyans, and rutin (quercetin-3-O-rutinoside) for flavonoids	HPLC-ESI-MS/HPLC-UV/VIS	*Anthocyanins* Delphinidin-3-O-glucoside Cyanidin-3-O-glucoside Petunidin-3-O-glucoside Peonidin-3-O-glucoside Malvidin-3-O-glucoside Delphinidin-3-O-arabinoside Petunidin-3-O-arabinoside Malvidin-3-O-arabinoside *Flavonoids* Myricetin-3-O-galactoside Myricetin-3-O-rhamnoside Myricetin-3-O-arabinoside Quercetin-3-O-glucoside Quercetin-3-O-rhamnoside Myricetin	[15]
Italy (Sardinia)	- Berries extracted by maceration with ethanol, for six weeks, in the dark at 4 °C.	HPLC-MS/MS and	*Ethanol extract* Gallic acid derivatives—352.2 Gallic acid—111.5 Elagic acid—76.5 Other gallic acid derivatives—164.2 Anthocyanins—2195.0 Delphinidin-3-O-glucoside—494.8 Petunidin 3-O-glucoside—425.9 Malvidin-3-O-glucoside—840.9 Other anthocyanins—433.4 Flavonols—1492.8 Myricetin-3-O-galactoside—450.5 Myricetin-3-O-rhamnoside—441.2 Myricetin—342.2 Quercetin—36.2 Other flavonols—222.7 *Total*—4040.0 mg/mL *Water extract*	[110]

Table 2. *Cont.*

Origin	Type of Extract	Identification/Quantification	Compounds	Reference
	- Berries extracted by maceration with water, for six weeks, in the dark at 4 °C.		Gallic acid derivatives—195.9 Gallic acid—76.0 Elagic acid—8.4 Other gallic acid derivatives—111.5 Anthocyanins—74.7 Delphinidin-3-O-glucoside—7.4 Petunidin-3-O-glucoside—11.2 Malvidin-3-O-glucoside—39.1 Other anthocyanins—17.0 Flavonols—103.0 Myricetin-3-O-galactoside- 23.4 Myricetin-3-O-rhamnoside- 52.9 Myricetin— Quercetin— Other flavonols—26.7 *Total*—373.6 (mg/mL)	
	- Berries extracted by maceration with ethyl acetate, for six weeks, in the dark at 4 °C. For quantitative determination: HPLC-DAD using calibration curves built with the method of external standard		*Ethyl acetate extract* Gallic acid derivatives—600.5 Gallic acid—361.7 Elagic acid—104.7 Other gallic acid derivatives—134.1 Anthocyanins—36.4 Delphinidin-3-O-glucoside—0.9 Petunidin 3-O-glucoside—1.7 Malvidin-3-O-glucoside—10.7 Other anthocyanins—1389.0 Flavonols—4.9 Myricetin-3-O-galactoside—216.9 Myricetin-3-O-rhamnoside—942.2 Myricetin—139.9 Quercetin—85.1 Other flavonols—26.7 *Total*—2025.9 (mg/L)	

Table 2. *Cont.*

Origin	Type of Extract	Identification/Quantification	Compounds	Reference
Italy (Sardinia)	Obtained directly from producer and with known industrial processes	HPLC-MS/MS and HPLC-DAD	Hydroxybenzoic acids—18 Gallic acid—12 Gallic acid derivatives—6 Flavanols—25 (+)-Catechin—25 Flavonols—124 Myricetin-3-O-arabinoside—51 Myricetin-3-O-galactoside—34 Myricetin-3-O-rhamnoside—3 Quercetin-3-O-glucoside—7 Quercetin-3-O-rhamnoside—6 Myricetin—20 Quercetin—3 Anthocyanins—110 Delphinidin-3-O-glucoside—20 Cyanidin-3-O-glucoside—5 Petunidin-3-O-glucoside—22 Peonidin-3-O-glucoside—5 Malvidin-3-O-glucoside—57 Anthocyanins arabinoside—11 *Total*—277 (mg/L)	[102]
Italy (Sardinia)	Maceration in an ethanol–water mixture for four months. After separation of the berries of the macerates, the liqueurs were produced by adding sucrose and water to obtain a final percentage of 28% *v/v* (alcohol) and 32% *w/v* (sugar).	HPLC-MS/MS and	Hydroxybenzoic acids—408.2 Gallic acid—294.2 Ellagic acid—55.8 Flavonols—58.1 Myricetin-3-O-galactoside—2.1 Myricetin-3-O-rhamnoside—23.0 Myricetin—25.6 Other flavonols—7.4 Anthocyanins—not detected *Total*—466.4 (mg/L)	[103]

Table 2. Cont.

Origin	Type of Extract	Identification/Quantification	Compounds	Reference
Tunisia	Berries extracted by maceration with mixtures of ethanol/water (90:10—60:40) ethanol, for 40 days	HPLC/ESMS and HPLC/UV/Vis	Myricetin-3-O-arabinoside Myricetin-3-O-galactoside Myricetin-3-O-rhamnoside Quercetin-3-O-glucoside Quercetin-3-O-rhamnoside Myricetin Quercetin Kaempferol Delphinidin-3-O-glucoside Cyanidin-3-O-glucoside Petunidin-3-O-glucoside Delphinidin-3-O-arabinoside Petunidin-3-O-glucoside Peonidin-3-O-glucoside Malvidin-3-O-glucoside Petunidin-3-O-arabinoside Malvidin-3-O-arabinoside	[101]
Tunisia	Extraction with 70% MeOH for 24 h in a H$_2$O bath shaker	HPLC/UV/Vis	*Dark blue fruits* Delphinidin-3-O-glucoside—172 Cyanidin-3-O-glucoside—25.2 Petunidin-3-O-glucoside—103.7 Delphinidin-3-O-arabinoside—28.3 Peonidin-3-O-glucoside—11.8 Malvidin-3-O-glucoside—257.6 Petunidin-3-O-arabinoside—18.8 Malvidin-3-O-arabinoside—8.6 *Total*—625.8 (mg malvidin-3-O-glucoside equivalent/100 mL) *White fruits* Delphinidin-3-O-glucoside—1.7 Cyanidin-3-O-glucoside—0.3 Petunidin-3-O-glucoside—0.9 Delphinidin-3-O-arabinoside—0.2 Peonidin-3-O-glucoside—0.2 Malvidin-3-O-glucoside—1.9 Petunidin-3-O-arabinoside—0.2 Malvidin-3-O-arabinoside—0.1 *Total*—5.4 (mg malvidin-3-O-glucoside equivalent/100 mL)	[106]

Table 2. Cont.

Origin	Type of Extract	Identification/Quantification	Compounds	Reference
Tunisia	Maceration	HPLC-DAD	*Whole fruit* (mg/g) Phenolic acids—1.03 Gallic acid—1.03 Hydrolysable tannins—0.69 Gallotannins—0.69 Flavonols—0.33 Quercetin-3-O-rutinoside—0.01 Myricetin-3-O-galactoside—0.08 Quercetin-3-O-galactoside—0.12 Myricetin-3-O-rhamnoside—0.07 Quercetin-3-O-rhamnoside—0.05 Anthocyanins—4.64 Delphinidin-3-O-glucoside—0.66 Cyanidin-3-O-glucoside—0.29 Petunidin-3-O-glucoside—0.89 Malvidin-3-O-glucoside—1.42 Petunidin-3-O-arabinoside—0.87 Malvidin-3-O-arabinoside—0.51 *Total*—6.69 mg/g *Seed* (mg/g) Phenolic acids—2.22 Gallic acid—2.22 Hydrolysable tannins—8.99 Gallotannins—8.99 Flavonols— Quercetin-3-O-rutinoside— Myricetin-3-O-galactoside— Quercetin-3-O-galactoside— Myricetin-3-O-rhamnoside— Quercetin-3-O-rhamnoside— Anthocyanins— Delphinidin-3-O-glucoside— Cyanidin-3-O-glucoside— Petunidin-3-O-glucoside— Malvidin-3-O-glucoside— Petunidin-3-O-arabinoside— Malvidin-3-O-arabinoside— *Total*—11.11 mg/g *Pericarp* (mg/g)	[107]

Table 2. Cont.

Origin	Type of Extract	Identification/Quantification	Compounds	Reference
Tunisia	Sonication followed by maceration with	HPLC-DAD	Phenolic acids—0.89 Gallic acid—0.89 Hydrolysable tannins— Gallotannins— Flavonols—0.33 Quercetin-3-O-rutinoside—0.01 Myricetin-3-O-galactoside—0.08 Quercetin-3-O-galactoside—0.12 Myricetin-3-O-rhamnoside—0.07 Quercetin-3-O-rhamnoside—0.05 Anthocyanins—3.74 Delphinidin-3-O-glucoside—0.66 Cyanidin-3-O-glucoside—0.19 Petunidin-3-O-glucoside—0.39 Malvidin-3-O-glucoside—1.12 Petunidin-3-O-arabinoside—0.87 Malvidin-3-O-arabinoside—0.51 *Total*—4.96 mg/g *Leaves-September (aq—met/aq) (g/kg)* Gallic acid—16.90; 9.33 Delphinidin-3-O-glucoside—nd; nd Myricetin-3-O-rhamnoside—18.26; 23.13 Quercetin-3-O-galactoside—0.24; 0.21 Quercetin-3-O-rutinoside—0.41; 0.45 Malvidin-3-O-glucoside—nd; nd Myricetin—0.41; 0.41 Ellagic acid—5.15; 2.76 Quercetin—0.05; 0.09 Kaempferol—0.14; 0.14 *Total*—41.56; 36.52 *Leaves-December (aq—met/aq) (g/kg)* Gallic acid—11.37; 0.79	[109]

Table 2. *Cont.*

Origin	Type of Extract	Identification/Quantification	Compounds	Reference
			Delphinidin-3-O-glucoside—nd; nd Myricetin-3-O-rhamnoside—20.93; 18.95 Quercetin-3-O-galactoside—0.27, 0.29 Quercetin-3-O-rutinoside—0.51; 0.32 Malvidin-3-O-glucoside—nd; nd Myricetin—4.20; 0.50 Ellagic acid—7.27; 3.52 Quercetin—0.16; 0.10 Kaempferol—0.22; 0.21 *Total*—44.93; 24.68	
			Berries-September (aq—met/aq) (g/kg) Gallic acid—16.32; 5.00 Delphinidin-3-O-glucoside—nd; nd Myricetin-3-O-rhamnoside—9.67; 9.80 Quercetin-3-O-galactoside—1.92, 2.05 Quercetin-3-O-rutinoside—together with quercetin-3-O-galactoside in both cases Malvidin-3-O-glucoside—nd; nd Myricetin—0.27; 0.31 Ellagic acid—19.10; 8.34 Quercetin—0.32; 0.28 Kaempferol—0.17; 0.11 *Total*—47.77; 25.89	
			Berries-December (aq—met/aq) (g/kg) Gallic acid—4.54; 1.21 Delphinidin-3-O-glucoside—0.21; 0.16 Myricetin-3-O-rhamnoside—4.02; 5.69 Quercetin-3-O-galactoside—1.01, 1.22	

Table 2. Cont.

Origin	Type of Extract	Identification/Quantification	Compounds	Reference
			Quercetin-3-O-rutinoside—together with quercetin-3-O-galactoside in both cases Malvidin-3-O-glucoside—0.30; 0.32 Myricetin—0.31; 0.18 Ellagic acid—4.92; 2.99 Quercetin—0.04; 0.11 Kaempferol—0.09; 0.05 *Total*—15.44; 11.93	
			Pericarps-December (aq—met/aq) (g/kg) Gallic acid—1.72; 0.24 Delphinidin-3-O-glucoside—0.22; 0.39 Myricetin-3-O-rhamnoside—3.10; 3.51 Quercetin-3-O-galactoside—0.40; 0.59 Quercetin-3-O-rutinoside—together with quercetin-3-O-galactoside in both cases Malvidin-3-O-glucoside—0.42; 0.43 Myricetin—0.08; 0.08 Ellagic acid—0.69; 0.73 Quercetin—0.01; 0.02 Kaempferol—nd; 0.01 *Total*—6.64; 6.00	
			Seeds-December (aq—met/aq) (g/kg) Gallic acid—16.62; 15.98 Delphinidin-3-O-glucoside—nd; nd Myricetin-3-O-rhamnoside—2.25; 4.85 Quercetin-3-O-galactoside—0.33; 5.30	

Table 2. *Cont.*

Origin	Type of Extract	Identification/Quantification	Compounds	Reference
			Quercetin-3-O-rutinoside—2.51; together with quercetin-3-O-galactoside in both cases Malvidin-3-O-glucoside—nd; nd Myricetin—1.90; 0.94 Ellagic acid—29.35; 21.18 Quercetin—0.18; 1.40 Kaempferol—0.19; 0.49 *Total*—53.33; 50.14	
Portugal	Sonication for 30 min, followed by maceration with water for 24 h, in the dark	HPLC–DAD–ESI-MS/MS	*Berries* Oenothein B Galloyl-HHDP-glucose Digalloyl HHDP-glucose Quinic acid 3,5-di-O-gallate Delphinidin-3-O-glucoside—1.33 mg/g Cyanidin-3-O-glucoside—1.33 mg/g Petunidin-3-O-glucoside—1.33 mg/g Malvidin-3-O-monoglucoside—1.67 mg/g Peonidin-3-O-monoglucoside—1.67 mg/g Petunidin-3-O-pentoside—0.977 mg/g Malvidin-3-O-pentoside—0.977 mg/g Myricetin galactoside-gallate Myricetin galactoside—0.00171 mg/g Myricetin rhamnoside—0.00236 mg/g Quercetin rhamnoside—0.000698 mg/g *Leaves* Myricetin galactoside-gallate—0.00261 mg/g	[112]

Table 2. Cont.

Origin	Type of Extract	Identification/Quantification	Compounds	Reference
Portugal	Liquid phase extraction (LPE) Supercritical fluid extraction (SFE)	HPLC-DAD-ESI-MS/MS	Myricetin galactoside—0.00261 mg/g Myricetin rhamnoside—0.000255 mg/g Myricetin—0.000075 mg/g Quercetin galactoside-gallate—0.0136 mg/g *Leaves and berries* (LPE) Gallic acid Myricetin-3-O-rhamnoside V Ellagic acid Quercetin-O-rhamnoside Myricetin Kaempferol-O-rhamnoside Quercetin *Leaves* (SFE) Myricetin-galactoside Myricetin-rhamnoside Quercetin-rhamnoside *Berries* (SFE) Myricetin-galactoside Myricetin-3-O-rhamnoside Quercetin-O-rhamnoside Delphinidin-3-O-glucoside Petunidin-3-O-glucoside Malvidin-3-O-glucoside	[111]
Italy (Sardinia)	Maceration in methanol	HPLC/UV	*Control* Phenolic acids (mg/g) Gallic acid—0.17 Vanillic acid—0.10 Syringic acid—0.14 Ellagic acid—1.44 Flavonols/flavanols Myricetin—1.11	[121]

Table 2. Cont.

Origin	Type of Extract	Identification/Quantification	Compounds	Reference
			Quercetin—0.20	
			Catechin—1.12	
			Fermented homogenate	
			Phenolic acids (mg/g)	
			Gallic acid—0.55	
			Vanillic acid—0.28	
			Syringic acid—0.28	
			Ellagic acid—2.78	
			Flavonols/flavanols	
			Myricetin—2.56	
			Quercetin—0.79	
			Catechin—1.26	
Tunisia	Maceration in water	HPLC-DAD-ESI-MS/MS	Hydroxybenzoic acid hexose	[32]
			Delphinidin-3-O-galactoside	
			Delphinidin-3-O-glucoside	
			Quercetin hexoside	
			Delphinidin-3-O-rhamnoside	
			Delphinidin rutinoside	
			Delphinidin-3-(6 coumaroyl)-glucoside	
			Petunidin-3-O-glucoside	
			Petunidin diglucoside	
			Petunidin malonylglucoside	
			Petunidin-3-O-rutinoside	
			Isorhamnetin-O-rhamnoside	
			Malvidin-O-galactoside	
			Malvidin-O-glucoside	
			Peonidin diglucoside	
			Petunidin methyl pentose	

Table 2. Cont.

Origin	Type of Extract	Identification/Quantification	Compounds	Reference
Tunisia	Maceration in water	HPLC–DAD–ESI-MS/MS	Hydroxybenzoic acid hexose Delphinidin-3-O-galactoside Delphinidin-3-O-glucoside Quercetin hexoside Delphinidin-3-O-rhamnoside Delphinidin rutinoside Delphinidin-3-(6 coumaroyl)-glucoside Petunidin-3-O-glucoside Petunidin diglucoside Petunidin malonylglucoside Petunidin-3-O-rutinoside Isorhamnetin-O-rhamnoside Malvidin-O-galactoside Malvidin-O-glucoside Peonidin diglucoside Petunidin methyl pentose	[73]
Italy	Flavoured sea salts	HPLC–DAD and 1H-NMR	*Phenols* (mg/100 g) Ellagic acid—11.7 Gallic acid—69.4 Myricetin—0.9 Myricetin-3-galactoside—7.3 Myricitrin—13.3 Quercetin-3-galactoside—0.9 Quercetin-3-glucoside Quercitrin—1.1 Vitexin—0.7	[122]

nd: not detected.

3. *Myrtus communis*: Leaves

3.1. Antioxidant Activity

The antioxidant activity of leaf extracts of myrtle has also been deeply studied as well as their phenolic profiles that are somehow different from those of berries (red and dark blue ones), at least in the absence of anthocyanins. This was already reported in the previous section [109,111,112,114].

The effect of various factors on the antioxidant activity of myrtle leaves has deeply studied. The chemical profile and biological properties of plants can be affected by climatic conditions, harvesting time, abiotic stress, genotype among other factors [123]. For this reason, the authors [123] studied the effect of different NaCl concentrations (control, 2, 4, and 6 dS/m) and three harvesting times in different seasons including spring, summer, and fall on the phenolic, flavonoid content, and antioxidant activity (DPPH radical scavenging activity, reducing power, and β-carotene/linoleic acid bleaching test) of myrtle extracts. The highest antioxidant activity was found in plants harvested in summer and spring and in high stress condition. In the DPPH test, the lowest IC_{50} values were obtained in 6 dS/m in summer (249.41 μg/mL), followed by spring (375.23 μg/mL), and fall (618.38 μg/mL). The chemical composition is described in Table 3. After the sum of the compounds identified in the myrtle extracts, it is possible to verify an increase of phenols plus flavonoids since spring (131.26 mg/100 g) up to the fall (260.87 mg/100 g). The contribution of phenols on the antioxidant activity was not determined by the authors, but strong correlation between phenol and flavonoid contents and the DPPH test, reducing power, and β-carotene/linoleic acid bleaching test was detected. Sacchetti et al. [124] after harvesting myrtle plants at different places of Sardinia also reported the different capacity of myrtle extracts to scavenge the DPPH free radicals.

The identification of the compounds that constituted the essential oils and methanolic extracts isolated from leaf, flower, and stems of Tunisian *M. communis* var. *italica* and the antioxidant activity (DPPH radical scavenging, β-carotene-linoleic acid bleaching, reducing power, and metal chelating activity assays) were determined by [125]. The amounts of total phenols, and condensed tannins and flavonoids were different according to the plant part from where they were extracted (Table 3). The analysis indicated that the main phenolic class was hydrolysable tannins (gallotannins) in leaf (8.90 mg/g) and flower (3.50 mg/g) while in the stem predominated flavonoid class (1.86 mg/g) due to the high presence of catechin (1.12 mg/g) (Table 3). In almost all antioxidant tests, leaf extracts had the best activity, presenting the lowest IC_{50} values, the exception was in DPPH method that flower extract had the lowest IC_{50} value. For DPPH assays, the IC_{50} values for leaf, stem and flower were 8 μg/mL, 90 μg/mL, and 3 μg/mL, respectively. For β-carotene-linoleic bleaching test, the IC_{50} values were: 70 μg/mL, 124 μg/mL, and 78 μg/mL, respectively. For chelating activity, the IC_{50} values were 5 μg/mL, 10 μg/mL, and 46 μg/mL, respectively, whereas for reducing power, such values were 10 μg/mL, 150 μg/mL, and 50 μg/mL, respectively. In comparison with essential oils, the methanolic extracts exhibited higher antioxidant activity, showing the importance of the presence of phenols in the samples [125].

3.2. Comparison of Antioxidant Activity of Myrtle Leaves with Other Plant Species

In several works, the authors compare the antioxidant activities of extracts obtained from myrtle leaves with those obtained from other species and the results can be sometimes quite different, as described below.

The antioxidant activity of selected medicinal plants from the North-West of Morocco (*Origanum compactum* Benth., *Cistus crispus* L., *Centaurium erythraea* Rafin., *Myrtus communis* L., and *Arbutus unedo* L.) were tested for their anticancer and antioxidant activities. The antioxidant activity was evaluated using the reducing power activity and the capacity for scavenging the ABTS free radicals. The authors also evaluated the effect of extraction solvent on the activities (methanol, ethanol, and *n*-hexane) [60]. All extracts were able to scavenge the free radicals and have ferric-reducing power, nevertheless dependent on the plant and type of extracts. The methanol and *n*-hexane extracts of myrtle and the methanolic extract of *C. erythraea* showed important antioxidant capacity to scavenge ABTS free radicals (IC_{50} = 57.83, 48.42, 63.48 µg/mL, respectively), and to reduce ferric to ferrous ions (IC_{50} = 16.59, 23.8, 27.28 µg/mL, respectively), but their IC_{50} values were inferior than the positive controls used (Trolox and ascorbic acid), therefore, showed better antioxidant activity [60].

The antioxidant activity, measured through the capacity for scavenging the DPPH and nitric oxide (NO) free radicals, β-carotene-bleaching test and metal chelating power, of six plants (*M. communis*, *Eryngium maritimum*, *Pistacia lentiscus*, *Globularia alypum*, *Marrubium vulgare*, and *Scilla maritima*) was determined by [126]. The total phenols, total flavonoids, flavonols, proanthocyanidins, and total tannins were also evaluated. The authors observed that methanol extracts of *M. communis* (leaves) (285.73 mg gallic acid equivalent/g), *P. lentiscus* (leaves) (238.33 mg gallic acid equivalent/g), and *G. alypum* (flowers) (156.97 mg gallic acid equivalent/g) presented the highest amounts of total phenolic compounds while the concentrations of total flavonoids, flavonols, proanthocyanidins, and total tannins varied with plant species. In the DPPH assay, *P. lentiscus* (IC_{50} = 0.008 mg/mL) and *M. communis* (IC_{50} = 0.003 mg/mL) had the best activity and their inhibitions were similar. In the β-carotene assay, leaf and fruits extracts of *M. communis* and *P. lentiscus* leaves were the most potent with 63.60%, 47.61%, and 43.02%, respectively. Metal chelating activity assay showed that *E. maritimum* leaves and stems and *M. communis* leaves had the best chelating power, 49.78%, 32.32%, and 35.98%, respectively. These results indicate that *M. communis* extracts present good antioxidant activity, being even better than other plants from Algeria [126]. Myrtle extracts did not exhibit any anti-inflammatory activity when determined through the inhibition of cyclooxygenase-1-inhibition, nevertheless, it was the best extract for inhibiting acetylcholinesterase activity along with the *P. lentiscus* with IC_{50} values of 0.03 and 0.01 mg/mL, respectively [126].

The best antioxidant activity of myrtle extracts amongst two sets of sixteen and four plant extracts was also previously reported by [127,128], regardless the extraction solvent (hexane or methanol). β-Carotene-bleaching test was used for determining the antioxidant activity and the results were presented as antioxidant activity coefficients. In the set of sixteen samples, the antioxidant activity coefficients for hexane and methanol extracts obtained from fresh leaves were 641 and 260, respectively, whereas for dried leaves, the values were 12.2 and 51.5, respectively [127]. In both fresh and dried material, myrtle extracts were the most active, nevertheless in the second set of extracts [128], the highest antioxidant activity coefficient was observed for fresh extract of *Myrtus communis* (AAC = 635), whereas in dried material, *Thymus vulgaris* was the most active (antioxidant activity coefficient = 34). The good antioxidant activity of hexane extracts can be partly or wholly assigned to the presence of nonpolar phenolic compounds such as tocopherols. Demo et al. [129] detected and quantified α-tocopherol in hexane extracts of myrtle leaves (2.144%).

Mothana et al. [35] studied the antimicrobial, anticancer, and antioxidant activity of 32 Yemeni plants. Concerning the antixoxidant activity and within this set of samples, only six had high DPPH free radical scavenging activity: methanolic extracts of *Achillea biebersteinii*, *Chrozophora oblongifolia*, *Myrtus communis*, *Oxalis corniculata*, *Phragmanthera regularis*, and *Tecoma stans* at 50 µg/mL. In contrast, Özcan et al. [130] did not find similar results for Turkish myrtle, although the methods (ABTS radical scavenging activity and capacity for oxidizing ferrous ion to ferric ion by various types of peroxides within the plasma) and the species used were different (anise, bitter fennel fruits and flowers, basil, laurel, oregano, and pickling herb). The peroxide value and the Trolox equivalent of methanolic extracts were 0.6866 µmol H_2O_2 and 0.3189 Trolox equivalent/g, respectively, although presenting higher amounts of total phenols (9.9761 mg gallic acid equivalent/g) than the other species (1.3175–10.5832 mg gallic acid equivalent/g). Only oregano extracts presented higher concentration of total phenols than myrtle leaves. The authors [130] also evaluated the antioxidant activity of the essential oils. These ones had better capacity for reducing ferrous ions, since they showed higher peroxide values, than the methanolic extracts, nevertheless poorer capacity for scavenging the ABTS free radicals.

Gião et al. [131] determined the antiradical activity (ABTS free radicals) of aqueous extracts of 32 plants from Portugal. Two types of extraction were used: boiling water added to the sample and left during 5 min at rom temperature (infusion), and water added to the sample and the mixture heated until boiling, which was maintained for 5 min. The authors detected that the antiradicalar activity was dependent on the species as well as of the method of extraction. The highest antioxidant activity was observed for avocado (0.157 mg equivalent ascorbic acid/g), followed by agrimony (0.067 g equivalent ascorbic acid/g), eucalyptus (0.149 g equivalent ascorbic acid/g), yarrow (0.118 g equivalent ascorbic acid/g), myrtle (0.141 g equivalent ascorbic acid/g), thyme (0.142 g equivalent ascorbic acid/g), and heath (0.065 g equivalent ascorbic acid/g). In addition, powder infusion was the best method for obtaining the most active extracts which also possessed the highest amounts of phenols. The authors found a positive correlation between the phenol content and the antiradicalr activity [131]. Later on, Gião et al. [132] studied the effect of different stages of processing (fresh, frozen, dehumidified/packed in two consecutive years, and storage after dehumidification under controlled relative humidity, maintained for one year in a dark room) on the antiradicalar activity of ten species (agrimony (*Agrimonia eupatoria*), eucalyptus (*Eucalyptus globulus*), walnut-tree (*Juglans regia*), myrtle (*Myrtus communis*), raspberry (*Rubus idaeus*), sage (*Salvia* sp.), savory (*Satureja montana*), sweet-amber (*Hypericum androsaemum*), thyme (*Thymus vulgaris*), and yarrow (*Achillea millefolium*)). The samples used were infusions and the antiradicalar method used was based on the abilty for scavenging ABTS free radicals. According to the authors [132], antioxidant activity and total phenolic content decreased by ca. 30–80%, between fresh and frozen forms, whereas from the frozen stage to the packaged form the variations observed were not statistically significant. The highest difference was observed for myrtle, which means that this species is sensitive to the technological processing and, therefore, for preserving their properties during processing conditions after harvest and throughout storage, other techniques must be thought and assayed in the near future.

Gonçalves et al. [133] compared the antioxidant activity of ten plant species from Portugal, including *M. communis*, measured through diverse methods (DPPH and hydroxyl radical scavenging activity, reducing and chelatin power, and inhibition of lipid peroxidation in mouse brain homogenates using thiobarbituric acid reactive substances). The extracts obtained were aqueous obtained by maceration at room temperature, for 2 h, or extraction in hot water (90 °C), for 5 min. *Pistacia lentiscus* L. and *M. communis* in cold and hot aqueous extracts were the most effective for scavenging the DPPH free radicals (377.30 and 319.81 mmol Trolox equivalent/g and 230.36 and 246.51 mmol Trolox equivalent/g, respectively). The same extracts were also the best ones for chelating iron ions without significant differences between the hot and cold extracts. However, the capacity for scavenging hydroxyl radicals was better in hot extracts, nevertheless never exceeding 50%, even at higher extract concentration (1.6 mg/mL extract). With the exception of this activity, the authors found a positive correlation between the total phenolic content and the antioxidant activity [133]. Concerning the capacity for preventing lipid peroxidation, all samples had activity, although those of *Centaurea erythraea*, *Paronychia argentea*, and *Ruscus aculeatus* were significantly less active than the other aqueous extracts.

3.3. Effect of Extraction Method and Extraction Solvent on the Antioxidant Activity of Myrtle Leaves

The antiradicalar activity of leaf extracts measured through the capacity for scavenging DPPH as well as the total antioxidant power were evaluated by Belmimoun et al. [134]. The authors used diverse methods and extraction solvents: decoction, maceration with ethanol, and extraction with solvents of increasing polarity by Soxhlet (dichloromethane and methanol). The IC_{50} value for the aqueous extract was 29 µg/mL, whereas the total antioxidant power was 68.05 mg/g, better when compared to the essential oils obtained by hydrodistillation (615 µg/mL and 36 mg/g, respectively), explained by the absence of phenol compounds in the essential oils [134].

Romani et al. [135] also evaluated the influence of different solvents on the antioxidant activity of leaf myrtle extracts obtained by liquid–liquid extraction. The authors also evaluated the role of pure compounds and group of compounds found in the myrtle extracts on the antioxidant activity found in the work. As expected, different solvents extracted diverse phenolic compounds. Hydroalcoholic extracts had galloylglucosides, ellagitannins, galloyl-quinic acids, and flavonol glycosides; whereas ethyl acetate extract and aqueous residues after liquid–liquid extraction were enriched in flavonol glycosides and hydrolysable tannins (galloyl-glucosides, ellagitannins, and galloyl-quinic acids), respectively (Table 3). The antioxidant activity of extracts was determined evaluating the capacity of extracts to prevent the formation of MDA and conjugated dienes after exposing human LDL to copper ions. Hydroalcoholic extract was mainly constituted by galloyl-glucosides and ellagitannins and was the most active in inhibiting LDL oxidation (IC_{50} = 0.36 µM) followed by the aqueous residue after liquid–liquid extraction (IC_{50} = 2.88 µM), also mainly constituted by galloyl-glucosides and ellagitannins, and ethyl acetate extract (IC_{50} = 2.27 µM), mainly constituted by myricetin glucosides and galloylquinic acids. The capacity for preventing MDA accumulation was also determined using pure compounds such as gallic acid, 3,5-di-O-galloylquinic acid, myricitrin, and rutin, and the IC_{50} values found were 20, 2.2,7.8, and 3.7 µM, respectively, showing that 3,5-di-O-galloylquinic acid was the most active. In addition, the authors [135] also determined the IC_{50} values considering the total polyphenol concentration and the concentration of the single compound present in each extract and it was possible to find that the copresence of different polyphenols increased the antioxidant activity. Two examples are the aqueous residue in which was practically constituted by galloyl-glucosides and had a IC_{50} value close to that of 3,5-di-O-galloylquinic acid, and the other example is that of the ethyl acetate extract that had a ratio between galloyl derivatives and flavonols of about 1:1, and the IC_{50} value is very similar to that of 3,5-di-O-galloylquinic acid. This last result indicates that flavonols do not play an important role in the antioxidant activity when they are mixed with hydrolysable tannins, but a ratio of 9:1, such as observed in the hydroalcoholic extract, the IC_{50} decreased drastically, that is, the activity increased. The authors [135] concluded that the antioxidant activity was dependent on the ratio between the sum of galloylglucosides, ellagitannins, and flavonols and also of the ratio between these galloyl derivatives vs. galloyl-quinic acids.

The effect of different solvents (water, hexane, chloroform, ethyl acetate, methanol, and a total flavonoids oligomer fraction) and essential oils on the capacity for scavenging DPPH free radicals revealed that the aqueous extract was the most active (IC_{50} = 1.9 µg/mL), even better than the total flavonoids oligomer fraction (IC_{50} = 3 µg/mL). Chloroform, hexane extracts, and essential oils were significantly less active than those extracts [66]. Later on, Hayder et al. [64] evaluated the capacity of myricetin-3-O-galactoside and myricetin-3-O-rhamnoside (flavonoids), isolated from the leaves of *Myrtus communis*, to inhibit xanthine oxidase activity, lipid peroxidation, and to scavenge the free radical DPPH. Both flavonoids were able to scavenge the free radicals with IC_{50} values of 1.4 µg/mL and 3.1 µg/mL for myricetin-3-O-rhamnoside and myricetin-3-O-galactoside, respectively, comparable than to that of the positive control (vitamin E) (IC_{50} = 3 µg/mL). Both flavonoids were able to inhibit xanthine oxidase (in the catalysis process there is production of superoxide radical anions). At 100 µg/mL, myricetin-3-O-rhamnoside and myricetin-3-O-galactoside showed percentages of inhibitory activities of 59% and 57%, respectively. However, when higher concentrations of myricetin-3-O-rhamnoside (300 µg/mL) and myricetin-3-O-galactoside (200 and 300 µg/mL) were used, there was an increase of xanthine oxidase activity, that is, a pro-oxidant activity. The inhibition of the malondialdehyde formation by K562 (human chronic myelogenous leukemia) cell line, induced by hydrogen peroxide, was also assayed, and the authors [64] found that the IC_{50} values for myricetin-3-O-galactoside and myricetin-3-O-rhamnoside were 160 and 220 µg/mL, respectively, measured through the thiobarbituric acid test. These concentrations did not involve a decrease of cell viability.

The evaluation of antioxidant activity of pure compounds isolated from myrtle leaves was also reported previously [65]. In this case, the compound studied was 3,5-O-digalloylquinic acid and the antioxidant activity was determined by its ability for inhibiting lipid peroxidation induced by hydrogen peroxide in the K562 cell line. The pure molecule displayed an important malondialdehyde formation inhibition percentage (82.2%) and low IC_{50} value = 180 µg/mL. This concentration did not induce a decrease of cell viability whereby the decrease of malondialdehyde amounts can only be attributed to the real antioxidant activity of 3,5-O-digalloylquinic acid [65] as reported for myricetin-3-O-galactoside and myricetin-3-O-rhamnoside [64].

Tumen et al. [136] studied the effect of dichloromethane, acetone, ethyl acetate, and methanol extracts of myrtle leaf and berries on the ability for scavenging DPPH and N,N-dimethyl-p-phenylenediamine (DMPD) radicals, reducing power, and chelating activity. The authors reported that the polar extracts (acetone, ethyl acetate, and methanol extracts) exerted strong scavenging effect against DPPH and DMPD as well as good reducing power. However, the dichloromethane extract of the berries possessed the best metal chelation ability. Berry extracts were better antioxidants than leaf extracts, maybe to the highest concentrations of phenols in those extracts, according to the Tumen et al. [136].

Yoshimura et al. [137], using different solvents in the extraction of phenols from leaves of myrtle from Japan, isolated, identified, and determined the capacity of every single compound for scavenging the DPPH free radicals. Among the compounds evaluated, the hydrolyzable tannins oenothein B, eugeniflorin D_2, tellimagrandin I, and tellimagrandin II exhibited the best activity (IC_{50} = 6.12, 4.56, 8.00, and 7.62 µM, respectively).

Previously, Dairi et al. [138] studied the scavenging capacity of the ABTS and peroxyl radicals by Algerian myrtle extracts obtained by microwave assisted extraction and maceration. In addition, the authors also evaluated the antioxidant activity of leaf extracts in lipid system models oxidized *in vitro*: human LDL Cu^{2+}-oxidation and AAPH-induced l-α phosphatidylcholine aqueous dispersion oxidation. The results showed that there were not differences in the amounts of phenols obtained by both methods and they presented strong ability for scavenging the ABTS free radicals, even better than BHA and α-tocopherol. The same extracts also exhibited higher capacity for scavenging the peroxyl free radicals than BHA but less effective activity than the references caffeic acid and myricetin 3-O-rhamnoside. In the lipid system (Cu^{2+}-induced LDL system), both myrtle extracts, as well as myricetin 3-O-rhamnoside, were able to inhibit the production of conjugated dienes in a dose-dependent manner and to prolong the lag phase. When the AAPH-induced l-α phosphatidylcholine aqueous dispersion was used, both myrtle extracts were effective to prevent lipid oxidation, but less than myricetin 3-O-rhamnoside. The possible synergic effect of myrtle extracts, caffeic acid, and myricetin 3-O-rhamnoside on α-tocopherol-enriched phospholipid aqueous dispersions was also evaluated by the authors and they observed that no synergic or additive effect was observed between α-tocopherol and myrtle extracts or caffeic acid, but myricetin 3-O-rhamnoside had an additive effect. According to the authors [138], myrtle extracts, in which myricetin 3-O-rhamnoside can be found, can improve the antioxidant activity of complex lipid systems, stabilizing them [138].

The absence of significant differences in the amounts of total phenols in the extracts obtained by microwave-assisted extraction and maceration, reported by Dairi et al. [138], such was also verified by Dahmoune et al. [139] when compared the total phenol amounts of leaf myrtle extracts obtained by microwave-assisted extraction (162.49 mg gallic acid equivalent/g), ultrasound-assisted extraction (147.77 mg gallic acid equivalent/g), and maceration (128.00 mg gallic acid equivalent/g). However, the amounts of total flavonoids and tannins observed in the extracts were different depending on the extraction procedures. Microwave-assisted extraction was able to extract more flavonoids (5.02 mg quercetin equivalent/g) and tannins (32.65 mg quercetin equivalent/g) than ultrasound-assisted extraction (3.88 mg quercetin equivalent/g and 23.32 mg/g, respectively) and maceration (4.15 mg quercetin equivalent/g and 17.15 mg/g, respectively). The capacity for scavenging ABTS (IC_{50} = 38.20 mg gallic acid equivalent/mL), DPPH (IC_{50} = 16.80 mg gallic acid equivalent/mL), and peroxyl radicals (757.77 µmol Trolox equivalent/g) was also more effective when myrtle extracts were obtained by microwave-assisted extraction, than by other extraction processes. However, optimal microwave-assisted extraction conditions were needed in order to achieve these values of phenols and antioxidant activity. Such conditions were 42% ethanol concentration, 500 W microwave power, 62 s irradiation time, and 32 mL/g solvent to material ratio. Microwave-assisted extraction of myrtle leaf allowed shortening the extraction time about 14 and 15 times when compared to the ultrasound-assisted extraction and maceration, respectively [139].

According to Pereira et al. [140], supercritical fluid extraction does not present disadvantages for extracting natural products, on the contrary, it can present the advantage to make selective extractions by varying pressure and temperature. Taking into account these premises, the authors used the response surface methodology to optimize the supercritical carbon dioxide fluid extraction conditions to obtain myrtle leaf extracts. The optimal conditions obtained were: 23 MPa, 45 °C, and CO_2 flow rate of 0.3 kg/h agreeing to those predicted by the response surface methodology model. The capacity for scavenging ABTS was inferior when compared to the ethanolic extracts of the same plant. Keeping those parameters constant, the authors [140] used ethanol as cosolvent and at different percentages to know if the increase of polarity of solvent could improve the antioxidant activity. The authors observed that the increase of ethanol content increased the antioxidant activity that could be by around 4 and 5 times for scavenging ABTS and peroxyl radicals, respectively, when the flow rate of ethanol was 0.09 kg/h.

As leaves and branches of myrtle are frequently consumed as an infusion and decoction, Messaoud et al. [141] studied the chemical composition, volatiles and phenols, and the antibacterial and antioxidant activities of leaf infusions prepared during three different times (5, 10, and 15 min). The phenolic compounds and their amounts found during those periods are depicted in Table 3. Phenolic acids and flavonol glycosides were the major group of infusions (7.64 to 14.28 µmol/g and 7.05 to 12.11 µmol/g, respectively), which variations depended on the time of heating (Table 3). Longer heating periods (15 min), higher was the amounts of phenols found in the myrtle infusion. The antioxidant activity was measured using four in vitro methods: DPPH (2,2-diphenyl-1-picrylhydrazyl) method, β-carotene bleaching test, chelating effect on ferrous ions, and ferric reducing power method. The results showed that the heating time influenced the antioxidant activity of myrtle infusions, independent on the method used. For DPPH method, the IC_{50} values found were: 356.14, 283.71, and 282.53 µg/mL in infusion samples after 5, 10, and 15 min of heating, respectively. For β-carotene bleaching test, the IC_{50} values found were: 247.91, 138.43, and 84.88 µg/mL in infusion samples after 5, 10, and 15 min of heating, respectively. For chelating effect on ferrous ions, the IC_{50} values found were: 223.56, 215.86, and 206.44 µg/mL in infusion samples after 5, 10, and 15 min of heating, respectively. For the ferric reducing power method, the values found were: 31.26, 35.81, and 38.93 mmol Fe^{2+}/mL in infusion samples after 5, 10, and 15 min of heating, respectively. As observed for phenols, the antioxidant capacity of infusions increases as heating time also increases. Such results suggest that phenolic compounds are responsible for the activities found. In fact, the authors [141] found a linear correlation between the phenols content and DPPH radical scavenging activity ($r^2 = 0.709$), β-carotene bleaching test ($r^2 = 0.831$), and ferric reducing power method ($r^2 = 0.858$).

3.4. Acylphloroglucinols on the Antioxidant Activity of Myrtle Leaves

Generally, the antioxidant leaf extracts of myrtle are assigned to phenols, particularly hydrolizable tannins and flavonoids, nevertheless the acylphloroglucinols semimyrtucommulone and myrtucommulone A are also described as antioxidants. Rosa et al. [142] reported that these acylphloroglucinols had antioxidant activity because they were able to prevent the thermal (140 °C), solvent-free oxidation of cholesterol. Myrtucommulone A at 5 nmol and 10 nmol exerted a complete inhibition of cholesterol degradation after 1 h or 2 h, showing a 90% protection at 2.5 nmol and 50% protection at 5 nmol at 1 and 2 h, respectively. Semimyrtucommulone was less active than myrtucommulone A. A complete inhibition of the oxidative process of cholesterol was observed from 5 nmol at 1 h and 20 nmol at 2 h, showing a 70% protection at 10 nmol at 2 h [142]. The lipid peroxidation was determined having LDL as lipid substrate and the oxidation was induced by Cu^{2+}. The results showed that both acylphloroglucinols preserved LDL from oxidative damage. In addition, a protective effect on the reduction of polyunsaturated fatty acids and cholesterol was also observed by inhibiting the increase of their oxidative products (conjugated dienes fatty acids hydroperoxides, 7β-hydroxycholesterol, and 7-ketocholesterol). According to these results, semimyrtucommulone and myrtucommulone A can be seen as dietary antioxidants with antiatherogenicity.

From the myrtle leaves, it was possible to isolate and identify myrtucommuacetalone, myrtucommulone M, myricetin, isousnic acid, growth regulator G3 factor, and myrtucommulone E. Myricetin was able to inhibit reactive oxygen species production on zymosan-stimulated whole blood phagocytes (IC_{50} = 1.6 µg/mL), in a dose-dependent manner. The J774.2 cells treated with phorbol 12-myristate 13-acetate (stimulant used to distinguish the activity of the oxidative burst from zymosan activation that is involved in phagocytosis) alone (positive control) or in combination with myrtucommuacetalone and myricetin for 30 min, showed that these compounds were able to inhibit the production of reactive oxygen species. Myricetin was able to inhibit the production of these reactive species in both stimulant processes, suggesting that this flavonoid is able to inhibit reactive oxygen species, mainly superoxide, by a myeloperoxidase independent pathway [143]. Myrtucommuacetalone and growth regulator G3 factor also inhibited the production of nitric oxide in mouse macrophages (82.3% and 59.36%, respectively), at 25 µg/mL concentration [143].

3.5. Complexity of Myrtle Extracts on the Antioxidant Activity

As aforementioned, several methods have been used for evaluating the antiradicalar activity and distinct results were obtained due to diverse factors. The substrates were complex mixtures that could also contribute for the diversity of results. Sanna et al. [144] compared two spectroscopic methods (ultraviolet-visible spectroscopy and electron paramagnetic resonance) or the antioxidant ability of myrtle leaf exctracts. In both cases, DPPH free radicals were used for evaluating the antiradicalar activity of extracts, in which the depletion of DPPH in the presence of an antoxidant is measured. Since the samples used in both assays were the same, all differences in the results could only be attributed to the method itself [144]. The results showed that for ultraviolet-visible spectroscopy method there was not proportionality between the extract concentration and absorbance, because for increasing extract concentrations, the colour changed from dark purple (DPPH solution colour) to dark brown, although the extract had been depleted all the DPPH present in the solution. However, the decrease in DPPH signal intensities measured by electron paramagnetic resonance was concentration dependent. The authors concluded that the estimation of radical scavenging ability performed by electron paramagnetic resonance is more trustworthy than ultraviolet-visible spectroscopy measurements. Though this conclusion, the utilization of the ultraviolet-visible spectroscopy for DPPH method is still largely used.

The complexity of sample matrix makes difficult to assign the biological activity to a compound or to a set of compounds. However, Romani et al. [145] were able to assign the antiradical activity of myrtle leaf, from Italy, to gallotannins which were predominant in myrtle extracts as well as in the commercial extract of chestnut bark used as reference. However the amounts of gallotannins varied significantly from one harvesting year to another harvesting year (Table 3), which makes difficult to have a final product with identical magnitude of activity. The establishment of standardized extracts is required to prevent such variability. The chemical composition of tannin aqueous and hydro-alcoholic extracts of myrtle leaf (Table 3) was evaluated by HPLC/DAD/ESI-MS methods.

3.6. Antioxidant Activity of the Leaf Foods

The capacity of myrtle extracts to retard food oxidation was evaluated by Turhan et al. [146] when the brining process of anchovies with sodium chloride (15 g/100 mL) was done with myrtle, rosemary and nettle extracts and stored at 4 °C, for 28 days. The lipid oxidation was followed by determining the peroxide value, thiobarbituric acid reactive substance (TBARS), and oxidative rancidity score. Myrtle and rosemary extracts were the most effective in slowing down the lipid oxidation because they decreased the peroxide value from 37.77 meq O_2/kg, in the control, to 11.48 meq O_2/kg, in rosemary extract; this value is not significantly different from the myrtle extract. These values were found after

28 days of storage. These extracts were also able to decrease the TBARS values from 1.89 mg MDA/kg (control) to 0.59 mg MDA/kg and 0.50 mg MDA/kg, in the case of brined anchovies with myrtle and rosemary extracts, after 28 days of storage. These values can be attributed to the highest amounts of total phenols in the myrtle (72.4 mg/g) and rosemary (52.6 mg/g) extracts, when compared to the lowest amounts of phenols in the nettle extract (7.2 mg/g). The capacity for scavenging the DPPH free radicals and the reducing power were also better for those extracts, which may explain the best capacity of myrtle and rosemary extracts for retarding the lipid oxidation of brined anchovies when stored during 28 days [146].

The application of myrtle extracts in food to prevent oxidation was also evaluated by Dairi et al. [147]. The nutritional quality of extra virgin olive oil can be lost when lipids oxidation occur, by losing its phenolic compounds, particularly during heating procedures. Due to the antioxidant properties of myrtle extracts, Dairi et al. [147] studied the effect of myrtle extract, obtained by two different methods (microwave-assisted extraction and maceration) on the preservation of nutritional quality of extra virgin olive oil, particularly of the phenolic compounds after heating processes (butane-air flame, oven and microwave). The evolution of the phenolic compounds content was monitoring by reversed phase dispersive liquid–liquid microextraction (RP-DLLME)-HPLCDAD-FLD method. The results showed that the addition of myrtle extracts not only preserved the endogenous phenolic compound of extra virgin olive oil (hydroxytyrosol, tyrosol, luteolin, apigenin, and secoiridoid 1) when compared with the control, in which myrtle extract was not added, but also reduced the specific extinction coefficient (K_{232}) values. This parameter checks the degree of a vegetal oil oxidation, being indicative of the formation of primary products of oxidation. However, these benefits induced by myrtle extract, mainly constituted by galloyl quinic acid, gallic acid, and myricitrin, were dependent on the type of heating of olive oil. In the phenol preservation, the most protective effect of the myrtle extract was found during flame and microwave heating, whereas in the prevention of primary oxidation products the most effective one occurred when sample oils were submitted to the flame heating. The myrtle extract did not exert any beneficial effect on the prevention of the formation of secondary products of oxidation, that is, it did not reduce the specific extinction coefficient (K_{270}) [147]. According to the authors, myrtle extracts may be a tool for improving the oxidative stability of olive oil, by improving its phenol composition.

After knowing that the enriched olive oil with myrtle extract prevented its oxidation [147], later on, Dairi et al. [148] wanted to know if the enriched oil would have better antioxidant properties acting against free radical attacks that can occur during lipid digestion. To reach the objectives, the authors studied the effect of myrtle extract, obtained by two different methods (microwave-assisted extraction and maceration), on egg yolk phosphatidylcholine/bile salts aqueous dispersion oxidation under simulated intestinal conditions (pH 7.4), that is, a model that would permit to know if such extracts could prevent lipid peroxidation that might occur in small intestine during lipids digestion. AAPH (2,2′-azobis (2-aminopropane) dihydrochloride) or a Fe^{3+}/ascorbic acid system were used to initialize the phospholipid peroxidation. In addition, the capacity for preventing DPPH and peroxyl radicals (ORAC) was also checked by the authors [148]. The phenolic composition of myrtle extracts is presented in Table 3, and the chemical composition was not greatly different in both extraction procedures. The extra virgin olive oil enriched with myrtle extract increased the neutralization of DPPH and peroxyl radicals, even better than the references α-tocopherol and butylated hydroxytoluene (BHT). When the lipidic model was used, the phospholipid stability increased by a factor of 33.6% and 34.8%, for myrtle microwave assisted extraction and maceration extraction when compared to the control (without myrtle extraction), when the lipid induction was performed with the Fe^{3+}/ascorbic acid system. However, when the induction was made with AAPH, the effect was very poor. This work allowed the authors to conclude that the capacity of extra virgin olive oil enriched with myrtle extract to inhibit phospholipid peroxidation under simulated intestinal conditions can be seen as a potential functional food [148].

The antioxidant activity of sea salts flavoured with Mediterranean herbs (myrtle, rosemary, and mixtures) was evaluated by Rosa et al. [122] in chemical models of lipid peroxidation and in cell cultures. Simultaneously, the authors compared the antioxidant activity of these samples with those of normal salt. The flavoured myrtle added to salt was constituted by a mixture of extract of myrtle berry juice, leaves, and myrtle essential oil. These flavoured salts preserved liposomes from Cu^{2+}-induced oxidation, decreasing the accumulation of malondialdehyde, by scavenging peroxyl radicals or chelating Cu^{2+} at the aqueous phase or at the liposome particle surface/core [122]. The methanolic extracts of flavoured salts also significantly reduced the reactive oxygen species generation in *tert*-butylhydroperoxide-induced intracellular Caco-2 cells. According to the authors this ability was correlated to the capacity of extract components to permeate cell membrane and scavenge reactive oxygen species inside cells [122].

Liposomes, resembling cell membranes, are lipid molecules that can encapsulate biologically both hydrophilic and lipophilic active substances or used as lipid substrate for evaluating the capacity of samples to preventing lipid peroxidation [54]. These authors evaluated the antioxidant ability of methanolic extracts obtained from the aerial parts of Greek myrtle before and after encapsulation. The activity was followed by three methods (Rancimat method, oxidative stability by DSC, and formation of malondialdehyde). The two first methods are based on the generation of volatiles and thermal release, respectively, indicating a terminal oxidation process, whereas the generation of malondialdehyde occurs at lower temperatures and at a different stage of oxidation. The encapsulation of the extract, for the same concentration, enhanced the antioxidant action more than the same extract in pure form [54]. Therefore, the encapsulation altered the activity of extract, improving it.

3.7. Anti-Inflammatory Activity of Leaf Extracts

Zaidi et al. [149] studied the effect of 24 selected Pakistani medicinal plants, including *M. communis*, which are traditionally prescribed for gastro-intestinal disorders. *Helicobacter pylori* infection is associated with gastritis, peptic ulcer, and gastric cancer. In these disorders oxidative stress is many times involved and, consequently, inflammatory processes. For this reason, the authors [149] evaluated the effect of plant extracts, such as aqueous myrtle extract, on the inhibition of secretion of IL-8 and inhibition or prevention of generation of reactive oxygen species (ROS) in clinically isolated *Helicobacter pylori* strain (193)-infected cells (human gastric cancer cell line AGS), in order to confirm the anti-inflammatory and cytoprotective effects in gastric epithelial cells attributed to those 24 plants. The authors observed that only four extracts (*Cinnamomum cassia*, *Myrtus communis*, *Syzygium aromaticum*, and *Terminalia chebula*) manifestly inhibited IL-8 secretion at both 50 and 100 µg/mL. In addition, only *Achillea millefolium*, *Berberis aristata*, *Coriandrum sativum*, *Foeniculum vulgare*, *Matricaria chamomilla*, and *Prunus domestica* were able to significantly suppression ROS generation (particularly superoxide anion radicals) from *Helicobacter pylori*-infected cells [149]. The ROS measurement generated was done by detecting the fluorescence emission, by flow cytometry, caused by the intercalation of oxidized hydroethidine, by superoxide, into DNA [59]. The chemical composition of the extracts was not determined by the authors and the results obtained were explained according to previous results. As so, they attributed the property for inhibiting IL-8 by myrtle extracts to the possible presence of myrtucommulone in the extract.

The anti-inflammatory activity of the aqueous and ethanolic extracts obtained from the aerial parts of *M. communis* was evaluated by Hosseinzadeh et al. [91] using xylene-induced ear oedema and a cotton pellet test, in mice. Antinociceptive activity was also performed using hot plate and writhing tests in mice. The ethanolic (0.05 g/kg) and aqueous extracts (0.005, 0.015, and 0.03 g/kg) demonstrated anti-inflammatory effects against chronic inflammation, whereas in the acute inflammatory activity (xylene-induced ear oedema study), the aqueous extract at doses 0.1, 0.2, and 0.03 g/kg showed significant anti-inflammatory activity. The ethanolic extract also had activity against acute inflammation in all doses (0.05, 0.15, and 0.35 g/kg), but was not dose-dependent. The aqueous and ethanolic extracts of the aerial parts of myrtle exhibited antinociceptive activity.

The authors suggested that this activity might be mediated by opioid receptors [91]. The chemical composition of the extracts was not performed but the authors attributed the antinociceptive and anti-inflammatory activities to flavonoids and/or tannins, according to the references consulted by them. The highest concentrations of extracts with anti-inflammatory and antinociceptive activities were lower than the LD_{50} (lethal dose 50) values found for aqueous and ethanolic extracts (0.473 and 0.79 g/kg, respectively) [91].

Generally, the antioxidant and anti-inflammatory activities of myrtle extracts have been attributed to the phenolic compounds. The higher activity of leaf extracts than berry extracts were attributed by some authors to the presence of hydrolysable tannins in leaf extracts at higher concentrations than in berry extracts, which means the weak influence of anthocyanins, present in coloured berries, in the antioxidant activity [103,135]. However, Feisst et al. [150] reported, for the first time, that two nonprenylated acylphloroglucinols, myrtucommulone and semimyrtucommulone, isolated from leaf extracts of myrtle, potently suppressed the biosynthesis of eicosanoids by inhibiting cyclooxygenase-1 (COX-1) and 5-lipoxygenase (5-LOX) *in vitro* and *in vivo* at IC_{50} values ranging from 1.8 to 29 μM. These enzymes are involved in the formation of the proinflammatory prostaglandins and leukotriens, respectively. At the same time, the authors showed that myrtucommulone and semimyrtucommulone were able to prevent the mobilization of Ca^{2+} in polymorphonuclear leukocytes at IC_{50} = 0.55 μM and 4.5 μM, respectively, mediated by G protein signaling pathways. This effect inhibited the generation of reactive oxygen species (peroxide) and the release of elastase at similar concentrations. However, the phenolic part of those acylphloroglucinols (isobutyrophenone) was much less effective or even not active [150]. However, the acylphloroglucinols only inhibited partially peroxide formation or failed to inhibit elastase release when ionomycin was added to polymorphonuclear leukocytes. According to these results, the authors suggest that the suppression of Ca^{2+} mobilization by the myrtle acylphloroglucinols is the main cause for the inhibition of peroxide formation and elastase release induced by fMLP (*N*-formylmethionyl-leucyl-phenilalanine), which is confirmed when ionomycin is added to the system that needs much higher concentrations of the acylphloroglucinols to produce biological effect. Ionomycin did not use the G protein signaling pathways for elevating internal Ca^{2+} [150].

The inhibition effect of myrtucommulone on COX-1 in human platelets, and 5-LOX in intact polymorphonuclear leukocytes, observed by Feisst et al. [150] led Koeberle et al. [151] to ascertain if this acylphloroglucinol was able to inhibit selectively prostaglandin E_2 (PGE_2) via microsomal PGE_2 synthase (mPGES)-1. For this purpose, the authors measured the effect of myrtucommulone in diverse systems (cell-free assay using microsomal preparations of interleukin-1β-stimulated A549 cells as the source of mPGES-1; intact A549 cells, and lipopolysaccharide stimulated human whole blood). The results observed by the authors were that myrtucommulone was able to inhibit the conversion of PGH_2 to PGE_2 (IC_{50} = 1 mmol/L) in the cell-free mPGES-1 system. In addition, the levels of PGE_2 also diminished in intact A549 cells and in human whole blood at low micromolar concentrations, nevertheless the inhibition of COX-2 by myrtucommulone in A549 cells or isolated human recombinant COX-2 was only observed for higher concentrations (>30 mmol/L). Concerning COX-1 inhibition, the authors observed IC_{50} > 15 mmol/L values, both in cellular or cell-free systems, that is, only presenting moderate activity. According to these results the anti-inflammatory activity of myrtucommulone is due to the suppression of PGE_2 formation and not so much to the inhibition of the COX enzymes [151].

The anti-inflammatory activity of myrtucommulone isolated from myrtle leaves was evaluated *in vivo* by Rossi et al. [152]. In this study, the authors induced inflammation in mice by the subplantar and intrapleural injection of carrageenan, respectively, that triggers the development paw oedema and pleurisy. The action of myrtucommulone was followed by administering the compound intraperitoneally. Myrtucommulone, at concentrations 0.5, 1.5, and 4.5 mg/kg i.p., reduced the development of mouse paw oedema and, at 4.5 mg/kg i.p., 30 min before and after carrageenan, showed anti-inflammatory activity in the pleurisy model. The mechanism involved in the anti-inflammatory activity of myrtucommulone was determined by the authors and they observed that carrageenan injection in the pleurisy test reduced the exudate volume and leukocyte number, myeloperoxidase activity, the lung intercellular adhesion molecule-1 and P-selectin. tumor necrosis factor-α (TNF-α) and interleukin-1β (IL-1β), leukotriene B4 (LTB$_4$), lung peroxidation (thiobarbituric acid-reactant substance), and nitrotyrosine and poly (ADP-ribose). Such results permitted to the authors to suggest that the mechanisms involved in the protection effect of myrtucommulone in lung injury include suppression of adhesion molecules, inhibition of LTB$_4$ generation and neutrophil infiltration [152].

The anti-inflammatory activity of natural compounds is sometimes attributed to their capacity for protecting tissues against oxidative damage. Chronic liver disease with fibrosis is a health problem that can be caused by duct obstruction which leads to cholestasis and liver damage. The oxidative stress seems to have an important role in the damage. Sen et al. [75] aimed at investigating the antioxidant and antifibrotic effect of *Myrtus communis* extracts against against liver injury and fibrosis occurring in rats with biliary obstruction in animal models. Glutathione and superoxide dismutase values that decreased in damaged liver, and malondialdehyde levels, myeloperoxidase activity, tissue luminol, lucigenin, transforming growth factor-beta (TGF-β), and hydroxyproline levels that increase in damaged liver, the treatment with myrtle extract reversed all of these parameters, that is, this extract protects the liver tissues against oxidative damage through its radical scavenging and antioxidant activities, decreasing the fibrotic activity by reducing the hepatic TGF-β and hydroxyproline contents [75]. Later on, Sen et al. [74] reported that ethanolic extracts obtained from myrtle leaves when supplemented to the diet of Wistar albino rats in which colitis was induced by acetic acid, on the fourth day, they decreased the levels of malondialdehyde, tissue luminol, lucigenin, nitric oxide, and peroxoxynitrite chemiluminescence, as well the myeloperoxidase activity, and increased the glutathione levels, when compared to those animals in which the disease was induced and any myrtle supplementation was given. The study showed that ethanol extract had significant antiiinflammatory activity protecting the tissues against oxidative damage [74].

Fekri et al. [89] evaluated the biochemical and histopathological effect of preventive and therapeutic doses of extracts of myrtle leaves against bleomycin-induced pulmonary fibrosis in an animal model. Inflammatory and oxidative processes are involved in the pulmonary fibrosis. For this reason, the authors [89] evaluated the effect of myrtle extract on the lipid peroxidation as well as on the activity of catalase in the animal submitted to bleomycin. The oxidation of lipids decreased and the activity of catalase increased, that is, the oxidative stress promoted by bleomycin was reversed with the myrtle treatment. Simultaneously, the methanolic extract of myrtle leaves decreased the hydroxyproline concentration in animals subjected to bleomycin-induced pulmonary fibrosis in early and late phases. Hydroxyproline is an indicator of collagen deposition in lungs in pulmonary fibrosis. The authors also reported the improvement in inflammation and fibrosis in myrtle group [89].

The anti-inflammatory activity of the aqueous and ethanolic extracts obtained from the aerial parts of *M. communis* was evaluated by Hosseinzadeh et al. [91] using xylene-induced ear oedema and a cotton pellet test, in mice. Antinociceptive activity was also performed using hot plate and writhing tests in mice. The ethanolic (0.05 g/kg) and aqueous extracts (0.005, 0.015, and 0.03 g/kg) demonstrated anti-inflammatory effects against chronic inflammation, whereas in the acute inflammatory activity (xylene-induced ear oedema study), the aqueous extract at doses 0.1, 0.2, and 0.03 g/kg showed significant anti-inflammatory activity. The ethanolic extract also had activity against acute inflammation in all doses (0.05, 0.15, and 0.35 g/kg), but was not dose-dependent. The aqueous and ethanolic extracts of the aerial parts of myrtle exhibited antinociceptive activity. The authors suggested that this activity might be mediated by opioid receptors [91]. The chemical composition of the extracts was not performed but the authors attributed the antinociceptive and anti-inflammatory activities to flavonoids and/or tannins, according to the references consulted by them. The highest concentrations of extracts with anti-inflammatory and antinociceptive activities were lower than the LD_{50} (lethal dose 50) values found for aqueous and ethanolic extracts (0.473 and 0.79 g/kg, respectively) [91].

One problem of the plant extracts is the heterogeneity in the concentration of the bioactive compounds. This fact may originate biological responses with different strength. For overcoming this problem, there is the possibility to obtain standardized extracts with well defined concentrations of the bioactive compounds. Fiorini-Puybaret et al. [153] used a standardized ethanolic extract (0.75% of myrtucommulones) obtained from myrtle leaves, with the trade name Myrtacine® (Ducray Laboratory, Lavaur, France) with the objective to ascertain if this extract is able to treat acne in its diverse aspects: antibacterial activity against *Propionibacterium acnes*; antiproliferative activity on human keratinocytes and anti-inflammatory properties using a cellular model of inflammation. These biological properties were also compared with myrtucommulones A and B', which are present in the standardized extract. This approach was based on the fact that the nonprenylated acylphloroglucinols of myrtle possessed antimicrobial, antioxidant, and anti-inflammatory activities [30,150,154]. Anti-inflammatory effect was determined through the measurement of 6-keto-prostaglandin F1α and [3H]-arachidonic acid metabolite production by A23187-stimulated human keratinocytes. COX and lipoxygenase LOX metabolite production from ionomycin-stimulated human keratinocytes was also evaluated as well as the lipase activity [153]. The results showed that A23187-stimulated keratinocytes in the presence of Myrtacine® at 10 µg/mL inhibited in 23% the production of 6-keto PGF1α compared to the control. Preincubation of SVK14 keratinocytes with 0.1 and 0.5 µg/mL myrtucommulone A also significantly reduced 6-keto PGF1α production in 21% and 17%, respectively, whereas myrtucommulone B' only lowered the production of 6-keto PGF1α in 9%. At 3 and 10 µg/mL, Myrtacine® significantly decreased all metabolite production from cyclooxygenase (6-keto PGF1α, PGE2, PGF2α, PGD2, and PGA2) and lipoxygenase (LTB4 and 12-hydroxyeicosatetraenoic acid or HETE). Moreover, Myrtacine® also exhibited anti-lipase activity: at 100 µg/mL and 1 mg/mL was able to inhibit the activity of lipase by 53% and 100%, respectively [153]. This anti-inflammatory activity along with the anti-*P. acnes* and antiproliferative activities can lead Myrtacine® to be used in the treatment of comedones and inflammatory acne lesions [153].

The mechanisms involved in the anti-inflammatory activity of myrtucommulone isolated from myrtle leaves have been cleared by diverse research teams as aforementioned; nevertheless there is no information about its bioavailability. Gerbeth et al. [155] proposed to study the metabolic stability of that acylphloroglucinol, obtained by synthesis, using rat and human liver microsomes and its oral availability in a pilot rat study. The study started by using Caco-2 cells and the results showed a high absorption of myrtucommulone. In rat model, the authors [155] reported that after 1 h of administrating 4 mg/kg myrtucommulone, an average plasma level of 258.67 ng/mL was observed. Physiologically-based pharmacokinetic modelling of myrtucommulone in the rat, it was observed that it was rapid and extensively distributed by plasma, skin, muscle, and brain. Moreover, myrtucommulone undergoes phase I biotransformation in human and rat liver microsomes, resulting hydroxylated and demethylated metabolites [155].

Table 3. Phenols, flavonoids, and acylphloroglucinols in leaf myrtle extracts.

Origin	Type of Extract	Identification/Quantification	Compounds	Reference
Italy	Hydroalcoholic extract, the remnant was fractionated by liquid–liquid extraction with ethyl acetate, and water residue	HPLC/MS and HPLC/DAD	*Hydroalcoholic extract* Galloyl derivatives (mg/mL) Gallic acid—0.259 Mono, di-galloyl glucosides and ellagitannins—10.06 5-O-galloyl quinic acid—traces 3,5-O-galloyl quinic acid—0.64 Flavonols (mg/mL) Myricitrin—0.91 Myricetin-3-O-galactoside—0.47 Myricetin-3-(6″-O-galloylgalactoside)—0.33 Myricetin glycosides—0.06 Quercitrin—0.02 *Ethyl acetate extract* Galloyl derivatives (mg/mL) Gallic acid—0.73 Mono, di-galloyl glucosides and ellagitannins—5.92 5-O-galloyl quinic acid—traces 3,5-O-galloyl quinic acid—1.49 Flavonols (mg/mL) Myricitrin—2.83 Myricetin-3-O-galactoside—1.54 Myricetin-3-(6″-O-galloylgalactoside)—1.07 Myricetin glycosides—0.23 Quercitrin—0.07 *Aqueous residue* Galloyl derivatives (mg/mL) Mono, di-galloyl glucosides and ellagitannins—0.30 Flavonols (mg/mL) Myricitrin—0.001	[135]
Tunisia	Acid hydrolysis with HCl 1 M,	HPLC/UV/Vis	*Leaf* Phenolic acids—1.40 (mg/g) Gallic acid—1.05 Caffeic acid—0.08 Syringic acid—0.08	[125]

Table 3. *Cont.*

Origin	Type of Extract	Identification/Quantification	Compounds	Reference
			Vanillic acid—0.04	
			Ferulic acid—0.05	
			Hydrolysable tannins—8.90 (mg/g)	
			Gallotannins—8.75	
			Flavonoids—0.91 (mg/g)	
			Quercetin-3-rutinoside—	
			Myricetin-3-O-galactoside—0.23	
			Quercetin-3-galactoside—0.13	
			Myricetin-3-O-rahmnoside—0.05	
			Quercetin-3-O-rahmnoside—0.29	
			Myricetin—0.10	
			Quercetin—0.11	
			Catechin—traces	
			Unknown—0.15 (mg/g)	
			Total—11.21 (mg/g)	
			Stem	
			Phenolic acids—1.17 (mg/g)	
			Gallic acid—1.02	
			Caffeic acid—	
			Syringic acid—0.08	
			Vanillic acid—0.02	
			Ferulic acid—0.05	
			Hydrolysable tannins—traces (mg/g)	
			Gallotannins—traces	
			Flavonoids—1.86 (mg/g)	
			Quercetin-3-rutinoside—0.08	
			Myricetin-3-O-galactoside—0.11	
			Quercetin-3-galactoside—0.12	
			Myricetin-3-O-rahmnoside—0.15	
			Quercetin-3-O-rahmnoside—0.09	
			Myricetin—0.19	
			Quercetin—	
			Catechin—1.12	
			Unknown—(mg/g)	
			Total—3.03 (mg/g)	
			Flower	
			Phenolic acids—2.34 (mg/g)	

Table 3. Cont.

Origin	Type of Extract	Identification/Quantification	Compounds	Reference
			Gallic acid—2.34	
			Caffeic acid—	
			Syringic acid—	
			Vanillic acid—	
			Ferulic acid—	
			Hydrolysable tannins—3.50 (mg/g)	
			Gallotannins—3.50	
			Flavonoids—traces (mg/g)	
			Quercetin-3-rutinoside—	
			Myricetin-3-O-galactoside—traces	
			Quercetin-3-galactoside—	
			Myricetin-3-O-rahmnoside—traces	
			Quercetin-3-O-rahmnoside—	
			Myricetin—	
			Quercetin—	
			Catechin—traces	
			Unknown—0.19 (mg/g)	
			Total—6.02 (mg/g)	
Algeria	- Maceration in hydroalcoholic solution (50:50) - Hydroalcoholic extract (50:50) irradiated by microwaves (700 w), for 1 min	HPLC-DAD	*Microwave assisted extraction* Galloylquinic acid—7.33 GAE mg/g Gallic acid—3.53 mg/g Myricetin-3-O-galactoside—2.38 mg MRE/g Myricetin-3-O-rhamnoside (MR)—12.26 mg/g Ellagic acid—0.84 mg MRE/g *Maceration* Galloylquinic acid—7.66 GAE mg/g Gallic acid—3.31 mg/g Myricetin-3-O-galactoside—2.37 mg MRE/g Myricetin-3-O-rhamnoside (MR)—11.78 mg/g Ellagic acid—0.88 mg MRE/g	[147]
Algeria	Microwave-assisted extraction	HPLC-DAD	Galloylquinic acid Gallic acid Gallotannin Myricetin-3-O-galactoside Digalloylquinic acid Trigalloylquinic HHDD-glucose Myricetin galloylgalactoside Myricetin-3-O-rhamnoside Quercetin-3-O-rhamnoside	[138]

Table 3. *Cont.*

Origin	Type of Extract	Identification/Quantification	Compounds	Reference
Iran	Maceration with methanol	HPLC	*Spring* (mg/100 g) Gallic acid—5.32 Chlorogenic acid—2.89 p-Coumaric acid—11.73 Ferulic acid—85.56 Rutin—10.87 Luteolin—2.21 Quercetin—5.23 Apigenin—7.45 *Summer* (mg/100 g) Gallic acid—6.72 Chlorogenic acid—3.79 p-Coumaric acid—14.13 Ferulic acid—94.71 Rutin—16.48 Luteolin—1.72 Quercetin—6.41 Apigenin—8.70 *Fall* (mg/100 g) Gallic acid—18.79 Chlorogenic acid—3.70 p-Coumaric acid—15.24 Ferulic acid—168.89 Rutin—35.38 Luteolin—3.40 Quercetin—5.70 Apigenin—10.07	[123]
Tunisia	Decoction in water: 5, 10, and 15 min	HPLC-UV/Vis	5 min (μmol/g) Gallic acid—6.47 Caffeic acid—0.71 Syringic acid—0.18 Ferulic acid—0.29 Myricetin-3-O-galactoside—0.59 Myricetin-3-O-rhamnoside—0.71 Myricetin-3-O-arabinoside—0.12 Quercetin-3-O-galactoside—5.35 Quercetin-3-O-rhamnoside—0.29	[141]

Table 3. *Cont.*

Origin	Type of Extract	Identification/Quantification	Compounds	Reference
			Myricetin—3.00 Quercetin—1.59 *Total*—19.28 *Phenolic acids*—7.64 *Flavonol glycosides*—7.05 *Flavonols*—4.58	
			10 min (µmol/g) Gallic acid—8.23 Caffeic acid—0.88 Syringic acid—0.29 Ferulic acid—0.41 Myricetin-3-O-galactoside—0.76 Myricetin-3-O-rhamnoside—0.82 Myricetin-3-O-arabinoside—0.18 Quercetin-3-O-galactoside—6.64 Quercetin-3-O-rhamnoside—0.29 Myricetin—3.82 Quercetin—2.41 *Total*—24.75 *Phenolic acids*—9.82 *Flavonol glycosides*—8.70 *Flavonols*—6.23	
			15 min (µmol/g) Gallic acid—11.82 Caffeic acid—1.41 Syringic acid—0.53 Ferulic acid—0.53 Myricetin-3-O-galactoside—1.06 Myricetin-3-O-rhamnoside—1.18 Myricetin-3-O-arabinoside—0.24 Quercetin-3-O-galactoside—9.11 Quercetin-3-O-rhamnoside—0.53 Myricetin—5.00 Quercetin—3.59 *Total*—34.98 *Phenolic acids*—14.28 *Flavonol glycosides*—12.11 *Flavonols*—8.58	

Table 3. Cont.

Origin	Type of Extract	Identification/Quantification	Compounds	Reference
Not reported	Not reported	Single-crystal X-ray diffraction 1H-NMR, high resolution electrospray ionization mass spectrometry, and Heteronuclear multiple-bond correlation spectroscopy	Myrtucommuacetalone Myrtucommulone M Myricetin Isousnic acid Growth regulator G3 factor Myrtucommulone E	[143]
Italy	Aqueous	HPLC/DAD/ESI-MS methods	Aqueous (2009–2010) fresh material (mmol/L) HHDP glucose—0.151–nd Monogalloyl-glucose—0.102–nd Galloylquinic acid—nd–0.169 Gallic acid—2.712–4.232 Gallotannin m/z 801—0.545–nd Gallotannin m/z 429—nd–nd Gallotannin m/z 633—0.249–0.300 Gallotannin m/z 633—0.134–nd Gallotannin m/z 801—0.338–0.335 Gallotannin m/z 633—0.484–nd Gallotannin m/z 1583—nd–nd Ellagitannin m/z 933—0.132–0.067 Galloylquinic acid—0.619–0.355 Gallotannin m/z 1565—3.378–0.400 Gallotannin m/z 1567—2.403–2.344 Gallotannin m/z 935—1.075–nd Digalloylquinic acid—nd–0.711 Trigalloyl HHDP-glucose—nd–0.423 Ellagitannin m/z 953—0.261–0.551 Gallotannin m/z 783—5.824–nd Ellagitannin m/z 1253—nd–0.254 Ellagitannin m/z 953—0.240–nd Ellagitannin m/z 1085—0.336–0.239 Myricetin galloylgalactoside—0.297–0.429 Myricetin 3-O-galactoside—0.274–0.754 Myricetin 3-O-rhamnoside—1.326–1.945 Ellagic acid—0.266–0.757 Quercetin-3-O-rhamnoside—1.326–1.945 Total polyphenols—21.148–14.266 Aqueous—hydroalcoholic (2010) dried material (mmol/L) HHDP glucose—nd–nd	[145]

Table 3. *Cont.*

Origin	Type of Extract	Identification/Quantification	Compounds	Reference
Japan	Aqueous acetone 70%	Preparative chromatography and comparison of spectroscopy data with those previously reported	Monogalloyl-glucose—nd-nd Galloylquinic acid—0.208–0.144 Gallic acid—4.489–0.268 Gallotannin *m/z* 801—nd–nd Gallotannin *m/z* 429—nd–0.144 Gallotannin *m/z* 633—0.435–0.265 Gallotannin *m/z* 633—nd–nd Gallotannin *m/z* 801—0.397–0.154 Gallotannin *m/z* 633—nd–nd Gallotannin *m/z* 1583—nd–7.050 Ellagitannin *m/z* 933—0.189–nd Galloylquinic acid—0.386–0.374 Gallotannin *m/z* 1565—0.606–0.495 Gallotannin *m/z* 1567—2.968–2.678 Gallotannin *m/z* 935—0.286–nd Digalloylquinic acid—0.559–1.574 Trigalloyl HHDP-glucose—nd–nd Ellagitannin *m/z* 953—nd–nd Gallotannin *m/z* 783—nd–nd Ellagitannin *m/z* 1253—0.407–0.416 Ellagitannin *m/z* 953—0.794–nd Ellagitannin *m/z* 1085—0.276–nd Myricetin galloylgalactoside—0.300–0.486 Myricetin 3-O-galactoside—0.620–1.084 Myricetin 3-O-rhamnoside—1.392–2.526 Ellagic acid—0.918–0.612 Quercetin-3-O-rhamnoside—nd–0.038 *Total polyphenols*—15.229–18.308 Oenothein B Eugeniflorin Tellimagrandin I Tellimagrandin II Gallic acid Quinic acid 3,5-di-O-gallate Myricetin-3-O-β-D-xyloside Myricetin-3-O-β-D-galactoside Myricetin-3-O-β-D-galactoside-6″-O-gallate Myricetin-3-O-β-L-rhamnoside	[122]

nd: not detected.

4. Myrtus nivellei

The antioxidant and anti-inflammatory activities of berries and/or leaves of *M. nivellei* are much fewer reported than those found for *M. communis*. Rached et al. [156] collected fifty two plants in different regions of Algeria and evaluated their antioxidant activity through two methods: DPPH and β-carotene-linoleic acid bleaching. Forty-eight active extracts were found from 38 Algerian species and *M. nivellei* leaves were in this group with IC_{50} value = 4.90 µg/mL (DPPH assay), in an aqueous extract, obtained by decoction, with total phenol concentration of 242.68 mg/gallic acid equivalent/g and total flavonoid content of 28.53 mg catechin equivalent/g. The IC_{50} value was close to that found for BHA (IC_{50} = 4.15 µg/mL) but higher and, therefore, poorer than quercetin (IC_{50} = 1.66 µg/mL) and ascorbic acid (IC_{50} = 2.66 µg/mL). A liquid–liquid fractionation assay from the aqueous extract was performed using solvents with increasing polarity (chloroform, ethyl acetate and *n*-butanol). In the DPPH assay, the IC_{50} values found for these extracts were: 53.50, 3.08, and 4.40 µg/mL, respectively. The remaining aqueous extract also had capacity for scavenging the DPPH free radicals (IC_{50} = 64.84 µg/mL). A good linear correlation was found between the antioxidant activity of the diverse fractions and total phenols and total flavonoids' contents [156].

Different extracts of leaves of *M. nevellei* were obtained (aqueous, ethanolic, and methanolic) and their antioxidant activities were evaluated by [157]. Ethanolic extract revealed to be the most effective for scavenging DPPH free radicals (EC_{50} = 0.59 µg/mL), closest to the reference, ascorbic acid (EC_{50} = 0.39 µg/mL). However, the aqueous extract more easily reduced ferric ion (64.86%) than the ethanolic extract (35.14%). The ethanolic extract possessed higher amounts of phenols (734.3 µg gallic acid equivalent/mg) and flavonoids (181.1 µg quercetin equivalent/mg) than the aqueous extract (466.5 µg gallic acid equivalent/mg and 135.5 µg quercetin equivalent/mg, respectively) [157].

The anti-inflammatory activity of methanolic extract of the aerial parts of *M. nivellei* was evaluated for the first time by Touaibia and Chaouch [158] using the carrageenan-induced paw oedema test. The authors revealed that the dose of 400 mg/kg was able to reduce significantly the paw oedema (80.41%). This inhibition percentage was similar to that of diclofenac, but at 50 mg/kg. Oral lethal dose 50 (LD_{50}) of the methanolic extract was higher than 1000 mg/kg, and therefore, the authors considered this dose as being highly safe [158].

M. nivellei is a Sahara-endemic plant used in folk medicine. In the absence of any preservation programmes can originate its disappearance very quickly. Touaibia and Chaouch [19] obtained in vitro calli from this species, evaluated their antioxidant activity and compared to those obtained from leaf extracts. Total phenol and total flavonoid' contents of calli extracts were inferior (73 µg gallic acid equivalent/g and 91 µg quercetin equivalent/g) when those obtained from leaf extracts (in situ): 348 µg gallic acid equivalent/g and 152.25 µg quercetin equivalent/g. These lower amounts of phenols might be responsible for the lowest capacity of calli for scavenging the DPPH free radicals (EC_{50} = 1.44 mg/mL). EC_{50} value for leaf samples (in situ) was 0.98 mg/mL. Nevertheless, calli extract exhibited higher capacity for preventing lipid peroxidation and reducing power than leaf extracts [19].

The chemical composition of Saharan myrtle only very recently was unravelled [20,22]. The biological properties of these extracts and their compounds were also reported [20]. From leaves of *M. nivellei*, Mansour et al. [20] obtained aqueous extracts by decoction and infusion that were analysed by ultrahigh-performance liquid chromatography photodiode array high-resolution mass spectrometry (UHPLC-PDA-HRMS) and then confirmed by nuclear magnetic resonance (NMR) spectroscopy. The phenolic compounds present in the infusion and decoction were also quantified by HPLC-UV-PDA. The fourteen compounds identified are depicted in Table 4. Myricetin 3-*O*-β-D-(6″-galloyl)glucopyranoside, isomyricitrin, and myricitrin were the major compounds present in the aqueous extracts of *M. nivellei*. Decoction extracted more phenols (150.5 mg/g) than the infusion (102.6 mg/g), corresponding to 73.8 and 23.6 mg/100 mL of a single tea cup, respectively. The capacity of decoction, infusion, and isolated compounds for scavenging the DPPH free radicals were analysed by the authors [20] and compared with green and black teas. The EC_{50} values for decoction and infusion of black and green teas were:

EC_{50} = 10.2, 18.6, 22.9, and 18.0 µg/mL, respectively. The activities of isolated compounds were better than those of infusion and decoction. The EC_{50} values for 3,4,5-*tri*-*O*-galloyl-quinic acid, myricetin-3-*O*-β-D-(6″-galloyl)glucopyranoside, *iso*myricitrin, 1,2,3,6-tetra-*O*-galloyl glucose, myricitrin, quercetin-3-*O*-β-D-(6″-galloyl)glucopyranoside, myricetin-3-*O*-β-xyloside, myricetin, and quercitrin were: 3.8, 5.6, 6.7, 4.0, 4.3, 8.8, 7.0, 3.5, and 5.9 µg/mL, respectively. Myricetin, 3,4,5-*tri*-*O*-galloyl-quinic acid and 1,2,3,6-tetra-*O*-galloyl glucose had a similar capacity for scavenging the free radicals of that of the reference, ascorbic acid, that is a powerful natural soluble antioxidant. These results indicate that the effective antioxidant capacity of *M. nivellei* teas can be attributed to flavonoids, their glycosides and polygalloyl derivatives [20]. Nevertheless, it seems that when in combination with the other phenolic compounds, some antagonism may occur among them, since the antioxidant activity of the whole tea is lower than the isolated compounds.

The chemical composition of crude aqueous extract, ethyl acetate and butanol fractions of Saharan myrtle leaves conducted by liquid chromatography with diode array detection, coupled to mass spectrometry (ion trap) with electrospray ionization (HPLC-DAD−ESI/MSn) permitted to identify 17, 25, and 19 compounds, respectively (Table 4) [22]. The ethyl acetate fraction had the highest concentration of phenol compounds, followed by the butanol fraction and the crude aqueous extract. The antioxidant activities of the extracts were evaluated through three methods: DPPH, reducing power, inhibition of β-carotene bleaching, and thiobarbituric acid reactive substance methods. The results showed that the ethyl acetate fraction exhibited better activity than the remaining extracts or fraction. In the DPPH method, the EC_{50} values found for ethyl acetate, butanol fractions and crude aqueous extracts were: 3.27, 4.6, and 7.1 µg/mL, respectively; in the reducing power, the EC_{50} values were: 3.15, 3.93, and 6.23 µg/mL, respectively; in the inhibition of β-carotene bleaching, EC_{50} values were: 82, 92.9, and 112 µg/mL, respectively; and in the thiobarbituric acid reactive substance, the EC_{50} values were: 0.46, 0.74, and 0.87, respectively. According to the authors, the best activity of the ethyl fraction can be attributed to the presence of some compounds, such as myricetin-hexosyl-gallate, myricetin-3-*O*-rhamnoside, gallocatechin-gallate-dimer, digalloyl, trigalloyl-HHDP-glucoside, tetragalloylglucoside, and of the quercetin and kaempferol derivatives. Such results are in line with those already reported by Pereira et al. [111,112] in which the authors found a good correlation between antioxidant activity and flavonol glycosides in *M. communis* extracts. With the exception of the inhibition of β-carotene bleaching method, all samples had better activity than the reference used, Trolox. The anti-inflammatory activity was measured through the capacity of samples to suppress the NO production by LPS (lipopolysaccharide)-induced murine macrophage-like RAW 264.7 cells. Such as observed for the antioxidant activity, ethyl acetate was also the best sample (EC_{50} = 104 µg/mL) for suppressing NO production and, therefore, best anti-inflammatory activity, followed by the butanol fraction (EC_{50} = 127 µg/mL) and the crude aqueous sample (EC_{50} = 149 µg/mL), however all of them presenting much lower activity than the reference, dexamethasone (EC_{50} = 16 µg/mL). The authors also attributed the anti-inflammatory activity to the presence of flavonols, ellagitannins and phenolic acids. The authors [22] also evaluated the cytotoxic properties of Saharan myrtle extract and fraction against diverse tumor cell lines (breast cancer MCF-7, lung cancer NCI-H460, cervical cancer HeLa, and liver cancer HepG2 lines). The ethyl acetate fraction showed a significant higher potential against all cancer cell lines, followed by the butanol fraction and the crude aqueous extract, nevertheless the same fraction was also that exhibited the lowest cytotoxicity on non-tumor cells (porcin liver primary cells, PLP2). According to the authors [22], ellagic acid, ellagitannins, quercetin, and its derivatives may have a crucial role in the cytotoxicity activity.

Table 4. Phenols and flavonoids in Saharan myrtle extracts.

Origin	Type of Extract	Identification/Quantification	Compounds	Reference
Algeria (Sahara)	Infusion and decoction	UHPLC-PDA-HRMS, NMR and HPLC-UV-PDA	Roseoside 2-Hydroxy-1,8-cineole-β-D-glucopyranoside 2-Hydroxy-1,8-cineole 2-O-α-l-arabinofuranosyl (1→6)-β-D-glucopyranoside 3,4,5-Tri-O-galloyl-quinic acid Myricetin-3-O-β-D(6″-galloyl)glucopyranoside Isomyricitrin 1,2,3,6-Tetra-O-galloyl glucose Myricitrin Quercetin-3-O-β-D-(6″-galloyl)glucopyranoside Myricetin-3-O-β-xyloside Isoquercitrin 3-Oxo-α-ionol-9-O-β-D-glucopyranoside Myricetin Quercitrin	[20]
Algeria	Decoction water Fractionation: ethyl acetate and butanol	Liquid chromatography diode array detection, coupled to mass spectrometry (ion trap) with electrospray ionization (HPLC-DAD−ESI/MSn)	Crude aqueous extract (mg/g) Galloyl-HHDP-glucoside—nd Galloyl-HHDP-glucoside—29.0 Digalloylquinic acid—nd Digalloyl-HHDP-glucoside—14.5 Trigalloylglucose—3.0 Rugosin B—5.4 Digalloyl-HHDP-glucoside—8.9 Trigalloylquinic acid—11.2 Trigalloylglucose—nd Digalloyl-HHDP-glucoside—7.22 Gallocatechin-gallate-dimer—10.9 Valoneic acid dilactone—nd Myricetin-hhexosyl-gallate—13.4 Trigalloyl-HHDP-glucoside—4.63 Myricetin-3-O-glucoside—8.48 Tetragalloylglucose—nd Rugosin A—4.9 Tetragalloylglucose—4.02 Quercetin-hexoxyl-gallate—1.88 Myricetin-3-O-rhamnoside—11.3 Quercetin-3-O-glucoside—1.64	[22]

Table 4. *Cont.*

Origin	Type of Extract	Identification/Quantification	Compounds	Reference
			Ellagic acid—nd	
			Kaempferol-hexosyl-gallate—4.3	
			Kaempferol-3-O-glucoside—nd	
			Quercetin-3-O-rhamnoside—nd	
			Myricetin—nd	
			Myricetin-coumaroylhexoside—nd	
			Total hydrosable tannins—93 (mg/g)	
			Total phenolic acids—	
			Total flavonoids—45	
			Total phenolic compounds—138	
			Ethyl acetate fraction (mg/g)	
			Galloyl-HHDP-glucoside—nd	
			Galloyl-HHDP-glucoside—nd	
			Digalloylquinic acid—6.41	
			Digalloyl-HHDP-glucoside—19.28	
			Trigalloylglucoside—7.1	
			Rugosin B—7.0	
			Digalloyl-HHDP-glucoside—20.72	
			Trigalloylquinic acid—22.2	
			Trigalloylglucoside—12.3	
			Digalloyl-HHDP-glucoside—11.1	
			Gallocatechin-gallate-dimer—35.6	
			Valoneic acid dilactone—9.5	
			Myricetin-hhexosyl-gallate—37.0	
			Trigalloyl-HHDP-glucoside—17.1	
			Myricetin-3-O-glucoside—19.88	
			Tetragalloylglucose—16.3	
			Rugosin A—9.7	
			Tetragalloylglucose—13.2	
			Quercetin-hexoxyl-gallate—10.54	
			Myricetin-3-O-rhamnoside—85.75	
			Quercetin-3-O-glucoside—3.1	
			Ellagic acid—27.1	
			Kaempferol-hexoxyl-gallate—8.34	
			Kaempferol-3-O-glucoside—3.3	
			Quercetin-3-O-rhamnoside—3.2	

Table 4. *Cont.*

Origin	Type of Extract	Identification/Quantification	Compounds	Reference
			Myricetin—5.5	
			Myricetin-coumaroylhexoside—2.12	
			Total hydrosable tannins—172 (mg/g)	
			Total phenolic acids—27.08	
			Total flavonoids—200	
			Total phenolic compounds—398	
			Butanol fraction (mg/g)	
			Galloyl-HHDP-glucoside—10.01	
			Galloyl-HHDP-glucoside—17.4	
			Digalloylquinic acid—14.3	
			Digalloyl-HHDP-glucoside—26.7	
			Trigalloylglucoside—6.18	
			Rugosin B—9.4	
			Digalloyl-HHDP-glucoside—16.9	
			Trigalloylquinic acid—31.3	
			Trigalloylglucoside—12.2	
			Digalloyl-HHDP-glucoside—6.6	
			Gallocatechin-gallate-dimer—13.2	
			Valoneic acid dilactone—8.47	
			Myricetin-hhexosyl-gallate—17.8	
			Trigalloyl-HHDP-glucoside—nd	
			Myricetin-3-O-glucoside—23.6	
			Tetragalloylglucose—nd	
			Rugosin A—7.8	
			Tetragalloylglucose—nd	
			Quercetin-hexoxyl-gallate—1.99	
			Myricetin-3-O-rhamnoside—12.4	
			Quercetin-3-O-glucoside—2.18	
			Ellagic acid—6.4	
			Kaempferol-hexosyl-gallate—nd	
			Kaempferol-3-O-glucoside—nd	
			Quercetin-3-O-rhamnoside—nd	
			Myricetin—nd	
			Myricetin-coumaroylhexoside—nd	
			Total hydrosable tannins—167.5 (mg/g)	
			Total phenolic acids—6.4	
			Total flavonoids—62.9	
			Total phenolic compounds—236.8	

nd: not detected

5. Conclusions

The myrtle berries are mainly used for doing liqueur; nevertheless berries can also be used for making jam, preserving their biological properties, such as the liposome oxidation. The antioxidant activity of berries, due to the presence of phenols, also seems to be a possibility to use the berries' pulp as prebiotics in some food formulations, such as probiotic-enriched ice-creams. For a myrtle liqueur of high quality it is also required that berries must be processed immediately after harvest. Two approaches can be followed: to store fruits in adequate conditions, such as controlled atmospheres; or to process the berries and store the hydro-alcoholic extracts. For the former case, the results showed that berries held at 80% O_2 at 2 °C preserve their quality of phenolic and anthocyanins contents, and antioxidant activity, for at least 20 days. When fruits are immediately submitted to maceration, the extract obtained is stable for three months, being flavonoids and, particularly, anthocyanins the most instable compounds. The antioxidant activity of berry extracts can only be poorly attributed to the anthocyanins, since white berries, in some cases, exhibit stronger antioxidant activity than dark blue berries. Some type of flavonoids and gallic acid and their derivatives may be responsible for the antioxidant activities found in berry extracts. Beyond the maceration, several other methods of extraction (e.g., supercritical fluid extraction, ultrasound-assisted extraction, and decoction) may be used, nevertheless did not provide much better phenol content or antioxidant activity. The type of solvent of solvent mixtures used revealed also to be important on the capacity for extracting higher amounts of some types of phenol compounds and, therefore, on the antioxidant activity, nevertheless sometimes the results are dissimilar, depending on the research team and conditions of work. Seeds revealed to be best antioxidants than the remaining parts of the fruit, probably due to the presence of higher concentrations of galloyl derivatives. When leaf and berry extracts of myrtle were compared in terms of antioxidant capacity, leaf extracts revealed to be those that exhibited higher antioxidant activity, not only to the highest amounts of total phenols but also for the highest concentrations of hydroxybenzoic acids and flavonols and their derivatives although the most important factor in the relevant activity of leaf myrtle extracts is the ratio between the sum of galloylglucosides, ellagitannins, and flavonols and also of the ratio between these galloyl derivatives and galloyl-quinic acids. The utilization of leaf extracts for stabilizing complex lipid systems, olive oil, and brined anchovies revealed to be possible, particularly when myricetin 3-*O*-rhamnoside is present, due to its antioxidant activity. The anti-inflammatory activity was also reported for both berry and leaf extracts of myrtle. In some cases such activity was attributed to the flavonoids and/or hydrolysable tannins, nevertheless nonprenylated acylphloroglucinols (e.g., myrtucommulone and semimyrtucommulone) were revealed to have also a remarkable role in that activity.

The chemical composition and antioxidant activity of Saharan myrtle is much less studied, most likely to its restricted distribution, which only appears in specific places of the Sahara. Only very recently, a detailed chemical composition of their extracts was performed as well as their antioxidant, anti-inflammatory, cytotoxic, and antibacterial activities. In the aerial parts or leaves were possible to find compounds belonging to the galloyl derivatives, flavonols, and flavonols derivatives, and phenolic acids as reported for myrtle extracts, nevertheless, some new compounds were found, such as 2-hydroxy-1,8-cineole-β-D-glucopyranoside, 2-hydroxy-1,8-cineole 2-*O*-α-L-arabinofuranosyl (1→6)-β-D-glucopyranoside, rugosin A, rugosin B, and valoneic acid dilactone, which were not reported in myrtle extracts. The effective antioxidant capacity of *M. nivellei* teas can be attributed to flavonoids, their glycosides, and polygalloyl derivatives.

Funding: This study was partially funded by Fundação para a Ciência e a Tecnologia (FCT), under the projects UID/BIA/04325/2013—MEDTBIO.

Conflicts of Interest: The authors declare no conflicts of interest.

References

1. Migliore, J.; Baumel, A.; Juin, M.; Médail, F. From Mediterranean shores to central Saharan mountains: Key phylogeographical insights from the genus *Myrtus*. *J. Biogeogr.* **2012**, *39*, 942–956. [CrossRef]
2. Thornhill, A.H.; Ho, S.Y.W.; Külheim, C.; Crisp, M.D. Interpreting the modern distribution of Myrtaceae using a dated molecular phylogeny. *Mol. Phylogenet. Evol.* **2015**, *93*, 29–43. [CrossRef] [PubMed]
3. Vasconcelos, T.N.C.; Proença, C.E.B.; Ahmad, B.; Aguilar, D.S.; Aguilar, R.; Amorim, B.S.; Campbell, K.; Costa, I.R.; de Carvalho, P.S.; Faria, J.E.Q.; et al. Myrteae phylogeny, calibration, biogeography and diversification patterns: Increased understanding in the most species rich tribe of Myrtaceae. *Mol. Phylogenet. Evol.* **2017**, *109*, 113–137. [CrossRef] [PubMed]
4. Alipour, G.; Dashti, S.; Hosseinzadeh, H. Review of pharmacological effects of *Myrtus communis* L. and its active constituents. *Phytother. Res.* **2014**, *28*, 1125–1136. [CrossRef] [PubMed]
5. Bouzabata, A.; Casanova, J.; Bighelli, A.; Cavaleiro, C.; Salgueiro, L.; Tomi, F. The genus *Myrtus* L. in Algeria: Composition and biological aspects of essential oils from *M. communis* and *M. nivellei*: A review. *Chem. Biodivers.* **2016**, *13*, 672–680. [CrossRef] [PubMed]
6. Melito, S.; la Bella, S.; Martinelli, F.; Cammalleri, I.; Tuttolomondo, T.; Leto, C.; Fadda, A.; Molinu, M.G.; Mulas, M. Morphological, chemical, and genetic diversity of wild myrtle (*Myrtus communis* L.) populations in Sicily. *Turk. J. Agric. For.* **2016**, *40*, 249–261. [CrossRef]
7. Mobli, M.; Qaraaty, M.; Amin, G.; Haririan, I.; Hajimahmoodi, M.; Rahimi, R. Scientific evolution of medicinal plants used for the treatment of abnormal uterine bleeding by Avicenna. *Arch. Gynecol. Obstet.* **2015**, *292*, 21–35. [CrossRef] [PubMed]
8. Mulas, M.; Cani, M.R. Germaplasm evaluation of spontaneous myrtle (*Myrtus communis* L.) for cultivar selection and crop development. *J. Herbs Spices Med. Plants* **1999**, *63*, 31–49. [CrossRef]
9. Hajiaghaee, R.; Faizi, M.; Shahmohammadi, Z.; Abdollahnejad, F.; Naghdibadi, H.; Najafi, F.; Razmi, A. Hydroalcoholic extract of *Myrtus communis* can alter anxiety and sleep parameters: A behavioural and EEG sleep pattern study in mice and rats. *Pharm. Biol.* **2016**, *54*, 2141–2148. [CrossRef] [PubMed]
10. Sisay, M.; Gashaw, T. Ethnobotanical, ethnopharmacological, and phytochemical studies of *Myrtus communis* Linn: A popular herb in Unani system of medicine. *J. Evid. Based Complement. Altern. Med.* **2017**, *22*, 1035–1043. [CrossRef] [PubMed]
11. Mahboubi, M. Effectiveness of *Myrtus communis* in the treatment of hemorrhoids. *J. Integr. Med.* **2017**, *15*, 351–358. [CrossRef]
12. Rahimi, R.; Abdollahi, M. Evidence-based review of medicinal plants used for the treatment of hemorrhoids. *Int. J. Pharmacol.* **2013**, *9*, 1–11.
13. Safavi, M.; Shams-Ardakani, M.; Foroumadi, A. Medicinal plants in the treatment of *Helicobacter pylori* infections. *Pharm. Biol.* **2015**, *53*, 939–960. [CrossRef] [PubMed]
14. Fadda, A.; Palma, A.; d'Aquino, S.; Mulas, M. Effects of myrtle (*Myrtus communis* L.) fruit cold storage under modified atmosphere on liqueur quality. *J. Food Process. Preserv.* **2017**, *41*, e12776. [CrossRef]
15. Montoro, P.; Tuberoso, C.L.; Piacente, S.; Perrone, A. Stability and antioxidant activity of polyphenols in extracts of *Myrtus communis* L. berries used for the preparation of myrtle liqueur. *J. Pharm. Biomed. Anal.* **2006**, *41*, 1614–1619. [CrossRef] [PubMed]
16. Bouzabata, A.; Bazzali, O.; Cabral, C.; Gonçalves, M.J.; Cruz, M.T.; Bighelli, A.; Cavaleiro, C.; Casanova, J.; Salgueiro, L.; Tomi, F. New compounds, chemical composition, antifungal activity and cytotoxicity of the essential oil from *Myrtus nivellei* Batt. & Trab., an endemic species of Central Sahara. *J. Ethnopharmacol.* **2013**, *149*, 613–620. [PubMed]
17. Hammiche, V.; Maiza, K. Traditional medicine in Central Sahara: Pharmacopoeia of Tassili N'ajjer. *J. Ethnopharmacol.* **2006**, *105*, 358–367. [CrossRef] [PubMed]
18. Sahki, A.; Boutamine Sahki, R. *Le Hoggar: Promenade botanique*; Editions Esope: Lyon, France, 2004.
19. Touaibia, M.; Chaouch, F.Z. Propriétés antioxydantes et antimicrobiennes des extraits de *Myrtus nivellei* Batt et Trab. obtenus in situ et in vitro. *Phytothér.* **2017**, *15*, 16–22. [CrossRef]
20. Mansour, A.; Celano, R.; Mencherini, T.; Picerno, P.; Piccinelli, A.L.; Foudil-Cherif, Y.; Csupor, D.; Rahili, G.; Yahi, N.; Nabavi, S.M.; et al. A new cineol derivative, polyphenols and norterpenoids from Saharan myrtle tea (*Myrtus nivellei*): Isolation, structure determination, quantitative determination and antioxidant activity. *Fitoterapia* **2017**, *119*, 32–39. [CrossRef] [PubMed]

21. Touaibia, M.; Chaouch, F.Z. Composition de l'huile essentielle et des extraits alcooliques de l'espèce Saharo-endemique *Myrtus nivellei* Batt et Trab (Myrtaceae). *Rev. Bioressour.* **2014**, *4*, 13–20. [CrossRef]
22. Rached, W.; Bennaceur, M.; Barros, L.; Calhelha, R.C.; Heleno, S.; Alves, M.J.; Carvalho, A.M.; Marouf, A.; Ferreira, I.C.F.R. Detailed phytochemical characterization and bioactive properties of *Myrtus nivelli* Batt & Trab. *Food Funct.* **2017**, *20*, 3111–3119.
23. Masoudi, M.; Kopaei, M.R.; Miraj, S. A comparison of the efficacy of metronidazole vaginal gel and Myrtus (*Myrtus communis*) extract combination and metronidazole vaginal gel alone in the treatment of recurrent bacterial vaginosis. *Avicenna J. Phytomed.* **2017**, *7*, 129–136. [PubMed]
24. Feuillolay, C.; Pecastaings, S.; le Gac, C.; Fiorini-Puybaret, C.; Luc, J.; Joulia, P.; Roques, C. A *Myrtus communis* extract enriched in myrtucummulones and ursolic acid reduces resistance of *Propionibacterium acnes* biofilms to antibiotics used in acne vulgaris. *Phytomedicine* **2016**, *23*, 307–315. [CrossRef] [PubMed]
25. Amensour, M.; Bouhdid, S.; Fernández-López, J.; Senhaji, N.S.; Abrini, J. Antibacterial activity of extracts of *Myrtus communis* against foodborne pathogenic and spoilage bacteria. *Int. J. Food Prop.* **2010**, *13*, 1215–1224. [CrossRef]
26. Saeide, S.; Boroujeni, N.A.; Ahmadi, H.; Hassanshahian, M. Antibacterial activity of some plant extracts against extended-spectrum beta-lactamase producing *Escherichia coli* isolates. *Jundishapur J. Microbiol.* **2015**, *8*, e15434. [CrossRef] [PubMed]
27. Mansouri, S.; Foroumadi, A.; Ghaneie, T.; Najar, A.G. Antibacterial activity of the crude extracts and fractionated constituents of *Myrtus communis*. *Pharm. Biol.* **2001**, *39*, 399–401. [CrossRef]
28. Al Laham, S.A.; Al Fadel, F.M. Antibacterial activity of various plants extracts against antibiotic-resistant *Aeromonas hydrophila*. *Jundishapur J. Microbiol.* **2014**, *7*, 211370. [CrossRef] [PubMed]
29. Eslami, G.; Hashemi, A.; Yazdi, M.M.K.; Benvidi, M.E.; Rad, P.K.; Moradi, S.L.; Fallah, F.; Dadashi, M. Antibacterial effects of *Zataria multiflora*, *Ziziphus*, chamolime and *Myrtus communis* methanolic extracts on IMP-type metallo-beta-lactamase-producing *Pseudomonas aeruginosa*. *Arch. Clin. Infect. Dis.* **2016**, *11*, e32413. [CrossRef]
30. Appendino, G.; Maxia, L.; Bettoni, P.; Locatelli, M.; Valdivia, C.; Ballero, M.; Stavri, M.; Gibbons, S.; Sterner, O. Antibacterial galloyllated alkylphloroglucinol glucosides from myrtle (*Myrtus communis*). *J. Nat. Prod.* **2006**, *69*, 251–254. [CrossRef] [PubMed]
31. Bonjar, G.H.S. Antibacterial screening of plants used in Iranian folkloric medicine. *Fitoterapia* **2004**, *75*, 231–235. [CrossRef] [PubMed]
32. Jabri, M.-A.; Tounsi, H.; Rtibi, K.; Ben-Said, A.; Aouadhi, C.; Hosni, K.; Sakly, M.; Sebai, H. Antidiarrhoeal, antimicrobial and antioxidant effects of myrtle berries (*Myrtus communis* L.) seeds extract. *J. Pharm. Pharmacol.* **2016**, *68*, 264–274. [CrossRef] [PubMed]
33. Abdoli, A.; Borazjani, J.M.; Roohi, P. Antimicrobial activity of aqueous and ethanolic extracts of *Heracleum persicum*, *Myrtus* and *Lemon verbena* against *Streptococcus mutans*. *Biosci. Biotechnol. Res. Commun.* **2017**, *10*, 205–212.
34. Pirbalouti, A.G.; Jahanbazi, P.; Enteshari, S.; Malekpoor, F.M.; Hamedi, B. Antimicrobial activity of some Iranian medicinal plants. *Arch. Biol. Belgrade* **2010**, *62*, 633–642.
35. Mothana, R.A.A.; Kriegisch, S.; Harms, M.; Wende, K.; Lindequist, U. Assessement of selected Yemeni medicinal plants for their in vitro antimicrobial, anticancer, and antioxidant activities. *Pharm. Bull.* **2011**, *49*, 200–210.
36. Salvagnini, L.E.; Oliveira, J.R.S.; dos Santos, L.E.; Moreira, R.R.D.; Pietro, R.C.F.R. Avaliação da atividade antibacteriana de folhas de *Myrtus communis* L: (Myrtaceae). *Braz. J. Pharmacogn.* **2008**, *18*, 241–244. [CrossRef]
37. Cottiglia, F.; Casu, L.; Leonti, M.; Caboni, P.; Floris, C.; Busonera, B.; Farci, P.; Ouhtit, A.; Sanna, G. Cytotoxic phloroglucinols from the leaves of *Myrtus communis*. *J. Nat. Prod.* **2012**, *75*, 225–229. [CrossRef] [PubMed]
38. Nourzadeh, M.; Amini, A.; Fakoor, F.; Raoof, M.; Sharififar, F. Comparative antimicrobial efficacy of *Eucalyptus galbie* and *Myrtus communis* L. extracts, chlorhexidine and sodium hypochlorite against *Enterococcus faecalis*. *Iran. Endod. J.* **2017**, *12*, 205–210. [PubMed]
39. Masoudi, M.; Miraj, S.; Rafieian-Kopaei, M. Comparison of the effects of *Myrtus communis* L., *Berberis vulgaris* and metronidazole vaginal gel alone for the treatment of bacterial vaginosis. *J. Clin. Diagn. Res.* **2016**, *10*, QC04–QC07. [CrossRef] [PubMed]

40. Al-Saimary, I.E.; Bakr, S.S.; Jaffar, T.; Al-Saimary, A.E.; Salim, H.; Al-Muosawi, R. Effects of some plant extracts and antibiotics on *Pseudomonas aeruginosa* isolated from various burn cases. *Saudi Med. J.* **2002**, *23*, 802–805. [PubMed]
41. Mehrabani, M.; Kazemi, A.; Mousavi, S.A.A.; Rezaifar, M.; Alikhah, H.; Nosky, A. Evaluation of antifungal activities of *Myrtus communis* L. by bioautography method. *Jundishapur J. Microbiol.* **2013**, *6*, e8316. [CrossRef]
42. Mousavi, S.A.A.; Kazemi, A. In vitro and in vivo antidermatophytic activities of some Iranian medicinal plants. *Med. Mycol.* **2015**, *53*, 852–859. [CrossRef] [PubMed]
43. Al-Mariri, A.; Safi, M. In vitro antibacterial activity of several plant extracts and oils against some Gram-negative bacteria. *Iran. J. Med. Sci.* **2014**, *39*, 36–43. [PubMed]
44. Atapour, M.; Zahedi, M.J.; Mehrabani, M.; Safavi, M.; Keyvanfard, V.; Foroughi, A.; Siavoshi, F.; Foroumadi, A. In vitro susceptibility of the Gram-negative bacterium *Helicobacter pylori* to extracts of Iranian medicinal plants. *Pharm. Biol.* **2009**, *47*, 77–80. [CrossRef]
45. Mansouri, S. Inhibition of Staphylococcus aureus mediated by extracts of Iranian plants. *Pharm. Biol.* **1999**, *37*, 375–377. [CrossRef]
46. Hamdy, A.A.; Kassem, H.A.; Awad, G.E.A.; El-Kady, S.M.; Benito, M.T.; Doyagüez, E.G.; Jimeno, M.L.; Lall, N.; Hussein, A.A. In-vitro evaluation of certain Egyptian traditional medicinal plants against *Propionibacterium acnes*. *S. Afr. J. Bot.* **2017**, *109*, 90–95. [CrossRef]
47. Rotstein, A.; Lifshitz, A.; Kashman, Y. Isolation and antibacterial activity of acylphloroglucinols from *Myrtus communis*. *Antimicrob. Agents Chemother.* **1974**, *6*, 539–542. [CrossRef] [PubMed]
48. Nabati, F.; Majob, F.; Habibi-Rezaei, M.; Bagherzadeh, K.; Amanlou, M.; Yousefi, B. Large scale screening of commonly used Iranian traditional medicnal plants against urease activity. *DARU J. Pharm. Sci.* **2012**, *20*, 72. [CrossRef] [PubMed]
49. Chen, M.; Chen, L.-F.; Li, M.-M.; Li, N.-P.; Cao, J.-Q.; Wang, Y.; Li, Y.-L.; Wang, L.; Ye, W.-C. Myrtucomvalones A–C, three unusual triketone-sesquiterpene adducts from the leaves of *Myrtus communis* 'Variegata'. *RSC Adv.* **2017**, *7*, 22735. [CrossRef]
50. Shaheen, F.; Ahmad, M.; Khan, S.N.; Hussain, S.S.; Anjum, S.; Tashkhodjaev, B.; Turgunov, K.; Sultankhodzhaev, M.N.; Choudhary, M.I. Atta-ur-Rahman New α-glucosidase inhibitors and antibacterial compounds from *Myrtus communis* L. *Eur. J. Org. Chem.* **2006**, *2006*, 2371–2377. [CrossRef]
51. Appendino, G.; Bianchi, F.; Minassi, A.; Sterner, O.; Ballero, M.; Gibbons, S. Oligomeric acylphloroglucinols from myrtle (*Myrtus communis*). *J. Nat. Prod.* **2002**, *65*, 334–338. [CrossRef] [PubMed]
52. Tanaka, N.; Jia, Y.; Niwa, K.; Imabayashi, K.; Tatano, Y.; Yagi, H.; Kashiwada, Y. Phloroglucinol derivatives and a chromone glucoside from the leaves of *Myrtus communis*. *Tetrahedron* **2018**, *74*, 117–123. [CrossRef]
53. Ajdari, M.R.; Tondro, G.H.; Sattarahmady, N.; Parsa, A.; Heli, H. Phytosynthesis of silver nanoparticles using Myrtus communis L. leaf extract and invesrigation of bactericidal activity. *J. Electron. Mater.* **2017**, *46*, 6930–6935. [CrossRef]
54. Gortzi, O.; Lalas, S.; Chinou, I.; Tsaknis, J. Reevaluation of bioactivity and antioxidant activity of *Myrtus communis* extract before and after encapsulation in liposomes. *Eur. Food Res. Technol.* **2008**, *226*, 583–590. [CrossRef]
55. Mahmoudvand, H.; Ezzatkhah, F.; Sharififar, F.; Sharifi, I.; Dezaki, E.S. Antileishmanial and cytotoxic effects of essential oil nd methanolic extract of *Myrtus communis* L. *Korean J. Parasitol.* **2015**, *53*, 21–27. [CrossRef] [PubMed]
56. Sangian, H.; Faramarzi, H.; Yazdinezhad, A.; Mousavi, S.J.; Zamani, Z.; Noubarani, M.; Ramazani, A. Antiplasmodial activity of ethanolic extracts of some selected medicinal plants from the northwest of Iran. *Parasitol. Res.* **2013**, *112*, 3697–3701. [CrossRef] [PubMed]
57. Shahnazi, M.; Azadmehr, A.; Jondabeh, M.D.; Hajiaghaee, R.; Norian, R.; Aghaei, H.; Saraei, M.; Alipour, M. Evaluating the effect of *Myrtus communis* on programmed cell death in hydatid cyst protoscolices. *Asian Pac. J. Trop. Med.* **2017**, *10*, 1072–1076. [CrossRef] [PubMed]
58. Naghibi, F.; Esmaeili, S.; Abdullah, N.R.; Nateghpour, M.; Taghvai, M.; Kamkar, S.; Mosaddegh, M. In vitro and in vivo antimalarial evaluations of myrtle extract, a plant traditionally used for treatment of parasitic disorders. *BioMed Res. Int.* **2013**, 316185. [CrossRef]
59. Grandjenette, C.; Schnekenburger, M.; Morceau, F.; Mack, F.; Wiechmann, K.; Werz, O.; Dicato, M.; Diederich, M. Dual induction of mitochondrial apoptosis and senescence in chronic myelogenous leukemia by myrtucommulone. *Anti-Cancer Agent Med. Chem.* **2015**, *15*, 363–373. [CrossRef]

60. Bouyahya, A.; Bakri, Y.; Et-Touys, A.; Assemian, I.C.C.; Abrini, J.; Dakka, N. In vitro antiproliferative activity of selected medicinal plants from the North-West of Morocco on several cancer cell lines. *Eur. J. Integr. Med.* **2018**, *18*, 23–29. [CrossRef]
61. Wiechmann, K.; Müller, H.; König, S.; Wielsch, N.; Svatoš, A.; Jauch, J.; Werz, O. Mitochondrial chaperonin HSP60 is the apoptosis-related target for myrtucommulone. *Cell Chem. Biol.* **2017**, *24*, 614–623. [CrossRef] [PubMed]
62. Tretiakova, I.; Blaaesius, D.; Maxia, L.; Wesselborg, S.; Schulze-Osthoff, K.; Cinalt, J., Jr.; Michaelis, M.; Werz, O. Myrtucommulone from *Myrtus communis* induces apoptosis in cancer cells via the mitochondrial pathway involving caspase-9. *Apoptosis* **2008**, *13*, 119–131. [CrossRef] [PubMed]
63. Izgi, K.; Iskender, B.; Jauch, J.; Sezen, S.; Cakir, M.; Charpentier, H.; Canatan, H.; Sakalar, C. Myrtucommulone-A induces both extrinsic and intrinsic apoptotic pathways in cancer cells. *J. Biochem. Mol. Toxicol.* **2015**, *29*, 432–439. [CrossRef] [PubMed]
64. Hayder, N.; Bouhlel, I.; Skandrani, I.; Kadri, M.; Steiman, R.; Guiraud, P.; Mariotte, A.-M.; Chedira, K.; Dijoux-Franca, M.-G.; Chekir-Ghedira, L. In vitro antioxidant and antigenotoxic potentials of myricetin-3-O-galactoside and myricetin-3-O-rhamnoside from *Myrtus communis*: Modulation of expression of genes involved in cell defence system using cDNA microarray. *Toxicol. In Vitro* **2008**, *22*, 567–581. [CrossRef] [PubMed]
65. Ines, S.; Ines, B.; Wissem, B.; Mohamed, B.S.; Nawel, H.; Dijoux-Franca, M.-G.; Kamel, G.; Leïla, C.-G. In vitro antioxidant and antigenotoxic potentials of 3,5-O-di-galloylquinic acid extracted from *Myrtus communis* leaves and modulation of cell gene expression by H_2O_2. *J. Appl. Toxicol.* **2012**, *32*, 333–341. [CrossRef] [PubMed]
66. Hayder, N.; Abdelwahed, A.; Kilani, S.; Ben Ammar, R.; Mahmoud, A.; Ghedira, K.; Chekir-Ghedira, L. Anti-genotoxic and free-radical scavenging activities of extracts from (Tunisina) *Myrtus communis*. *Mutat. Res.* **2004**, *564*, 89–95. [CrossRef] [PubMed]
67. Hayder, N.; Skandrani, I.; Kilani, S.; Bouhlel, I.; Abdelwahed, A.; Ammar, R.B.; Mahmoud, A.; Ghedira, K.; Chekir-Ghedira, L. Antimutagenic activity of *Myrtus communis* L. using the *Salmomella* microsome assay. *S. Afr. J. Bot.* **2008**, *74*, 121–125. [CrossRef]
68. Hayder, N.; Kilani, S.; Abdelwahed, A.; Mahmoud, A.; Meftahi, K.; Chibani, J.B.; Ghedira, K.; Chekir-Ghedira, L. Antimutagenic activity of aqueous extracts and essential oil isolated from *Myrtus communis*. *Pharmazie* **2003**, *58*, 523–524. [PubMed]
69. Sisay, M.; Engidawork, E.; Shibeshi, W. Evaluation of the antidiarrheal activity of the leaf extracts of *Myrtus communis* Linn (Myrtaceae) in mice model. *BMC Complement. Antern. Med.* **2017**, *17*, 103. [CrossRef] [PubMed]
70. Sumbul, S.; Ahmad, M.A.; Asif, M.; Saud, I.; Aktar, M. Evaluation of *Myrtus communis* Linn. berries (common myrtle) in experimental ulcer models in rats. *Hum. Exp. Toxicol.* **2010**, *29*, 935–944. [CrossRef] [PubMed]
71. Hashemipour, M.A.; Lofti, S.; Torabi, M.; Sharifi, F.; Ansari, M.; Ghassemi, A.; Sheikhshoaie, S. Evaluation of the effects of three plant species (*Myrtus communis* L., *Camellia sinensis* L., *Zataria multiflora* Boiss.) on the healing process of intraoral ulcers in rats. *J. Dent. Shiraz Univ. Med. Sci.* **2017**, *18*, 127–135.
72. Jabri, M.-A.; Rtibi, K.; Tounsi, H.; Hosni, K.; Marzouki, L.; Sakly, M.; Sebai, H. Fatty acids composition and mechanism of protective effects of myrtle berries seeds aqueous extract against alcohol-induced peptic ulcer in rat. *Can. J. Physiol. Pharmacol.* **2017**, *95*, 510–521. [CrossRef] [PubMed]
73. Jabri, M.-A.; Rtibi, K.; Tounsi, H.; Hosni, K.; Souli, A.; El-Benna, J.; Marzouki, L.; Sakly, M.; Sebai, H. Myrtle berries seeds aqueous extract inhibits in vitro human neutrophils myeloperoxidase and attenuates acetic acid-induced ulcerative colitis in rat. *RSC Adv.* **2015**. [CrossRef]
74. Sen, A.; Yuksel, M.; Bulut, G.; Bitis, L.; Ercan, F.; Ozyilmaz-Yay, N.; Akbulut, O.; Cobanoğlu, H.; Ozkan, S.; Sener, G. Therapeutic potential of *Myrtus communis* subsp. *communis* extract against acetic acid-induced colonic inflammation in rats. *J. Food Biochem.* **2017**, *41*, e12297. [CrossRef]
75. Sen, A.; Ozkan, S.; Recebova, K.; Cevik, O.; Ercan, F.; Demirci, E.K.; Bitis, L.; Sener, G. Effects of *Myrtus communis* extract treatment in bile duct ligated rats. *J. Surg. Res.* **2016**, *205*, 359–367. [CrossRef] [PubMed]

76. Zohalinezhad, M.E.; Hossini-Asl, M.K.; Akrami, R.; Nimrouzi, M.; Salehi, A.; Zarshenas, M.M. *Myrtus communis* L. freeze-dried aqueous extract versus omeprazol in gastrointestinal reflux disease: A double-blind randomized controlled clinical trial. *J. Evid. Based Complement. Altern. Med.* **2016**, *21*, 23–29. [CrossRef] [PubMed]
77. Salehi, M.; Azizkhani, M.; Mobli, M.; Shakeri, R.; Saberi-Firoozi, M.; Rahimi, R.; Karimi, M. The effect of *Myetus communis* L. syrup in reducing the recurrence of gastroesophageal reflux disease: A double-blind randomized controlled trial. *Iran. Red Crescent Med. J.* **2017**. [CrossRef]
78. Babaee, N.; Mansourian, A.; Momen-Heravi, F.; Moghadamnia, A.; Momen-Beitollahi, J. The efficacy of a paste containing *Myrtus communis* (myrtle) in the management of recurrent aphthous stomatitis: A randomized controlled trial. *Clin. Oral Investig.* **2010**, *14*, 65–70. [CrossRef] [PubMed]
79. Mortazavi, H.; Namazi, F.; Badiei, M.-R.; Mahin, B. Evaluation of therapeutic effects of adcortyl and *Myrtus communis* (myrtle) in patients with recurrent aphthous stomatitis: A clinical trial study. *HealthMed* **2012**, *6*, 1693–1698.
80. Safari, R.; Hoseinifar, S.H.; van Doan, H.; Dadar, M. The effects of dietary myrtle (*Myrtus communis*) on skin mucus immune parameters and mRNA levels of growth, antioxidant and immune related genes in zebrafish (*Danio rerio*). *Fish Sellfish Immunol.* **2017**, *66*, 264–269. [CrossRef] [PubMed]
81. Janbaz, K.H.; Nisa, M.; Saqib, F.; Imran, I.; Zia-Ul-Haq, M.; de Feo, V. Bronchodilator, vasodilator and spasmolytic activities of methanolic extract of *Myrtus communis*. *J. Physiol. Pharmacol.* **2013**, *64*, 479–484. [PubMed]
82. Gholamhoseinian, A.; Shahouzehi, B.; Sharifi-Far, F. Inhibitory activity of some plant methanol extracts on 3-hydroxy-3-methylglutaryl coenzyme A reductase. *Int. J. Pharmacol.* **2010**, *6*, 705–711.
83. Ahmed, A.H. Flavonoid content and antiobesity activity of leaves of *Myrtus communis*. *Asian J. Chem.* **2013**, *25*, 6818–6822.
84. Elfellah, M.S.; Akhter, M.H.; Khan, M.T. Anti-hyperglycaemic effect of an extract of *Myrtus communis* in streptozotocin-induced diabetes in mice. *J. Ethnopharmacol.* **1984**, *11*, 275–281. [CrossRef]
85. Baz, H.; Gulaboglu, M.; Gozcu, L.; Demir, M.; Canayakin, D.; Suleyman, H.; Halici, Z.; Baygutalp, K. Effects of aqueous extract of *Myrtus communis* L. leaves on streptozotocin-induced diabetic rats. *J. Res. Med. Dent. Sci.* **2016**, *4*, 214–218.
86. Önal, S.; Timur, S.; Okutucu, B.; Zihnioğlu, F. Inhibition of α-glucosidase by aqueous extracts of some potent antidiabetic medicinal herbs. *Prep. Biochem. Biotechnol.* **2005**, *35*, 29–36. [CrossRef] [PubMed]
87. Ozkol, H.; Tuluce, Y.; Dilsiz, N.; Koyuncu, I. Therapeutic potential of some plant extracts used in Turkish traditional medicine on streptozotocin-induced type 1 diabetes mellitus in rats. *J. Membr. Biol.* **2013**, *246*, 47–55. [CrossRef] [PubMed]
88. Abrishamkar, M.; Kamalinejad, M.; Jafari, R.; Chaibakhsh, S.; Karimi, M.; Ghorbani, J.; Jafari, Z.; Emtiazy, M. Effect of *Myrtus communis* L. syrup on chronic rhinosinusitis: A randomized double-blind, placebo-controlled pilot study. *Iran. Red Crescent Med. J.* **2017**, *19*, e57511. [CrossRef]
89. Fekri, M.S.; Mandegary, A.; Sharififar, F.; Poursalehi, H.R.; Nematollahi, M.H.; Izadi, A.; Mehdipour, M.; Asadi, A.; Fekri, M.S. Protective effect of standardized extract of *Myrtus communis* L. (myrtle) on experimentally bleomycin-induced pulmonary fibrosis: Biochemical and histopathological study. *Drug Chem. Toxicol.* **2018**, *11*, 1–7. [CrossRef] [PubMed]
90. Begum, S.; Ali, M.; Gul, H.; Ahmad, W.; Alam, S.; Khan, M. In vitro enzyme inhibition activities of *Myrtus communis* L. *Afr. J. Pharm. Pharmacol.* **2012**, *6*, 1083–1087.
91. Hosseinzadeh, H.; Khoshdel, M.; Ghorbani, M. Antinociceptive, anti-inflammatory effects and acute toxicity of aqueous and ethanolic extracts of *Myrtus communis* L. aerial parts in mice. *J. Acupunct. Meridian Stud.* **2011**, *4*, 242–247. [CrossRef] [PubMed]
92. Minaei, M.B.; Yazdi, E.G.; Ardakani, M.E.Z.; Dabaghian, F.H.; Ranjbar, A.M.; Yazdi, A.G. First case report: Treatment of the facial warts by using *Myrtus communis* L. topically on the other part of the body. *Iran. Red Crescent Med. J.* **2014**, *16*, e13565. [CrossRef] [PubMed]
93. Chaijan, M.R.; Handjani, F.; Zarshenas, M.; Rahimabadi, M.S.; Tavakkoli, A. The *Myrtus communis* L. solution versus ketoconazole shampoo in treatment of dandruff: A double blinded randomized clinical trial. *J. Pak. Med. Assoc.* **2018**, *68*, 715–720. [PubMed]

94. Qaraaty, M.; Kamali, S.H.; Dabaghian, F.H.; Zafarghandi, N.; Mokaberinejad, R.; Mobli, M.; Amin, G.; Nasei, M.; Kamalinejad, M. Effect of myrtle fruit syrup on abnormal uterine bledding: A randomized double-blind, placebo-controlled pilot study. *DARU J. Pharm. Sci.* **2014**, *22*, 45. [CrossRef] [PubMed]
95. Ergen, N.; Hoşbaş, S.; Orhan, D.D.; Aslan, M.; Sezik, E.; Atalay, A. Evaluation of the lifespan extension effects of several Turkish medicinal plants in *Caenorhabditis elegans*. *Turk. J. Biol.* **2018**, *42*, 163–173. [CrossRef]
96. Sanjust, E.; Mocci, G.; Zucca, P.; Rescigno, A. Mediterranean shrubs as potential antioxidant sources. *Nat. Prod. Res.* **2008**, *22*, 689–708. [CrossRef] [PubMed]
97. Alamanni, M.C.; Cossu, M. Radical scavenging activity and antioxidant activity of liquors of myrtle (*Myrtus communis* L.) berries and leaves. *Ital. J. Food Sci.* **2004**, *16*, 197–208.
98. Vacca, V.; Piga, A.; del Caro, A.; Fenu, P.A.M.; Agabbio, M. Changes in phenolic compounds, colour and antioxidant activity in industrial red myrtle liqueurs during storage. *Z. Naturforsch.* **2003**, *47*, 442–447. [CrossRef] [PubMed]
99. Tuberoso, C.I.G.; Barra, A.; Cabras, P. Effect of different technological processes on the chemical composition of myrtle (*Myrtus communis* L.) alcoholic extracts. *Eur. Food Res. Technol.* **2008**, *226*, 801–808. [CrossRef]
100. Zam, W.; Ali, A.; Ibrahim, W. Improvement of polyphenolic content and antioxidant activity of Syrian myrtle berries (*Myrtus communis* L.) hydro-alcoholic extracts using flavouring additives. *Prog. Nutr.* **2017**, *19*, 112–120.
101. Snoussi, A.; Hayet, B.H.K.; Essaidi, I.; Zgoulli, S.; Moncef, C.M.; Thonart, P.; Bouzouita, N. Improvement of the composition of Tunisian myrtle berries (*Myrtus communis* L.) alcohol extracts. *J. Agric. Food Chem.* **2012**, *60*, 608–614. [CrossRef] [PubMed]
102. Tuberoso, C.I.G.; Boban, M.; Bifulco, E.; Budimir, D.; Pirisi, F.M. Antioxidant capacity and vasodilatory properties of Mediterranean food: The case of Cannonau wine, myrtle berries liqueur and strawberry-tree honey. *Food Chem.* **2013**, *140*, 686–691. [CrossRef] [PubMed]
103. Serreli, G.; Jerković, I.; Gil, K.A.; Marijanović, Z.; Pacini, V.; Tuberoso, C.I.G. Phenolic compounds, volatiles and antioxidant capacity of white myrtle berry liqueurs. *Plant Foods Hum. Nutr.* **2017**, *72*, 205–210. [CrossRef] [PubMed]
104. Serce, S.; Ercisli, S.; Sengul, M.; Gunduz, K.; Orhan, E. Antioxidant activities and fatty acid composition of wild grown myrtle (*Myrtus communis* L.) fruits. *Pharmacogn. Mag.* **2010**, *6*. [CrossRef] [PubMed]
105. Polat, B.; Oba, S.; Karaman, K.; Arici, M.; Sagdic, O. Comparison of different solvent types for determination biological activities of myrtle berries collected from Turkey. *Qual. Assur. Saf. Crops* **2014**, *6*, 221–227. [CrossRef]
106. Messaoud, C.; Boussaid, M. *Myrtus communis* berry color morphs: A comparative analysis of essential oils, fatty acids, phenolic compounds, and antioxidant activities. *Chem. Biodivers.* **2011**, *8*, 300–310. [CrossRef] [PubMed]
107. Wannes, W.A.; Marzouk, B. Differences between myrtle fruit parts (*Myrtus communis* var. *italica*) in phenolics and antioxidant contents. *J. Food Biochem.* **2013**, *37*, 585–594.
108. Wannes, W.A.; Marzouk, B. Characterization of myrtle seed (*Myrtus communis* var. *baetica*) as a source of lipids, phenolics, and antioxidant activities. *J. Food Drug Anal.* **2016**, *24*, 316–323. [CrossRef] [PubMed]
109. Babou, L.; Hadidi, L.; Grosso, C.; Zaidi, F.; Valentão, P.; Andrade, P.B. Study of phenolic composition and antioxidant activity of myrtle leaves and fruits as a function of maturation. *Eur. Food Res. Technol.* **2016**, *242*, 1447–1457. [CrossRef]
110. Tuberoso, C.I.G.; Rosa, A.; Bifulco, E.; Melis, M.P.; Atzeri, A.; Pirisi, F.M.; Dessì, M.A. Chemical composition and antioxidant activities of *Myrtus communis* L. berries extracts. *Food Chem.* **2010**, *123*, 1242–1251. [CrossRef]
111. Pereira, P.; Cebola, M.-J.; Oliveira, M.C.; Gil, M.G.B. Supercritical fluid extraction vs conventional extraction of myrtle leaves and berries: Comparison of antioxidant activity and identification of bioactive compounds. *J. Supercrit. Fluids* **2016**, *113*, 1–9. [CrossRef]
112. Pereira, P.; Cebola, M.-J.; Oliveira, M.C.; Gil, M.G.B. Antioxidant capacity and identification of bioactive compounds of *Myrtus communis* L. extract obtained by ultrasound-assisted extraction. *J. Food Sci. Technol.* **2017**, *54*, 4362–4369. [CrossRef] [PubMed]
113. Amensour, M.; Sendra, E.; Abrini, J.; Bouhdid, S.; Pérez-Alvarez, J.A.; Fernández-López, J. Total phenolic content and antioxidant activity of myrtle (*Myrtus communis*) extracts. *Nat. Prod. Commun.* **2009**, *4*, 819–824. [PubMed]

114. Amensour, M.; Sendra, E.; Abrini, J.; Pérez-Alvarez, J.A.; Fernández-López, J. Antioxidant activity and total phenolic compounds of myrtle extracts. *CyTA J. Food* **2010**, *8*, 95–101. [CrossRef]
115. Serio, A.; Chaves-López, C.; Martuscelli, M.; Mazzarrino, G.; Mattia, C.; Paparella, A. Application of Central Composite Design to evaluate the antilisterial activity of hydro-alcohol berry extract of *Myrtus communis* L. *LWT Food Sci. Technol.* **2014**, *58*, 116–123. [CrossRef]
116. Amira, S.; Dade, M.; Schinella, G.; Rios, J.-L. Anti-inflammatory, anti-oxidant, and apoptotic activities of four plant species used in folk medicine in the Mediterranean basin. *Pak. J. Pharm. Sci.* **2012**, *25*, 65–72. [PubMed]
117. Jabri, M.-A.; Tounsi, H.; Rtibi, K.; Marzouki, L.; Sakly, M.; Sebai, H. Ameliorative and antioxidant effects of myrtle berry seeds (*Myrtus communis*) extract during reflux-induced esophagitis in rats. *Pharm. Biol.* **2016**, *54*, 1575–1585. [CrossRef] [PubMed]
118. Yoshida, N. Inflammation and oxidative stress in gastroesophageal reflux disease. *J. Clin. Biochem. Nutr.* **2007**, *40*, 13–23. [CrossRef] [PubMed]
119. Rosa, A.; Atzeri, A.; Deiana, M.; Scano, P.; Incani, A.; Piras, C.; Marincola, F.C. Comparative antioxidant activity and ^{1}H-NMR profiling of Mediterranean fruit products. *Food Res. Int.* **2015**, *69*, 322–330. [CrossRef]
120. Öztürk, H.I.; Demirci, T.; Akin, N. Production of functional probiotic ice creams with white and dark blue fruits of *Myrtus communis*: The comparison of the prebiotic potentials on *Lactobacillus casei* 431 and functional characteristics. *LWT Food Sci. Technol.* **2018**, *90*, 339–345. [CrossRef]
121. Curiel, J.A.; Pinto, D.; Marzani, B.; Filannino, P.; Farris, G.A.; Gobbeti, M.; Rizzello, C.G. Lactic acid fermentation as a tool to enhance the antioxidant properties of *Myrtus communis* berries. *Microb. Cell Fact.* **2015**, *14*, 67. [CrossRef] [PubMed]
122. Rosa, A.; Putzu, D.; Arzeri, A.; Marincola, F.C.; Sarais, G. Sea salts flavoured with Mediterranean herbs and fruits prevent cholesterol and phospholipid membrane oxidation and cell free radical generation. *Eur. Lip. Sci. Technol.* **2018**, *120*, 1700323. [CrossRef]
123. Shoshtari, Z.V.; Rahimmalek, M.; Sabzalian, M.R.; Hosseini, H. Essential oil and bioactive compounds variation in myrtle (*Myrtus communis* L.) as affected by seasonal variation and salt stress. *Chem. Biodivers.* **2017**, *14*, e1600365. [CrossRef] [PubMed]
124. Sacchetti, G.; Muzzoli, M.; Statti, G.A.; Conforti, F.; Bianchi, A.; Agrimonti, C.; Ballero, M.; Poli, F. Intra-specific biodiversity of Italian myrtle (*Myrtus communis*) through chemical markers profile and biological activities of leaf methanolic extracts. *Nat. Prod. Res.* **2007**, *21*, 167–179. [CrossRef] [PubMed]
125. Wannes, W.A.; Mhamdi, B.; Sriti, J.; Jemia, M.B.; Ouchikh, O.; Hamdaoui, G.; Kchouk, M.E.; Marzouk, B. Antioxidant activities of the essential oils and methanol extracts from myrtle (*Myrtus communis* var. *italica* L.) leaf, stem and flower. *Food Chem. Toxicol.* **2010**, *48*, 1362–1370.
126. Amessis-Ouchemoukh, N.; Madani, K.; Falé, P.L.V.; Serralheiro, M.L.; Araújo, M.E.M. Antioxidant capacity and phenolic contents of some Mediterranean medicinal plants and their potential role in the inhibition of cyclooxygenase-1 and acetylcholinesterase activities. *Ind. Crops Prod.* **2014**, *53*, 6–15. [CrossRef]
127. Chevolleau, S.; Mallet, J.F.; Ucciani, E.; Gamisans, J.; Gruber, M. Antioxidant activity in leaves of some Mediterranean plants. *J. Am. Oil Chem. Soc.* **1992**, *69*, 1269–1271. [CrossRef]
128. Chevolleau, S.; Debal, A.; Ucciani, E. Determination of the antioxidant activity of plant extracts. *Rev. Française Corps Gras* **1992**, *39*, 120–126.
129. Demo, A.; Petrakis, C.; Kefalas, P.; Boskou, D. Nutrient antioxidants in some herbs and Mediterranean plant leaves. *Food Res. Int.* **1998**, *31*, 351–354. [CrossRef]
130. Özcan, M.M.; Erel, Ö.; Herken, E.E. Antioxidant, phenolic content, and peroxide value of essential oil and extracts of some medicinal and aromatic plants used as condiments and herbal teas in Turkey. *J. Med. Food* **2009**, *12*, 198–202. [CrossRef] [PubMed]
131. Gião, M.S.; González-Sanjosé, M.L.; Rivero-Pérez, M.D.; Pereira, C.I.; Pintado, M.E.; Malcata, F.X. Infusions of Portuguese medicinal plants: Dependence of final antioxidant capacity and phenolic content on extraction features. *J. Sci. Food Agric.* **2007**, *87*, 2638–2647. [CrossRef] [PubMed]
132. Gião, M.S.; Pereira, I.C.; Pintado, M.E.; Malcata, F.X. Effect of technological processing upon the antioxidant capacity of aromatic and medicinal plant infusions: From harvest to packaging. *LWT Food Sci. Technol.* **2012**, *50*, 320–325. [CrossRef]
133. Gonçalves, S.; Gomes, D.; Costa, P.; Romano, A. The phenolic content and antioxidant activity of infusions from Mediterranean medicinal plants. *Ind. Crops Prod.* **2013**, *43*, 465–471. [CrossRef]

134. Belmimoun, A.; Meddah, B.; Meddah, A.T.; Sonnet, P. Antibacterial and antioxidant activities of the essential oils and phenolic extracts of *Myrtus communis* and *Zygophylum album* from Algeria. *J. Fund. Appl. Sci.* **2016**, *8*, 510–524. [CrossRef]
135. Romani, A.; Coinu, R.; Carta, S.; Pinelli, P.; Galardi, C.; Vincieri, F.; Franconi, F. Evaluation of antioxidant effect of different extracts of *Myrtus communis* L. *Free Rad. Res.* **2004**, *38*, 97–103. [CrossRef]
136. Tumen, I.; Senol, F.S.; Orhan, I.E. Inhibitory potential of the leaves and berries of *Myrtus communis* L. (myrtle) against enzymes linked to neurodegenerative diseases and their antioxidant actions. *Int J. Food Sci. Nutr.* **2012**, *63*, 387–392. [CrossRef] [PubMed]
137. Yoshimura, M.; Amakura, Y.; Tokuhara, M.; Yoshida, T. Polyphenolic compounds isolated from the leaves of *Myrtus communis*. *J. Nat. Med.* **2008**, *62*, 366–368. [CrossRef] [PubMed]
138. Dairi, S.; Madani, K.; Aoun, M.; Him, J.L.K.; Bron, P.; Lauret, C.; Cristol, J.-P.; Carbonneau, M.-A. Antioxidative properties and ability of phenolic compounds of *Myrtus communis* leaves to counteract in vitro LDL and phospholipid aqueous dispersion oxidation. *J. Food Sci.* **2014**, *79*, C1260–C1270. [CrossRef] [PubMed]
139. Dahmoune, F.; Nayak, B.; Moussi, K.; Remini, H.; Madani, K. Optimization of microwave-assisted extraction of polyphenols from *Myrtus communis* L. leaves. *Food Chem.* **2015**, *166*, 585–595. [CrossRef] [PubMed]
140. Pereira, P.; Bernardo-Gil, M.G.; Cebola, M.J.; Maurício, E.; Romano, A. Supercritical fluid extracts with antioxidant and antimicrobial activities from myrtle (*Myrtus communis* L.) leaves. Response surface optimization. *J. Supercrit. Fluids* **2013**, *83*, 57–64. [CrossRef]
141. Messaoud, C.; Laabidi, A.; Boussaid, M. *Myrtus communis* L. infusions: The effect of infusion time on phytochemical composition, antioxidant, and antimicrobial activities. *J. Food Sci.* **2012**, *77*, C941–C947. [CrossRef] [PubMed]
142. Rosa, A.; Melis, M.P.; Deiana, M.; Atzeri, A.; Appendino, G.; Corona, G.; Incani, A.; Loru, D.; Dessì, M.A. Protective effect of the oligomeric acylphloroglucinols from *Myrtus communis* on cholesterol and human low density lipoprotein oxidation. *Chem. Phys. Lip.* **2008**, *155*, 16–23. [CrossRef] [PubMed]
143. Choudhary, M.I.; Khan, M.; Ahmad, M.; Uousuf, S.; Fun, H.-K.; Soomro, S.; Mesaik, M.A.; Shaheen, F. New inhibitors of ROS generation and T-cell proliferation from *Myrtus communis*. *Org. Lett.* **2013**, *15*, 1862–1865. [CrossRef] [PubMed]
144. Sanna, D.; Delogu, G.; Mulas, M.; Schirra, M.; Fadda, A. Determination of free radical scavenging activity of plant extracts through DPPH assay: An EPR and UV-Vis study. *Food Anal. Methods* **2012**, *5*, 759–766. [CrossRef]
145. Romani, A.; Campo, M.; Pinelli, P. HPLC/DAD/ESI-ESI analyses and anti-radical activity of hydrolysable tannins from different vegetal species. *Food Chem.* **2012**, *130*, 214–221. [CrossRef]
146. Turhan, S.; Sagir, I.; Temiz, H. Oxidative stability of brined anchovies (*Engraulis encrasicholus*) with plant extracts. *Int. J. Food Sci. Technol.* **2009**, *44*, 386–393. [CrossRef]
147. Dairi, S.; Galeano-Díaz, T.; Acedo-Valenzuela, M.I.; Godoy-Caballero, M.P.; Dahmoune, F.; Remini, H.; Madani, K. Monitoring oxidative stability and phenolic compounds composition of myrtle-enriched extra virgin olive during heating treatment by flame, oven and microwave using reversed phase dispersive liquid-liquid microextraction (RP-DLLME)-HPLC-DAD-FLD method. *Ind. Crops Prod.* **2015**, *65*, 303–314. [CrossRef]
148. Dairi, S.; Carbonneau, M.-A.; Galeano-Diaz, T.; Remini, H.; Dahmoune, F.; Aoun, O.; Belbahi, A.; Lauret, C.; Cristol, J.-P.; Madani, K. Antioxidant effects of extra virgin olive oil enriched by myrtle phenolic extracts on iron-mediated lipid peroxidation under intestinal conditions model. *Food Chem.* **2017**, *237*, 297–304. [CrossRef] [PubMed]
149. Zaidi, S.F.; Muhammad, J.S.; Shahryar, S.; Usmanghani, K.; Gilani, A.-H.; Jafri, W.; Sugiyama, T. Anti-inflammatory and cytoprotective effects of selected Pakistani medicinal plants in *Helicobacter pylori*-infected gastric epithelial cells. *J. Ethnopharmacol.* **2012**, *141*, 403–410. [CrossRef] [PubMed]
150. Feisst, C.; Franke, L.; Appendino, G.; Werz, O. Identification of molecular targets of the oligomeric nonprenylated acylphloroglucinols from *Myrtus communis* and their implication as anti-inflammatory compounds. *J. Pharmacol. Exp. Ther.* **1995**, *315*, 389–396. [CrossRef] [PubMed]
151. Koeberle, A.; Pollastro, F.; Northoff, H.; Werz, O. Myrtucommulone, a natural acylphloroglucinol, inhibits microsomal prostaglandin E_2 synthase-1. *Br. J. Pharmacol.* **2009**, *156*, 952–961. [CrossRef] [PubMed]

152. Rossi, A.; di Paola, R.; Mazzon, E.; Genovese, T.; Caminiti, R.; Bramanti, P.; Pergola, C.; Koeberle, A.; Werz, O.; Sautebin, L.; et al. Myrtucommulone from *Myrtus communis* exhibits potent anti-inflammatory effectiveness in vivo. *J. Pharmacol. Exp. Ther.* **2009**, *329*, 76–86. [CrossRef] [PubMed]
153. Fiorini-Puybaret, C.; Aries, M.-F.; Fabre, B.; Mamatas, S.; Luc, J.; Degouy, A.; Ambonati, M.; Mejean, C.; Poli, F. Pharmacological properties of Myrtacine® and its potential value in acne treatment. *Planta Med.* **2011**, *77*, 1582–1589. [CrossRef] [PubMed]
154. Rosa, A.; Deiana, M.; Casu, V.; Corona, G.; Appendino, G.; Bianchi, F.; Ballero, M.; Dessì, M.A. Antioxidant activity of oligomeric acylphloroglucinols from *Myrtus communis* L. *Free Rad. Res.* **2003**, *37*, 1013–1019.
155. Gerbeth, K.; Hüsch, J.; Meins, J.; Rossi, A.; Sautebin, L.; Wiechmann, K.; Werz, O.; Skarke, C.; Barrett, J.S.; Schubert-Zsilavecz, M.; et al. Myrtucommulone from *Myrtus communis*: Metabolism, permeability, and systemic exposure in rats. *Planta Med.* **2012**, *78*, 1932–1938. [CrossRef] [PubMed]
156. Rached, W.; Benamar, H.; Bennaceur, M.; Marouf, A. Screening of the antioxidant potential of some Algerian indigenous plants. *J. Biol. Sci.* **2010**, *10*, 316–324. [CrossRef]
157. Touaibia, M.; Chaouch, F.Z. Evaluation de l'activité anti-oxydante des extraits aqueux, méthanolique et éthanolique de l'éspèce saharo-endémique *Myrtus nevelli* Batt et Trab. (Myrtaceae). *Int. J. Innov. Appl. Stud.* **2014**, *6*, 407–413.
158. Touaibia, M.; Chaouch, F.Z. Anti-inflammatory effect of *Myrtus nivellei* Batt & Trab (Myrtaceae) methanolic extract. *J. Fund. Appl. Sci.* **2015**, *7*, 77–82.

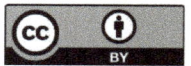

© 2018 by the authors. Licensee MDPI, Basel, Switzerland. This article is an open access article distributed under the terms and conditions of the Creative Commons Attribution (CC BY) license (http://creativecommons.org/licenses/by/4.0/).

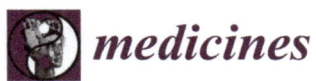

Review

Flavonoids from *Nelumbo nucifera* Gaertn., a Medicinal Plant: Uses in Traditional Medicine, Phytochemistry and Pharmacological Activities

Duangjai Tungmunnithum [1,*], Darawan Pinthong [2] and Christophe Hano [3,4]

[1] Department of Pharmaceutical Botany, Faculty of Pharmacy, Mahidol University, Bangkok 10400, Thailand
[2] Department of Pharmacology, Faculty of Science, Mahidol University, Bangkok 10400, Thailand; Darawan.pin@mahidol.ac.th
[3] Laboratoire de Biologie des Ligneux et des Grandes Cultures (LBLGC EA1207), INRA USC1328, Plant Lignans Team, Université d'Orléans, Pôle Universitaire d'Eure et Loir, 21 rue de Loigny la Bataille, 28000 Chartres, France; hano@univ-orleans.fr
[4] Bioactifs et Cosmétiques, GDR 3711 COSMACTIFS, CNRS/Université d'Orléans, 45067 Orléans CÉDEX 2, France
* Correspondence: duangjai.tun@mahidol.ac.th; Tel.: +66-264-486-96

Received: 31 October 2018; Accepted: 20 November 2018; Published: 23 November 2018

Abstract: *Nelumbo nucifera* Gaertn. has been used as an important ingredient for traditional medicines since ancient times, especially in Asian countries. Nowadays, many new or unknown phytochemical compounds from *N. nucifera* are still being discovered. Most of the current research about pharmacological activity focus on nuciferine, many other alkaloids, phenolic compounds, etc. However, there is no current review emphasizing on flavonoids, which is one of the potent secondary metabolites of this species and its pharmacological activities. Therefore, following a taxonomic description, we aim to illustrate and update the diversity of flavonoid phytochemical compounds from *N. nucifera*, the comparative analysis of flavonoid compositions and contents in various organs. The uses of this species in traditional medicine and the main pharmacological activities such as antioxidant, anti-inflammatory, anti-diabetic, anti-obesity, anti-angiogenic and anti-cancer activities are also illustrated in this works.

Keywords: *Nelumbo nucifera*; flavonoids; traditional medicine; pharmacological activities

1. Introduction

Nelumbo nucifera Gaertn. is an aquatic flowering plant belonging to the family nelumbonaceae. This perennial plant is well-known as various common names, e.g., sacred lotus, Indian lotus, Water lily and Chinese water lily. This species can be found mainly in Asian countries such as Thailand, China, Sri Lanka, India, Nepal, New Guinea or Japan [1–3]. Furthermore, *N. nucifera* is also distributed in Australia and Russia and was introduced to Western Europe and America long ago [4]. This plant is widely recognized by the beauty of its flowers, and has been considered a spiritual symbol for Buddhists, Hindus and Egyptians since ancient times. The flowers are very large and showy and considered sacred by Hindus, whereas the whole plant is holy according to Buddhists (Figure 1). Because of the beauty of its flower, it is also the national flower of India and Vietnam. Besides these considerations, there are also many advantages provided by this plant species such as being an ingredient for preparing various cuisines (such as its edible perianth, rhizomes and seeds) and also the important component for traditional medicines or herbal drugs [2,5–9], this latter point being the subject for many studies on phytochemical characterization and/or their bioactivities on this medicinal species, especially the leaves [1–44]. The present work highlights and updates on the comparative analysis of flavonoids and compositions in different organs of *N. nucifera* with an overview of main pharmacological activity from its flavonoid compounds. A proposed biosynthetic sequence of flavonoid *O*-glycosides (FOGs) as well as flavonoids *C*-glycosides (FCGs) derived flavonoids from this plant is also discussed. In addition, the taxonomic description and the uses in traditional medicine are also illustrated.

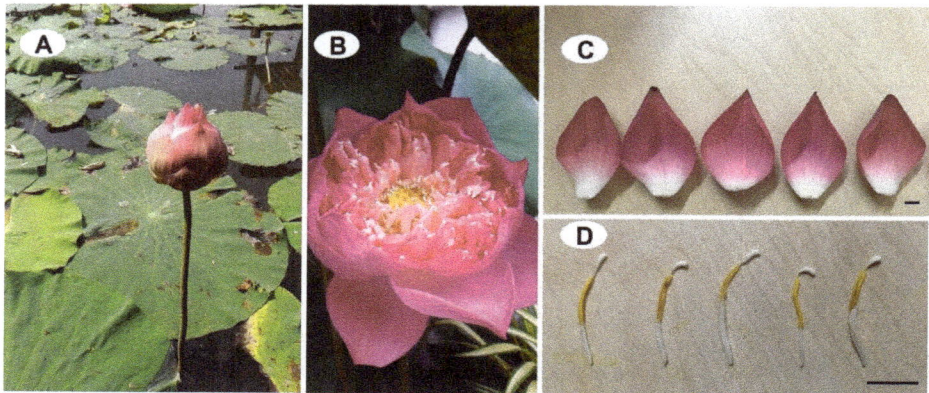

Figure 1. *Nelumbo nucifera* Gaertn.: (**A**) natural habitat; (**B**) flower; (**C**) perianth; and (**D**) dtamen. The photos were taken by D.T. Bar scale = 1 cm.

2. Taxonomic Description of *Nelumbo nucifera* Gaertn

Aquatic perennial, rhizomatous. Petiole 2–1.3 m, terete, glabrous or papillae hard and scattered. Leaf orbicular, blue-green, 28.5–90.5 cm in diam., glabrous, glaucous, water-repellent, margin entire. Flowers 9.52–4.5 cm in diam. Peduncles longer than petioles, glabrous or sparsely spinulate. Perianth caducous, oblong, oblong-elliptic or obovate, pink or white, 4.5–10.5 × 2.7–5.5 cm. Stamens longer than receptacle, filament slender; anther linear, 2–1.5 mm; connective appendage. Receptacle accrescent, turbinate, 4.5–9.5 cm in diam. Ovary Superior. Fruit oblong or ovoid, 3.2–5 × 6.5–15 cm, glabrous, pericarp thick, hardened. Many herbarium specimens both from the past and current collection have been cross-checked in the major herbaria of the country for species authentication.

3. *N. nucifera* is Used in Various Traditional Medicine

It is commonly known that *N. nucifera* or the lotus plant has been widely used as a component of traditional Chinese, Indian, Japanese, Thai, and Korean medicines and many others for several medicinal purposes [5,6]. The whole plant is used as an herbal medicine to cure diarrhea, insomnia, fever, body heat imbalance and gastritis [2,5,6,8]. In Korea, India and China, it is also used as a hemostatic [8]. Dry leaves and perianth of *N. nucifera* are consumed as health promoting teas. Yeon Yip Bap, a local food of Korea, also uses the leaves of *N. nucifera* as an ingredient [36]. Every part of this aquatic plant species—such as stamens, leaves, petioles, flowers, seeds and rhizomes—have been used for more than 1000 years in Chinese traditional medicines, and nowadays the production of *N. nucifera* leaves for traditional medicine usage and pharmaceutical industries is over 800,000 t/year in China [6,28]. The flowers and pedicels are used as both cardiac and hepatic tonics. The seeds are prepared to treat cutaneous diseases. They are also freshly eaten. The rhizome powder is used medicinally to promote the health balance (e.g., having positive effects on circulatory system). In China, leaves are used to fight against hyperlipidemia, hematemesis, metrorrhagia, fever treatment or to release skin inflammatory symptoms [6,8,28]. In addition, Asian people, practically in China and Taiwan, also prepare herbal tea from dry leaves of *N. nucifera* to lose weight and decrease body fat index [5,40]. In Thailand, the stamens constitute the necessary ingredient for preparing Thai traditional medicines. The herbal teas from stamens of *N. nucifera* are traditionally used by Thai people to improve the circulatory system, decrease blood glucose and blood lipid levels, and reduce oxidative stress substances in the body (Figure 2).

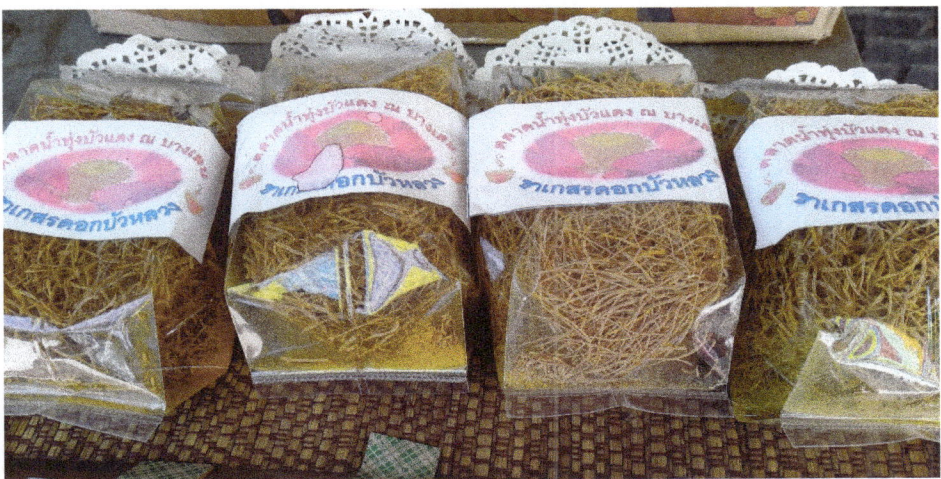

Figure 2. The herbal tea product from stamens of *Nelumbo nucifera* Gaertn. are sold in local markets. The photo was taken by D.T.

4. Flavonoids from *N. nucifera* and Their Pharmacological Activities

4.1. Phytochemical Diversity of N. nucifera *Flavonoids*

From a chemical point of view, flavonoids are phenylpropanoids with C6-C3-C6 backbone consisting in two phenyl rings (rings A and B) associated with one heterocyclic ring (ring C) (Figure 3). In plants, flavonoids are generally accumulated in the forms of glycosides. Glycosylation step results in changes in solubility, stability and/or toxic potential of these compounds but can also influence their cellular compartmentalization and biological activities [45]. In nature, flavonoids can be found in two distinct *O*- and *C*-glycoside forms with different actions both in plant and in human health [46]. The *O*-glycosylation of flavonoids leading to the production of flavonoid *O*-glycosides (FOGs), which widely occurs in the plant kingdom, has been well characterized and described [23]. On the contrary, flavonoid *C*-glycosides (FCGs) production has received much less attention and the *C*-glycosyltransferase enzymes catalyzing this step are far less studied than their *O*-glycosyltransferase cousins [11]. By definition, contrary to *O*-glycosylation that consists in the transfer of the sugar moieties to the oxygen atom of a hydroxyl group of the flavonoid, *C*-glycosylation leads to the creation of a very stable carbon–carbon bond between the sugar moieties and the carbon skeleton of the flavonoid. This less common glyosidic bound is much more resistant to hydrolysis occurring under acidic pH or from enzyme action, and is supposed to lead to important changes in the biological roles and activities of the resulting FCGs as compared to their FOG counterparts. From a pharmacological point of view, this specific glycosylation step drastically changes the disponibility, pharmacokinetics and biological activities of the flavonoids, including their antioxidant, anti-inflammatory, hepatoprotective, antiviral and anticancer actions [11,32]. Lotus is one of the richest sources of a wide variety of flavonoids mainly accumulated in the forms of FOGs and FCGs. The main FOGs and FCGs accumulated in lotus tissues are presented in Figure 3. Zhu et al. [27] reported on a higher antioxidant potential of FCGs than FOGs from distinct lotus extracts. However, the effect of *C*-glycosylation on biological activities of the resulting flavonoids have been scarcely investigated in lotus.

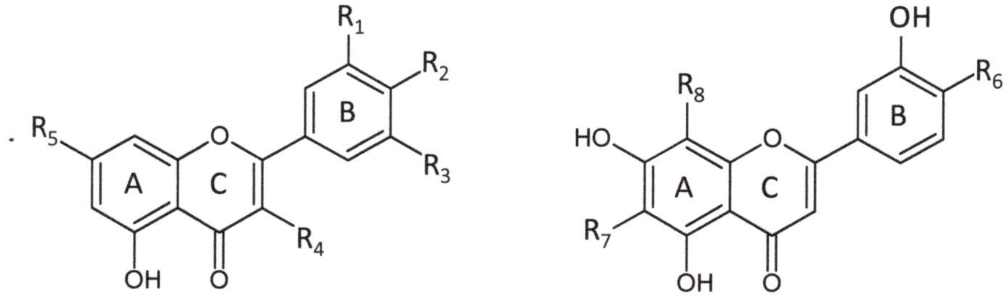

	Name	R_1	R_2	R_3	R_4	R_5
O1	Myr-3-Gal	OH	OH	OH	O-Gal	OH
O2	Myr-3-Glc	OH	OH	OH	O-Glc	OH
O3	Quer-3-Ara-Gal	OH	OH	H	O-Ara-Gal	OH
O4	Myr-3-Gln	OH	OH	OH	O-Gln	OH
O5	Rutin [1]	OH	OH	H	O-Rha-Glc	OH
O6	Hyperoside [2]	OH	OH	H	O-Gal	OH
O7	Isoquercitrin [3]	OH	OH	H	O-Glc	OH
O8	Kae-3-Rob	H	OH	H	O-Rob	OH
O9	Quer-3-Gln	OH	OH	H	O-Gln	OH
O10	Kae-3-Gal	H	OH	H	O-Gal	OH
O11	Iso-3-Rut	OCH_3	OH	H	O-Rut	OH
O12	Astragalin [4]	H	OH	H	O-Glc	OH
O13	Syr-3-Glc	OCH_3	OH	OCH_3	O-Glc	OH
O14	Iso-3-Glc	OCH_3	OH	H	O-Glc	OH
O15	Kae-3-Gln	H	OH	H	O-Gln	OH
O16	Kae-7-Glu	H	OH	H	OH	O-Glc
O17	Dio-7-Hex	OH	OCH_3	H	H	O-Hex
O18	Iso-3-Gln	OCH_3	OH	H	O-Gln	OH
19	Quer	OH	OH	H	OH	OH
20	Dio	OH	OCH_3	H	H	OH

	Name	R_6	R_7	R_8
C1	Orientin [5]	OH	H	C-Glc
C2	Isoorientin [6]	OH	C-Glc	H
C3	Vitexin [7]	H	H	C-Glc
C4	Isovitexin [8]	H	C-Glc	H
C5	Api-6-C-Glc-8-C-Glc	H	C-Glc	C-Glc
C6	Lut-6-C-Glc-8-C-Pen	OH	C-Glc	C-Pen
C7	Lut-6-C-Pen-8-C-Glc	OH	C-Pen	C-Glc
C8	Api-6-C-Glc-8-C-Xyl	H	C-Glc	C-Xyl
C9	Api-6-C-Xyl-8-C-Glc	H	C-Xyl	C-Glc
C10	Api-6-C-Glc-8-C-Ara	H	C-Glc	C-Ara
C11	Api-6-C-Ara-8-C-Glc	H	C-Ara	C-Glc
C12	Api-6-C-Glc-8-C-Rha	H	C-Glc	C-Rha
C13	Api-6-C-Rha-8-C-Glc	H	C-Rha	C-Glc

Figure 3. The chemical structures and names of the mains flavonoid O- (starting by O), C-glycosides (starting by C) and quercetin (Quer) and Diosmetin (Dio) aglycones from *Nelumbo nucifera* tissues. Flavonoid abbreviations used: Myr, myrycetin; Quer, quercetin; Kae, kaempferol; Iso, isorhamnetin; Syr, syringetin; Dio, diosmetin; Api, apigenin; Lut, luteolin. Sugar abbreviations used: Glc, glucoside; Gal, galactoside; Ara, arabionoside; Gln, glucuronide; Rut, rutinoside; Hex, hexoside; Xyl, xylose; Rha, rhamnose; Pen, pentose. [1] rutin, quercetin 3-O-rhamnopyranosyl-(1→6)-glucopyranoside; [2] hyperoside, quercetin 3-O-galactoside; [3] isoquercitrin, quercetin 3-O-glucoside; [4] Astragalin, kaempferol 3-O-glucoside; [5] orientin, luteolin 8-C-β-D-glucopyranoside; [6] isoorientin, luteolin 6-C-β-D-glucopyranoside; [7] vitexin, apigenin 8-C-β-D-glucopyranoside; [8] isovitexin, apigenin 6-C-β-D-glucopyranoside. Adapted from Chen et al. [25] and Li et al. [35].

Interestingly, in lotus, FOGs and FCGs present a different accumulation pattern with a preferential accumulation of FCGs in embryo (in which they represent more than 70% of the total flavonoid content), whereas leaves also accumulate high levels of flavonoids but exclusively FOGs [5,27,33] (Figure 4).

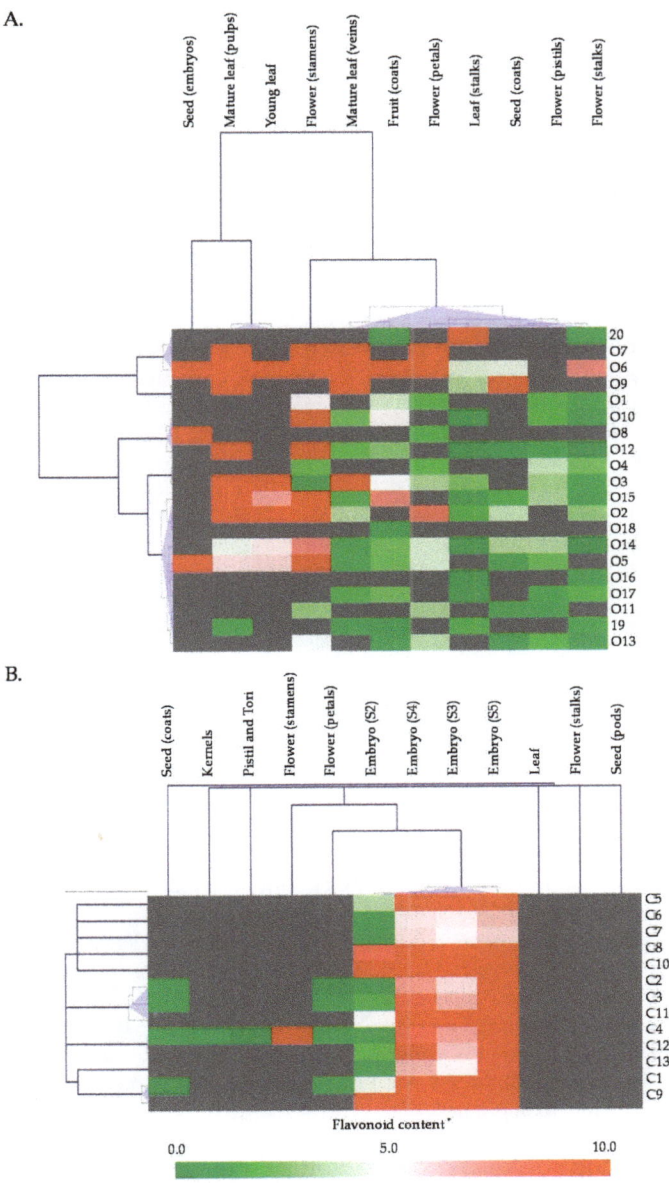

Figure 4. Comparative analysis of flavonoid contents and compositions different tissues of *Nelumbo nucifera*. Data were compiled from Chen et al. [33] and Li et al. [35]. (**A**) Comparative analysis of flavonoids aglycones and FOGs in 11 different tissues. (**B**) Comparative analysis of FCGs in 12 tissues and/or developmental stages including embryo (the major accumulation site of FCGs in *Nelumbo nucifera*) at five maturation stages. The names and structures of the flavonoids are presented in Figure 3. * Contents are expressed in mg.100 g^{-1} FW for all tissues except for seed embryo for which contents are expressed in mg.100 g^{-1} DW in (**A**)).

FOGs deriving from Quer **19** (hyperoside **O6**, isoquercitrin **O7** and Quer-3-Gln **O9**), Kae (astragalin **O12**) and Iso (Iso-3-Glc **O14**) were detected in all analyzed tissue with the exception of the embryo. A clear distinction between FOGs accumulation pattern in vegetative vs. reproductive tissues is observed. In leaves, FOGs derived from six different aglycones (Quer **19**, Kae, Iso, Lut, Dio **20** and Syr by order of abundance) with the Quer **19** derivatives rutin **O5**, hyperoside **O6** and isoquercitrin **O7** as main constituents [25,27,35]. In vegetative tissues, FOGs are accumulated at high levels, in particular in leaves tissues including young leaves, mature leaf pulps and mature leaf veins, in which the three Quer **19** derivatives hyperoside **O6**, Isoquercitrin **O7** and Quer-3-Gln **O9** account for more than 70% of the total flavonoid content [35]. We can note that the three Kae derivatives were dominant in floral tissues petals and stamens accounting for more than 60% of the total flavonoid content, indicating large differences in the biosynthesis and accumulation in these tissues that accumulate the lowest contents of flavonoids. FOGs deriving from Myr (Myr-3-Gal **O1**, Myr-3-Gln **O4**), Kae (Kae-3-Rob **O8**), Iso (Iso-3-Rut **O11**) and Syr (Syr-3-Glc **O13**) were detected in all reproductive tissues but not vegetative tissues. Quantitatively, we can note that, with the exception of seed coat (not surprisingly, considering the maternal origin of this tissue), all reproductive tissue accumulated far less FOGs than the vegetative tissues. Particularly, FOGs were far less represented in embryo than in other lotus tissue and were even almost undetected in seed kernels. However, embryo accumulated high levels of FCGs [25,27,35]. The main FCGs accumulated in embryo derived from Api and to a less extend from Lut, with the sole Api-6-C-Glc-8-C-Ara **C10** (schaftoside) accounting for more than 35% of the total flavonoids content in this tissue (Figure 4) [35]. Note that this very specific FCG accumulation in embryo might have taxonomic implications for possible authentication based on the association of these compounds as possible chemotaxonomic markers [47].

Besides these tissue-specific accumulations of FOGs vs. FCGs, the flavonoid composition and contents in lotus is also dependent of plant development. During development, an increase is observed in leaves, petals, stamens, pistils and tori for FOGs and embryo for both FOGs and FCGs. On the contrary, FOGs decreased during development in flower stalks, seed coats and kernels, whereas it remained constant in seed pods. In leaves, Quer-3-Gln **O9** is the major contributor of this variation during development. In embryo, the composition and content are extremely different with a continuous increase of Api-derived FCGs. We can also note that the variation observed in petals is much more complex with a global decrease during development but a very complex accumulation kinetics of the different constituents that need further studies [35].

The composition and contents of flavonoids also greatly vary according to the genetic background. Indeed, Chen et al. [25] reported on the differences in three lotus cultivars (Honglian, Baijian and Zhimahuoulian). Quer-3-Glc was the dominant FOG detected in the leaves of these cultivars but quantitative variations were observed. Honglian accumulated 1.8 times more isoquercitrin **O7** than Baijian, whereas this latter cultivar appeared as the richest source of flavonoids compared to the two other cultivars including Honglian. This could be explain by the fact that, contrary to the two other cultivars, Kae-3-O-Gal was absent in Honglian [25]. These observations could lead to the potential use of some flavonoids in authentication of *N. nucifera* cultivars for specific medicinal applications based on their flavonoid accumulation profiles [47].

Flavonoid biosynthetic pathway starts with the condensation of one *p*-coumaroyl-coA together with 3 malonyl-coA moieties catalyzed by chalcone synthase (CHS) leading to the synthesis of chalcone, the first committed flavonoid (Figure 5). Various hydroxylation, methylation and acetylation steps follow this first condensation and lead to a wide variety of derivatives including the flavonols and flavones accumulating in the louts tissues: Api, Dio **20**, Iso, Kae, Lut, Myr, Quer **19** and Syr. The aglycones could then be glycolsylated at different positions by a wide of glycosyltransferases branching a wide range of sugar moieties resulting in the great variety of FOGs and FCGs observed in lotus tissues. In lotus, two types of glycosyltransferases act with a very distinct distribution pattern [35]. Considering the FOGs distribution *O*-flavonoid glycosyltransferases must be highly active in leaves and much more ubiquitous than the *C*-flavonoid glycosyltransferases that are probably restricted to the embryo according to the high FCGs accumulation almost circumscribed to this tissue. These two tissues (leaves vs. embryo) constitute attractive starting materials to isolate these distinct classes of flavonoid glycosyltransferases from lotus for further characterization. Interestingly, from a structural point of view FCGs accumulated in embryo derived from Api and to a less extent from Lut, whereas FOGS accumulated in leaves derived from Quer **19** and to a less extent from Kae, Iso, Lut, Dio **20** and Syr. A regulation occurring at the level of the F3H enzyme (with the possible exception of Dio **20** if its biosynthetic sequence is conserved in lotus) could be responsible for these specific structural accumulation patterns (Figure 5). Once again, we can anticipate that the contrasting accumulation profiles of leaves vs. embryo could be used to elucidate these regulation flavonoid biosynthetic pathways at both molecular and biochemical levels to make the most potential of these compounds. We anticipate that future experiments using labeled compounds to elucidate the biosynthetic sequence of the different flavonoids and/or RNA sequencing technologies could be very informative.

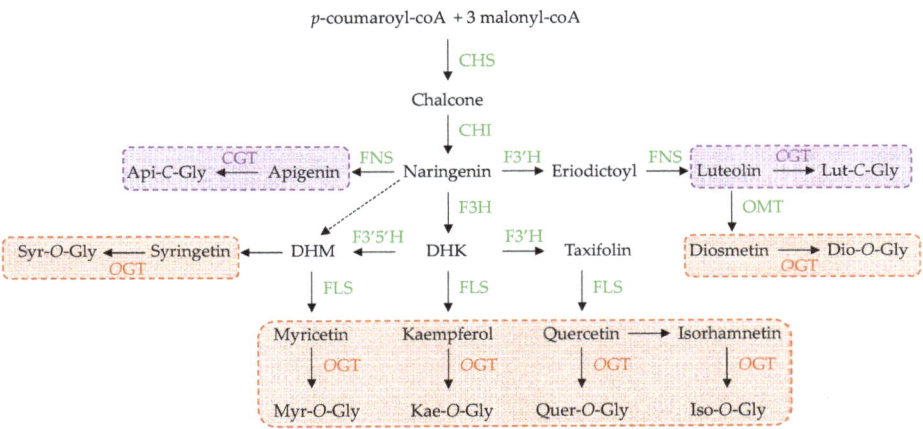

Figure 5. Proposed biosynthetic sequence of FOGs (orange) and FCGs (purple) derived flavonoids from *Nelumbo nucifera* adapted from Li et al. (2014). CHS, chalcone synthase; CHI, chalcone isomerase; FNS, flavone synthase; F3H, flavanone 3 hydroxylase; F3'H, flavonoid 3' hydroxylase; F3'5'H, flavonoid 3',5' hydroxylase; FLS, flavonol synthase; OGT, O-flavonoid glycosyltransferase; CGT, C-flavonoid glycosyltransferase; Api, apigenin; DHM, dihydromyricetin; DHK, dihydrokaempferol; Myr, myricetin; Kae, kaempferol; Quer, quercetin; Iso, isorhamnetin; Dio, diosmetin; Lut, luteolin; Syr, syringetin; Gly, glycoside(s).

4.2. Antioxidant Activities

It is well accepted that many degenerative diseases are the consequence of oxidative stress and caused by reactive oxygen species (ROS) and reactive nitrogen species (RNS). These ROS and RNS can damage many important organelles and molecules such as DNA, lipids and protein in the cells [6,7,48]. Jung et al. reported on the antioxidant potential from stamen methanolic extract of *N. nucifera* plant collected from Korea, investigating the main phytochemical compounds from this extract [8]. They evidenced the flavonoid Kae as the main contributor of the antioxidant potential of these extracts. For that, they used both in vitro DPPH assay and in vivo animal model, showing the inhibition of ROS generation from kidney homogenates of Wistar rats kidneys by using the 2',7'-dichlorodihydrofluorescein diacetate (DCHF-DA) probe [8]. This observation is in good agreement with the study of Rai et al. investigating both in vitro and in vivo antioxidant activity of a flavonoid-rich 50% (v/v) hydroalcoholic extract from *N. nucifera* seeds [7]. The absence of acute toxicity even at the highest oral administration dose of 1000 mg/kg body weight using Swiss Albino mice in vivo model of these extracts have also been described [6,7,48]. Besides, administration to Wistar rats in vivo model prior to carbon tetrachloride treatment produced a significant dose dependent increase in the level of superoxide dismutase, key enzyme scavenging the superoxide radicals [7]. Catechin, Quer **19**, Isoquercitrin **O7**, Quer-3-Gln **O9**, hyperoside **O6**, astragalin **O12** and Myr-3-Glc **O2** were isolated from the leaves extract of *N. nucifera* from Taiwan by Lin et al. [9]. They evidenced the first four as potent inhibitors of LDL oxidation, whereas Myr-3-Glc **O2** showed the more pronounced DPPH scavenging activity. Consequently, these results confirmed that the antioxidant activity of lotus leaves extract relied on both their flavonoid content and composition [9]. Interestingly, Chen et al. [49] studied antioxidant potential of the seed epicarp of *N. nucifera*, a flavonoid rich tissue considered as a byproduct, which displayed a strong in vitro antioxidant activity, as revealed by ABTS, DPPH and FRAP assays [49]. This byproduct could therefore be considered as a potential source for the functional food industry in the future. Furthermore, Liu et al. also examined the antioxidant activity from epicarp of *N. nucifera* seed in China at different ripening stages: green, half ripe and fully ripe stages [29]. They identified catechin, epicatechin, hyperoside **O6** and isoquercitrin **O7** at different levels depending on the ripening stages. The scavenging abilities revealed by the DPPH and ABTS in vitro assays were very effective but decreased during maturation [29]. Besides, Zhu et al. identified 14 flavonoids including four new compounds, Quer-3-O-Ara, Quer-3-O-Rha-(1→2)-Glc, Dio-7-Hex **O17**, and Iso-3-O-Ara-(1→2)-Glc, from their lotus leaves extract exhibiting a strong antioxidant potential [6]. Twenty flavonoids were identified in plumules extract of *N. nucifera* by Feng et al., and 14 flavonoids were under the form of FCGs [21]. In this study, the authors analyzed 38 different cultivars of lotus species, and evaluated their antioxidant activity by DPPH and FRAP in vitro assays. Their results clearly showed a significant positive correlation between the total polyphenol content and the antioxidant potential of the extract. Among these cultivars, four cultivars (Taikonglian, Yinqiu, Jinqi and Hongtailian) appeared as the most suitable cultivars for their use in healthcare products according to their strong antioxidant activity [21]. Additionally, eight FCGs and eight FOGs from embryos of *N. nucifera* were identified by Zhu et al. [27] and the FCGs were recognized as the major flavonoid forms found in these lotus seed embryo extract. Kae-7-Glc **O16** and luteolin 7-O-neohesperidoside were described for the first time in *N. nucifera* embryos. These authors also compared the antioxidant potential of extracts from seed embryos vs. leaves, and pointed that embryo extract exhibited at least a comparable or even higher antioxidant activity than leaves extracts. However, note that in lotus the total flavonoid content was lower in embryo than in leaves. Interestingly, these authors also pointed that the antioxidant potential of FCGs from *N. nucifera* embryo extracts was higher than that of FOGs from leaf extracts [26]. In addition, Jiang et al. identified four new FCGs (named nelumbosides A–D) from lotus embryo and evaluated their relative antioxidant activity using ABTS and DPPH assays [50]. They found that nelumbosides B exhibited the most promising radical scavenging activity [50].

4.3. Anti-Inflammatory Activities

Inflammation is part of a complex biological response of immune system to irritants, pathogens, damaged cells or other harmful stimuli. These complex processes deal with various biological pathways. Kim et al. investigated age-related effects of Kae, a flavonoid from *N. nucifera*, on ROS and GSH oxidative status in in vivo model [39]. Their results showed a reduction of ROS production and GSH level augmentation following Kae supply in a dose-dependent manner. They also evidenced a significant reduction in the levels of iNOS and TNF-α protein. The authors proposed that Kae may inhibit ROS generation by decreasing the gene expression of iNOS and TNF-α in aged gingival rat tissues via the NF-κB and mitogen-activated protein kinase (MAPK) signaling pathways. The authors also examined the hypothesis that Kae anti-inflammatory effects was mediated via glutathione and NF-κB levels modulation. Altogether, their results pointed out Kae as a potent anti-inflammatory compound [39]. The anti-inflammatory activity of Quer-3-Gln **O9** from *N. nucifera* leaves was also evaluated by Li et al. using lipopolysaccharide-treated RAW264.7 macrophages and showed that Quer-3-Gln **O9** inhibited LPS-induced NO release [40].

4.4. Anti-Diabetic and Anti-Obesity Activities

Aldose reductase (AR) is the key enzyme in polyol pathway and has been identified as a convenient drug target for type II diabetic treatment. Lim et al. showed that the flavonoids isolated from stamen methanolic extract from *N. nucifera* can inhibit rat lens AR activity with the highest inhibition degree observed for flavonoids with a 3-O-α-L-Rha-(1→6)-β-D-Glc substitution on their C rings (i.e., Kae-3-O-α-L-Rha-(1→6)-β-D-Glc and Iso-3-O-α-L-Rha-(1→6)-β-D-Glc) [22]. Ohkoshi et al. demonstrated that flavonoids extract from *N. nucifera* leaves stimulated lipolysis in white adipose tissue of in vivo mice model [38]. In addition, flavonoid-rich extracts from *N. nucifera* leaves was also able to regulate insulin secretion as well as blood glucose level [43] in both in vitro and in vivo models. The authors proposed a possible enhancement of the insulin secretion from β-cells through a Ca^{2+}-activated PKC-regulated ERK1/2 signaling pathway. They pointed out catechin as an active compound from this extract able to enhance insulin secretion in a dose-dependent manner. Indeed, oral administration of catechin at 100 mg/kg in fasted normal mice model 2 h before starch loading showed that catechin administration resulted in hypoglycemic effect on fasted mice. Furthermore, the same oral dose of catechin was able to reverse glucose intolerance in high-fat-diet-induced diabetic animal model. These results obtained from both in vitro and animal models showed that both *N. nucifera* leaves extract and catechin regulated glucose blood level and could improve postprandial hyperglycemia under diabetic conditions. These results strongly suggested that *N. nucifera* leaves extract and catechin are of particular interest to control hyperglycemia in non-insulin dependent diabetes mellitus [43]. However, the exact mechanism for the action of catechin on β-cells and glucose metabolism have to be further investigated and confirmed.

Obesity is considered as an important risk factor for many chronic diseases including type 2 diabetes. There are many attempts to find natural compounds that have anti-obesity abilities. Sergent et al. searched for pancreatic lipase inhibitors to prevent obesity, finding epigallocatechin-3-gallate, Kae and Quer 19 as effective pancreatic lipase natural inhibitors [18]. Ahn et al. also confirmed that flavonoid-rich *N. nucifera* leaves showed the anti-obesity potential to inhibit pancreatic lipase, but also adipocyte differentiation [35]. In the same direction, Liu et al. evaluated the inhibitory effects of total flavonoids *N. nucifera* leaves extract on α-glucosidase, α-amylase, pancreatic lipase and hypolipidemia activities [31]. Their results showed that a *N. nucifera* leaf extract containing flavonoids (mainly FOGs) could ameliorate hyperlipidemia by inhibiting these key enzymes related to the type 2 diabetes mellitus. You et al. proposed the rhizome extracts from *N. nucifera* as a nutraceutical component against obesity-related diseases, including diabetes mellitus thanks to their potent anti-adipogenic effect in human pre-adipocytes in vivo experiment and using rats fed with a high-fat diet [41]. Interestingly, Kae isolated from *N. nucifera* stamen inhibited lipogenic transcription factors and the accumulation of lipid through PPARα binding as well as the stimulation of fatty acid oxidation signaling in several adipocyte cells [12]. Besides, Sharma et al. also validated the traditional use of *N. nucifera* leaves for diabetes treatment and showed that *N. nucifera* leaf extract attenuated pancreatic β-cells toxicity induced by interleukin-1β and interferon-γ, and increased insulin secretion of pancreatic β-cells in streptozotocin-induced diabetic rats in vivo study [16]. Recently, Wang et al. demonstrated that *N. nucifera* leaf flavonoids could prevent diabetes type 2 through the inhibition of α-amylase [51]. In the same way, Liao et al. analyzed the binding affinity of ten flavonoids from *N. nucifera* leaf on α-amylase using spectroscopic methods [52]. They found that, among the tested flavonoids, Kae, Api and Iso displayed the most potent inhibiting potential on α-amylase activity. Their structure–function experiments also showed that the hydrogenation of the $C_2=C_3$ double bond of the flavonoid backbone of Quer and Api as well as the hydroxylation of 3 and 3' positions decreased the affinity of the flavonoids for this enzyme [52]. Additionally, the methanol extract from seed epicarp of *N. nucifera* revealed the significant α-amylase inhibiting activity, and was suggested to develop as potential anti-diabetic agents [49].

4.5. Anti-Angiogenic and Anti-Cancer Activities

One important approach for cancer therapy is to inhibit the angiogenesis. Lee et al. were the first to report on the potential *N. nucifera* leaves extract to inhibit vascular endothelial growth factor-induced angiogenesis using both in vitro and in vivo models [5]. Yang et al. also evaluated the anti-cancer effect of the flavonoids from *N. nucifera* leaves extracts (i.e., mainly FOGs) using human MCF-7 cell line and in vivo study using a xenograft nude mouse model [44]. Their results evidenced the anti-proliferative action of the flavonoids from *N. nucifera* leaf extracts on of breast cancer in both in vitro and in vivo models [44]. In addition, Wu et al. investigated the potential of *N. nucifera* leaves extract on breast cancer metastasis using both in vitro MDA-MB-231 and 4T-1 breast cancer cells and in vivo mice model through PKCα targeting [17]. Their result illustrated the effectiveness of the extracts for the development of potential chemopreventive agents to reduce breast cancer metastasis. The authors also showed the capacity of *N. nucifera* leaves extracts to inhibit the angiogenesis and metastasis of this breast cancer cells by down regulating the connective tissue growth factor mediated by PI3K/AKT/ERK signaling pathway. However, each cancer type resulting from many factors such as genetic or epigenetic factors, the chemopreventive agents or anti-cancer molecules here evidenced may possibly play distinct roles and regulate more than a single pathway. Thus, the anti-cancer actions of flavonoids from *N. nucifera* leaves extracts need to be investigate more specifically with different cancer types to gain more complete information.

5. Conclusions and Future Research Directions

Nelumbo nucifera Gaertn. is one of the most important medicinal plants used in various traditional medicines. *N. nucifera* is a natural source of many potent flavonoids exhibiting various effective pharmacological activities. Nowadays, many pharmacological activities such as anti-angiogenic, anti-cancer, anti-diabetic and anti-obesity activities of flavonoids isolated from this medicinal species have been described. However, most of these pharmacological activities still need further research investigations before leading to the discovery of potent drugs from the extracts of this plant species and their large-scale development.

In particular, from this literature review, several points appeared essential for future perspectives and research directions:

(1) To reach the maximum potential of this species as the raw plant material and the source of potential flavonoids, the cultivars, developmental stages, parts of plant, seasons and time to harvest are the major factors that should be considered.
(2) In the use of traditional medicines, there are many local names of this species depending on the areas and country. Some other plant may also be called by a similar name. Therefore, species authentication needs to be done before using it for medical and pharmaceutical applications.
(3) The geographic regions of the raw material should also be considered and compared in the future research from various Asian countries to determine the effect of environmental factors on the quality and quantity of phytochemicals.
(4) As a consequence of the last point, not only local medicinal plant species but also the wild and/or various local ecotypes are interesting for the future studies to discover novel phytochemical compounds to increase the alternative sources of raw material for medical and pharmaceutical applications. Research on the profiling and identification of new flavonoids is still a future challenge for the many unknown reported areas of Asia.
(5) For many pharmacological activities, the molecular mechanisms and/or signaling pathways need to be further clarified in the future research. In particular, there are few works to date on the biological activities of purified flavonoid C-glycosides (FCGs) from lotus.
(6) The indications of losing activity or adverse effects following prolonged exposure of extract or products should be investigated in future research studies.

Author Contributions: D.T. conceived and designed the review. D.T., D.P. and C.H. wrote the paper. D.T. and C.H. edited and improve the whole manuscript.

Funding: This research was funded by Mahidol University and Junior Research Fellowship Program 2018.

Acknowledgments: D.T. gratefully acknowledges the support of the French government via the French Embassy in Thailand in the form of Junior Research Fellowship Program 2018. This research project was supported by Mahidol University.

Conflicts of Interest: The authors declare no conflict of interest.

References

1. Chen, S.; Zheng, Y.; Fang, J.B.; Liu, Y.L.; Li, S.H. Flavonoids in lotus (Nelumbo) leaves evaluated by HPLC-MSnat the germplasm level. *Food Res. Int.* **2013**, *54*, 796–803. [CrossRef]
2. Sheikh, S.A. Ethno-medicinal uses and pharmacological activities of lotus (*Nelumbo nucifera*). *J. Med. Plants Stud.* **2014**, *2*, 42–46.
3. Deng, J.; Chen, S.; Yin, X.; Wang, K.; Liu, Y.; Li, S.; Yang, P. Systematic qualitative and quantitative assessment of anthocyanins, flavones and flavonols in the petals of 108 lotus (*Nelumbo nucifera*) cultivars. *Food Chem.* **2013**, *139*, 307–312. [CrossRef] [PubMed]
4. Paudel, K.R.; Panth, N. Phytochemical profile and biological activity of *Nelumbo nucifera*. *Evid.-Based Complement. Altern. Med.* **2015**, *2015*. [CrossRef] [PubMed]
5. Lee, J.S.; Shukla, S.; Kim, J.A.; Kim, M. Anti-angiogenic effect of *nelumbo nucifera* leaf extracts in human umbilical vein endothelial cells with antioxidant potential. *PLoS ONE* **2015**, *10*. [CrossRef] [PubMed]
6. Zhu, M.Z.; Wu, W.; Jiao, L.L.; Yang, P.F.; Guo, M.Q. Analysis of flavonoids in lotus (*Nelumbo nucifera*) leaves and their antioxidant activity using macroporous resin chromatography coupled with LC-MS/MS and antioxidant biochemical assays. *Molecules* **2015**, *20*, 10553–10565. [CrossRef] [PubMed]
7. Rai, S.; Wahile, A.; Mukherjee, K.; Saha, B.P.; Mukherjee, P.K. Antioxidant activity of *Nelumbo nucifera* (sacred lotus) seeds. *J. Ethnopharmacol.* **2006**, *104*, 322–327. [CrossRef] [PubMed]
8. Jung, H.A.; Kim, J.E.; Chung, H.Y.; Choi, J.S. Antioxidant principles of *Nelumbo nucifera* stamens. *Arch. Pharm. Res.* **2003**, *26*, 279–285. [CrossRef] [PubMed]
9. Lin, H.Y.; Kuo, Y.H.; Lin, Y.L.; Chiang, W. Antioxidative effect and active components from leaves of lotus (*Nelumbo nucifera*). *J. Agric. Food Chem.* **2009**, *57*, 6623–6629. [CrossRef] [PubMed]
10. Courts, F.L.; Williamson, G. The occurrence, fate and biological activities of c-glycosyl flavonoids in the human diet. *Crit. Rev. Food Sci. Nutr.* **2015**, *55*, 1352–1367. [CrossRef] [PubMed]
11. Lee, B.; Kwon, M.; Choi, J.S.; Jeong, H.O.; Chung, H.Y.; Kim, H.-R. Kaempferol Isolated from *Nelumbo nucifera* Inhibits Lipid Accumulation and Increases Fatty Acid Oxidation Signaling in Adipocytes. *J. Med. Food* **2015**, *18*, 1363–1370. [CrossRef] [PubMed]
12. Zhu, Y.T.; Jia, Y.W.; Liu, Y.M.; Liang, J.; Ding, L.S.; Liao, X. Lipase ligands in *nelumbo nucifera* leaves and study of their binding mechanism. *J. Agric. Food Chem.* **2014**, *62*, 10679–10686. [CrossRef] [PubMed]
13. Bin, X.; Jin, W.; Wenqing, W.; Chunyang, S.; Xiaolong, H.; Jianguo, F. *Nelumbo nucifera* alkaloid inhibits 3T3-L1 preadipocyte differentiation and improves high-fat diet-induced obesity and body fat accumulation in rats. *J. Med. Plant. Res.* **2011**, *5*, 2021–2028.
14. Chang, C.H.; Ou, T.T.; Yang, M.Y.; Huang, C.C.; Wang, C.J. *Nelumbo nucifera* Gaertn leaves extract inhibits the angiogenesis and metastasis of breast cancer cells by downregulation connective tissue growth factor (CTGF) mediated PI3K/AKT/ERK signaling. *J. Ethnopharmacol.* **2016**, *188*, 111–122. [CrossRef] [PubMed]
15. Sharma, B.R.; Kim, M.S.; Rhyu, D.Y. *Nelumbo Nucifera* leaf extract attenuated pancreatic beta-cells toxicity induced by interleukin-1beta and interferon-gamma, and increased insulin secrection of pancreatic beta-cells in streptozotocin-induced diabetic rats. *J. Tradit. Chin. Med.* **2016**, *36*, 71–77. [CrossRef]
16. Wu, C.H.; Yang, M.Y.; Lee, Y.J.; Wang, C.J. *Nelumbo nucifera* leaf polyphenol extract inhibits breast cancer cells metastasis in vitro and in vivo through PKCα targeting. *J. Funct. Foods* **2017**, *37*, 480–490. [CrossRef]
17. Sergent, T.; Vanderstraeten, J.; Winand, J.; Beguin, P.; Schneider, Y.J. Phenolic compounds and plant extracts as potential natural anti-obesity substances. *Food Chem.* **2012**, *135*, 68–73. [CrossRef]
18. Rajput, M.A.; Khan, R.A. Phytochemical screening, acute toxicity, anxiolytic and antidepressant activities of the *Nelumbo nucifera* fruit. *Metab. Brain Dis.* **2017**, *32*, 743–749. [CrossRef] [PubMed]

19. Mongkolrat, S.; Palanuvej, C.; Ruangrungsi, N. Quality assessment and liriodenine quantification of *Nelumbo nucifera* dried leaf in Thailand. *Pharmacogn. J.* **2012**, *4*, 24–28. [CrossRef]
20. Feng, C.Y.; Li, S.S.; Yin, D.D.; Zhang, H.J.; Tian, D.K.; Wu, Q.; Wang, L.J.; Su, S.; Wang, L.S. Rapid determination of flavonoids in plumules of sacred lotus cultivars and assessment of their antioxidant activities. *Ind. Crops Prod.* **2016**, *87*, 96–104. [CrossRef]
21. Lim, S.S.; Jung, Y.J.; Hyun, S.K.; Lee, Y.S.; Choi, J.S. Rat lens aldose reductase inhibitory constituents of *Nelumbo nucifera* stamens. *Phyther. Res.* **2006**, *20*, 825–830. [CrossRef] [PubMed]
22. Hofer, B. Recent developments in the enzymatic O-glycosylation of flavonoids. *Appl. Microbiol. Biotechnol.* **2016**, *100*, 4269–4281. [CrossRef] [PubMed]
23. Wu, H.M.; Kao, C.L.; Huang, S.C.; Li, W.J.; Li, H.T.; Chen, C.Y. Secondary Metabolites from the Stems of *Nelumbo nucifera* cv. Rosa-plena. *Chem. Nat. Compd.* **2017**, *53*, 797–798. [CrossRef]
24. Chen, S.; Fang, L.; Xi, H.; Guan, L.; Fang, J.; Liu, Y.; Wu, B.; Li, S. Simultaneous qualitative assessment and quantitative analysis of flavonoids in various tissues of lotus (*Nelumbo nucifera*) using high performance liquid chromatography coupled with triple quad mass spectrometry. *Anal. Chim. Acta* **2012**, *724*, 127–135. [CrossRef] [PubMed]
25. Zhu, F. Structures, properties, and applications of lotus starches. *Food Hydrocoll.* **2017**, *63*, 332–348. [CrossRef]
26. Zhu, M.; Liu, T.; Zhang, C.; Guo, M. Flavonoids of Lotus (*Nelumbo nucifera*) Seed Embryos and Their Antioxidant Potential. *J. Food Sci.* **2017**, *82*, 1834–1841. [CrossRef] [PubMed]
27. Huang, B.; Ban, X.; He, J.; Tong, J.; Tian, J.; Wang, Y. Hepatoprotective and antioxidant activity of ethanolic extracts of edible lotus (*Nelumbo nucifera* Gaertn.) leaves. *Food Chem.* **2010**, *120*, 873–878. [CrossRef]
28. Liu, Y.; Ma, S.S.; Ibrahim, S.A.; Li, E.H.; Yang, H.; Huang, W. Identification and antioxidant properties of polyphenols in lotus seed epicarp at different ripening stages. *Food Chem.* **2015**, *185*, 159–164. [CrossRef] [PubMed]
29. Huang, B.; Zhu, L.; Liu, S.; Li, D.; Chen, Y.; Ma, B.; Wang, Y. In vitro and in vivo evaluation of inhibition activity of lotus (*Nelumbo nucifera* Gaertn.) leaves against ultraviolet B-induced phototoxicity. *J. Photochem. Photobiol. B Biol.* **2013**, *121*, 1–5. [CrossRef] [PubMed]
30. Liu, S.; Li, D.; Huang, B.; Chen, Y.; Lu, X.; Wang, Y. Inhibition of pancreatic lipase, α-glucosidase, α-amylase, and hypolipidemic effects of the total flavonoids from *Nelumbo nucifera* leaves. *J. Ethnopharmacol.* **2013**, *149*, 263–269. [CrossRef] [PubMed]
31. Xiao, J.; Capanoglu, E.; Jassbi, A.R.; Miron, A. Advance on the Flavonoid C-glycosides and Health Benefits. *Crit. Rev. Food Sci. Nutr.* **2016**, *56*, S29–S45. [CrossRef] [PubMed]
32. Chen, S.; Wu, B.H.; Fang, J.B.; Liu, Y.L.; Zhang, H.H.; Fang, L.C.; Guan, L.; Li, S.H. Analysis of flavonoids from lotus (*Nelumbo nucifera*) leaves using high performance liquid chromatography/photodiode array detector tandem electrospray ionization mass spectrometry and an extraction method optimized by orthogonal design. *J. Chromatogr. A* **2012**, *1227*, 145–153. [CrossRef] [PubMed]
33. Charbe, N.B.; McCarron, P.A.; Lane, M.E.; Tambuwala, M.M. Application of three-dimensional printing for colon targeted drug delivery systems. *Int. J. Pharm. Investig.* **2017**, *7*, 47–59. [CrossRef] [PubMed]
34. Li, S.S.; Wu, J.; Chen, L.G.; Du, H.; Xu, Y.J.; Wang, L.J.; Zhang, H.J.; Zheng, X.C.; Wang, L.S. Biogenesis of C-glycosyl flavones and profiling of flavonoid glycosides in lotus (*Nelumbo nucifera*). *PLoS ONE* **2014**, *9*. [CrossRef] [PubMed]
35. Ahn, J.H.; Kim, E.S.; Lee, C.; Kim, S.; Cho, S.H.; Hwang, B.Y.; Lee, M.K. Chemical constituents from *Nelumbo nucifera* leaves and their anti-obesity effects. *Bioorganic Med. Chem. Lett.* **2013**, *23*, 3604–3608. [CrossRef] [PubMed]
36. Wang, H.M.; Yang, W.L.; Yang, S.C.; Chen, C.Y. Chemical constituents from the leaves of *Nelumbo nucifera* gaertn. cv. Rosa-plena. *Chem. Nat. Compd.* **2011**, *47*, 316–318. [CrossRef]
37. Ohkoshi, E.; Miyazaki, H.; Shindo, K.; Watanabe, H.; Yoshida, A.; Yajima, H. Constituents from the leaves of *Nelumbo nucifera* stimulate lipolysis in the white adipose tissue of mice. *Planta Med.* **2007**, *73*, 1255–1259. [CrossRef] [PubMed]
38. Kim, H.K.; Park, H.R.; Lee, J.S.; Chung, T.S.; Chung, H.Y.; Chung, J. Down-regulation of iNOS and TNF-α expression by kaempferol via NF-κB inactivation in aged rat gingival tissues. *Biogerontology* **2007**, *8*, 399–408. [CrossRef] [PubMed]

39. Li, F.; Sun, X.Y.; Li, X.W.; Yang, T.; Qi, L.W. Enrichment and separation of quercetin-3-O-β-D-glucuronide from lotus leaves (*nelumbo nucifera* gaertn.) and evaluation of its anti-inflammatory effect. *J. Chromatogr. B Anal. Technol. Biomed. Life Sci.* **2017**, *1040*, 186–191. [CrossRef] [PubMed]
40. You, J.S.; Lee, Y.J.; Kim, K.S.; Kim, S.H.; Chang, K.J. Ethanol extract of lotus (*Nelumbo nucifera*) root exhibits an anti-adipogenic effect in human pre-adipocytes and anti-obesity and anti-oxidant effects in rats fed a high-fat diet. *Nutr. Res.* **2014**, *34*, 258–267. [CrossRef] [PubMed]
41. Ho, H.H.; Hsu, L.S.; Chan, K.C.; Chen, H.M.; Wu, C.H.; Wang, C.J. Extract from the leaf of nucifera reduced the development of atherosclerosis via inhibition of vascular smooth muscle cell proliferation and migration. *Food Chem. Toxicol.* **2010**, *48*, 159–168. [CrossRef] [PubMed]
42. Huang, C.F.; Chen, Y.W.; Yang, C.Y.; Lin, H.Y.; Way, T. Der; Chiang, W.; Liu, S.H. Extract of lotus leaf (*Nelumbo nucifera*) and its active constituent catechin with insulin secretagogue activity. *J. Agric. Food Chem.* **2011**, *59*, 1087–1094. [CrossRef] [PubMed]
43. Yang, M.Y.; Chang, Y.C.; Chan, K.C.; Lee, Y.J.; Wang, C.J. Flavonoid-enriched extracts from *Nelumbo nucifera* leaves inhibits proliferation of breast cancer in vitro and in vivo. *Eur. J. Integr. Med.* **2011**, *3*. [CrossRef]
44. Ruvanthika, P.N.; Manikandan, S.; Lalitha, S. A comparative study on phytochemical screening of aerial parts of *Nelumbo nucifera* Gaertn. by gas chromatographic mass spectrometry. *Int. J. Pharm. Sci. Res.* **2017**, *8*, 2258–2266. [CrossRef]
45. Le Roy, J.; Huss, B.; Creach, A.; Hawkins, S.; Neutelings, G. Glycosylation Is a Major Regulator of Phenylpropanoid Availability and Biological Activity in Plants. *Front. Plant Sci.* **2016**, *7*. [CrossRef] [PubMed]
46. Ferreres, F.; Gil-Izquierdo, A.; Andrade, P.B.; Valentão, P.; Tomás-Barberán, F.A. Characterization of C-glycosyl flavones O-glycosylated by liquid chromatography-tandem mass spectrometry. *J. Chromatogr. A* **2007**, *1161*, 214–223. [CrossRef] [PubMed]
47. Drouet, S.; Garros, L.; Hano, C.; Tungmunnithum, D.; Renouard, S.; Hagège, D.; Maunit, B.; Lainé, É. A Critical View of Different Botanical, Molecular, and Chemical Techniques Used in Authentication of Plant Materials for Cosmetic Applications. *Cosmetics* **2018**, *5*, 30. [CrossRef]
48. Tungmunnithum, D.; Thongboonyou, A.; Pholboon, A.; Yangsabai, A. Flavonoids and Other Phenolic Compounds from Medicinal Plants for Pharmaceutical and Medical Aspects: An Overview. *Medicines* **2018**, *5*, 93. [CrossRef] [PubMed]
49. Chen, H.; Sun, K.; Yang, Z.; Guo, X.; Wei, S. Identification of Antioxidant and Anti- α -amylase Components in Lotus (*Nelumbo nucifera*, Gaertn.) Seed Epicarp. *Appl. Biochem. Biotechnol.* **2018**, 1–14. [CrossRef] [PubMed]
50. Jiang, X.L.; Wang, L.; Wang, E.J.; Zhang, G.L.; Chen, B.; Wang, M.K.; Li, F. Flavonoid glycosides and alkaloids from the embryos of *Nelumbo nucifera* seeds and their antioxidant activity. *Fitoterapia* **2018**, *125*, 184–190. [CrossRef] [PubMed]
51. Wang, M.; Shi, J.; Wang, L.; Hu, Y.; Ye, X.; Liu, D.; Chen, J. Inhibitory kinetics and mechanism of flavonoids from lotus (*Nelumbo nucifera* Gaertn.) leaf against pancreatic α-amylase. *Int. J. Biol. Macromol.* **2018**, *120*, 2589–2596. [CrossRef] [PubMed]
52. Liao, L.; Chen, J.; Liu, L.; Xiao, A. Screening and binding analysis of flavonoids with alpha-amylase inhibitory activity from lotus leaf. *J. Braz. Chem. Soc.* **2018**, *29*, 587–593. [CrossRef]

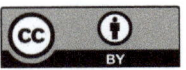

© 2018 by the authors. Licensee MDPI, Basel, Switzerland. This article is an open access article distributed under the terms and conditions of the Creative Commons Attribution (CC BY) license (http://creativecommons.org/licenses/by/4.0/).

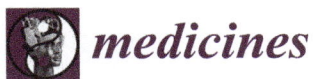

Article

Total Polyphenol Content and Antioxidant Capacity of Rosehips of Some *Rosa* Species

Noémi Koczka [1,*], Éva Stefanovits-Bányai [2] and Attila Ombódi [1]

1. Institute of Horticulture, Szent István University, Páter K. street 1, 2100 Gödöllő, Hungary; ombodi.attila@mkk.szie.hu
2. Department of Applied Chemistry, Szent István University, Villányi street 29-43, 1118 Budapest, Hungary; banyai.eva@etk.szie.hu
* Correspondence: koczka.noemi@mkk.szie.hu; Tel.: +36-28-522-000

Received: 30 June 2018; Accepted: 31 July 2018; Published: 4 August 2018

Abstract: Background: Rosehips, the fruits of *Rosa* species, are well known for their various health benefits like strengthening the immune system and treating digestive disorders. Antioxidant, anti-inflammatory, and cell regenerative effects are also among their health enhancing impacts. Rosehips are rich in compounds having antioxidant properties, like vitamin C, carotenoids, and phenolics. **Methods:** Total polyphenol content (Folin-Ciocalteu's method), and in vitro total antioxidant capacity (ferric-reducing ability of plasma, FRAP) in rosehips of four *Rosa* species (*R. canina*, *R. gallica*, *R. rugosa*, *R. spinosissima*) were determined and compared. Ripe fruits were harvested at two locations. Water and ethanolic extracts of dried fruit flesh were analyzed. **Results:** *R. spinosissima* had the highest total phenolic content and antioxidant capacity, significantly higher than the other investigated *Rosa* species. Both parameters were reported in decreasing order for *R. spinosissima* > *R. canina* > *R. rugosa* > *R. gallica*. Ethanolic extracts of rosehips showed higher phenolic content and antioxidant activity than water extracts. Antioxidant properties were influenced by the growing site of *Rosa* species. **Conclusions:** This study indicates that *R. spinosissima* exhibited the greatest phenolic and antioxidant content, and therefore can be used as a reliable source of natural antioxidants, and serve as a suitable species for further plant breeding activities. Furthermore, investigations of various *Rosa* species for their antioxidant properties may draw more attention to their potential as functional foods.

Keywords: phenolics; antioxidant activity; FRAP; *Rosa* spp.; rosehip

1. Introduction

The genus *Rosa* contains more than 100 species which are widely distributed across Europe, temperate Asia, and North America [1,2]. Roses have been cultivated since ancient times, but some of them can still be found growing in the wild. They are climbing or bushy woody perennials with thorny stems and attractive, sweetly scented flowers of various colors [3]. Fleshy red fruits varying in shape and size are known as rosehip. Rose leaves, flowers, and fruits have been used for thousands of years for their medicinal benefits. The leaves have antioxidant and anti-inflammatory properties. Rose flowers have antibacterial, astringent, tonic, and antioxidant effects used for mild inflammation of the skin or lining of the mouth and throat [4]. Fruits can be consumed fresh, but they are mostly prepared as herbal tea, jam, jelly, syrup or wine. Rosehip has traditionally been used against a wide range of ailments due to its biological activities like immunosuppressive, antioxidant, anti-inflammatory, anti-arthritic, analgesic, anti-diabetic, cardioprotective, antimicrobial, gastroprotective, and skin ameliorative effects [5–8].

Rosehip contains the highest amount of vitamin C among fruits and vegetables, and also contains vitamin A, B_1, B_2, B_6, D, E, and K [9–12]. Besides ascorbic acid, citric acid, and malic acid are the characteristic organic acids of the fruit [13,14]. Rosehip is also rich in carotenoids;

lycopene, ß-cryptoxanthin, ß-carotene, rubixanthin, gazaniaxanthin, and zeaxanthin are identified as its major components [5,10,15]. Active ingredients of rosehip are furthermore pectin and sugars, mainly glucose and fructose [5,11,14]. Rosehip's essential oil contains alcohols, aldehydes, monoterpenes, sesquiterpenes, and esters. The most abundant components are vitispiran, α-E-acaridial, hexadecanoic acid, docosane (C22), ß-ionone, 6-methyl-5-hepten-2-one, 2-heptanone, heptanal, and myristic acid [14,16]. Rosehip seeds have a high content of polyunsaturated fatty acids, the dominant compounds are linoleic acid (45–55%), followed by α-linolenic acid (18–32%) and oleic acid (13–20%) [17–19]. Rosehip contains different mineral nutrients, mainly phosphorus, potassium, calcium, magnesium, manganese, and zinc. The mineral composition of rosehips is highly dependent on species and environmental conditions [12].

Phenolic compounds including tannins, flavonoids, phenolic acids, and anthocyanins proved to be a very important group of biologically active ingredients present in rosehip [20]. Phenolics are well known for their antioxidant properties and there are a few studies analyzing the content and composition of polyphenols in different *Rosa* species, especially in *R. canina*. However, literature cites variable quantitative and qualitative descriptions of the phenolic profile of roses. Tumbas et al. [9] and Hosni et al. [21] identified quercetin and ellagic acid as the major phenolics of *R. canina*, while Türkben et al. [22] and Olsson et al. [23] reported quercetin and catechin to be the most important phenolic components in the species with an absence of ellagic acid or kaempferol. Demir et al. [14] and Elmastas et al. [24] identified phenolic acids in rosehip including gallic acid, 4-hydroxy benzoic acid, caftaric acid, 2,5-dihidroxy benzoic acid, chlorogenic acid, t-caffeic acid, p-coumaric acid, and ferrulic acid. Nadpal et al. [25] found protocatechuic acid in addition to the previously mentioned ones. The main flavonoids are methyl gallat, catechin [14,24], epicatechin [14,24,25], rutin, eriocitrin, quercetin, apigenin-7-*O*-glucoside, kaempferol, [14,24], quercitrin and, quinic acid [25].

Ercisli [12] reported a comprehensive study on the chemical composition of the species *R. canina*, *R. dumalis* subsp. *boissieri*, *R. dumalis* subsp. *antalyensis*, *R. villosa*, *R. pulverulenta*, and *R. pisiformis*, detecting the greatest total phenolic content in *R. canina*. Adamczak et al. [13] compared the flavonoid content of 11 *Rosa* species (*R. agrestis*, *R. canina*, *R. dumalis*, *R. glauca*, *R. inodora*, *R. jundzillii*, *R. rubiginosa*, *R. sherardii*, *R. tomentosa*, *R. villosa*, and *R. zalana*), finding a low average value of flavonoids for *R. canina*, the most common species, while flavonoids were the highest in *R. rubiginosa*. Demir et al. [14] investigated phenolic compounds of *R. canina*, *R. dumalis*, *R. gallica*, *R. dumalis* subsp. *boissieri*, and *R. hirtissima*, concluding that total phenolic contents of rosehips were significantly influenced by the species, whereas total flavonoid content was measured to be similar in all the examined species. Najda and Buczkowska [26] studied the chemical composition of *Rosa* species *R. californica*, *R.* × *damascena*, *R. rugosa*, *R. spinosissima*, and *R. villosa*. They found polyphenol content to be highly diverse in these species, with the highest total amount of phenolics measured in *R. rugosa* and *R. villosa*. Jimenez et al. [27] detected significant differences in total phenolic content among rosehips of *R. canina*, *R. corymbifera*, *R. glauca*, and *R. pouzinii* originating from different geographical zones. Nadpal et al. [25] found the total phenolics of *R. canina* to be significantly higher than that of *R. arvensis*.

Hence, although wild grown and cultivated *Rosa* species and cultivars differ in their chemical composition and health promoting benefits, they can be considered a potential raw material for functional foods [26]. The most abundant and studied species is *R. canina*, called dog rose. It is native to Europe and Asia and it is naturalized in North America. Fruits are smooth, bright red-orange and 15–30 mm long. They persist on the plant for several months and become black [28]. Being the most collected *Rosa* taxon, its hips or hip extracts are added to vitamin C tablets, food supplements, herbal remedies, and herbal teas. Specimens of the plant are used as rootstocks for grafting. The wild plant itself is widely used to stabilize soil in land reclamation and specialized landscaping schemes [3] (p. 346) [29].

R. gallica, French rose, or apothecary rose is indigenous to Southern and Central Europe and the Caucasus. An outstanding number of cultivars were bred from this species by means of crossing. The species is cultivated for the petals which are used to extract essential oil or to prepare herbal medicines [30]. Hips are globose to ovoid, 10–13 mm in diameter, bristly with a color of brick-red to brownish. Fruits are mainly used in Ayurvedic medicine [3] (p. 347).

R. rugosa, or Japanese rose is native to the Orient but the species has a wide range of adaptability. Due to the ability to hybridize with many other roses, and its high resistance to diseases like rose rust and rose black spot, it is a very important species for breeding processes. It is also remarkably tolerant to cold and salinity. Japanese rose is also a very popular plant material in landscaping as it is rather tolerant to environmental effects. Its rosehips are large, 20–30 mm in diameter and often slightly flat [31].

R. spinosissima, burnet rose, or Scots rose is endemic to Europe, and Western and Central Asia. Its hips are small (5–15 mm), globose or depressed globose with a black or dark purple color. Its cultivars are highly cold hardy and resistant to drought and diseases [32].

Several *in vitro* assays exist to measure the antioxidant capacity of food and biological samples. The sensitivity of these methods depends on some factors, such as pH, the presence of lipophilic and/or hydrophilic compounds. The ferric reducing ability of plasma (FRAP) assay is a simple and inexpensive method, however, effectively used for the detection of quantitative differences among samples. [33]. As reported earlier by several authors, the plant genotype, growing site, and extraction technique as well as differences in fruit ripeness, influence the total phenolic content and antioxidant activity of fruits [34–37].

The aim of this study was to determine and compare the total polyphenol content and total antioxidant capacity of rosehips of four *Rosa* species (*R. canina*, *R. gallica*, *R. rugosa*, and *R. spinosissima*). Total phenolics and FRAP values were evaluated both in water and ethanolic extracts of dried rosehips originating from two locations for each species.

2. Materials and Methods

2.1. Plant Material

Four *Rosa* species (*R. canina*, *R. gallica*, *R. rugosa*, and *R. spinosissima*) were selected for the study. Plants were located in Gödöllő (location 1, Northern Hungary) and in Szeged (location 2, Southern Hungary). Triplicated samples (100 g) of rosehips uniform in shape and color were collected randomly from different parts of the bushes at the ripe stage (with hard pericarp). Seeds were removed and analyses were carried out on fruit flesh. Samples were air-dried at 30 °C, then pulverized.

2.2. Extraction

Extraction was carried out according to Pharmacopoea Hungarica (Ph.Hg.) [38]. One hundred milliliters of distilled water was added to 1.00 g of dried material to prepare water extracts. Infusions were steeped for 24 h. The same sample weight and solvent volume were used for making ethanolic extracts with aqueous ethanol (water/ethanol 80/20 v/v, 20 °C), followed by a 72 h storage at room temperature. Extractions were replicated three times. Extracts were filtered and centrifuged at 1300 rpm for 10 min, then the supernatants were analyzed.

2.3. Determination of Total Polyphenols

For the determination of total phenolic content (TPC) by Folin-Ciocalteu reagent, the method described by Singleton and Rossi [39] was used. Briefly, 0.05 mL of diluted extract and 0.45 mL of distilled water were added to 2.5 mL of 1:10 diluted Folin-Ciocalteu's phenol reagent, followed by the addition of 2 mL of 7.5% (w/v) sodium carbonate. After storing the solutions for 5 min at 50 °C, their absorbance was determined by spectrophotometer at 760 nm. TPC was estimated from a standard curve of gallic acid. All measurements were repeated three times and results were expressed as mg gallic acid equivalent (GAE) per 100 g dry weight (DW).

2.4. Determination of Antioxidant Capacity

FRAP assay was carried out according to the method of Benzie and Strain [40] to characterize the antioxidant capacity of rosehip samples. This procedure is based on the reduction of ferric-tripyridyl-triazine (Fe^{3+}-TPTZ) complex to the ferrous (Fe^{2+}) form at low pH. Samples containing 100 μL of rosehip extract and 3 mL of FRAP solution were incubated at 37 °C for 4 min, then their absorbance was measured at 593 nm. Change in the absorbance compared to that of the standard solution of L-ascorbic acid (AA) was converted into a FRAP value, and the result was expressed as mmol AA per g DW.

2.5. Statistical Analysis

Data were analyzed using Microsoft Excel software. The effect of extraction method was investigated by paired *t*-tests. Effects of species and collection site were investigated by two-way analysis of variance performed separately for water extraction and for ethanol extraction data. Fisher's least significant difference test was applied as a post-hoc test.

3. Results

3.1. Total Polyphenol Content

The total phenolic content (TPC) was determined both from water and ethanolic extracts from hips of selected *Rosa* species. Results are summarized in Figure 1. Water soluble TPC values for analyzed rosehips ranged from 150.8 mg to 299.2 mg GAE/100 g DW. *R. spinosissima* was characterized by the highest phenolic content. Significantly lower values were found both for *R. canina* and *R. rugosa* which showed similar values. Significantly, the lowest TPC level was measured for *R. gallica*. In water extract of *R. canina*, TPC level proved to be significantly higher in the samples from Gödöllő (location 1) than in those from Szeged (location 2). However, there were no remarkable differences between the two sampling sites in the case of the other three species.

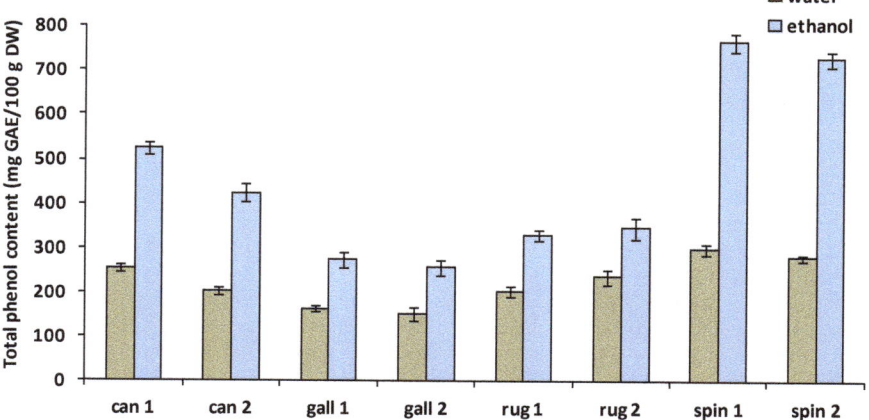

Figure 1. Total polyphenol content of water and ethanolic extracts of *R. canina* (can), *R. gallica* (gall), *R. rugosa* (rug) and *R. spinosissima* (spin); means ± SD; 1 = location 1 (Gödöllő), 2 = location 2 (Szeged). GAE: gallic acid equivalent; DW: dry weight.

The ethanolic extraction method resulted in significantly higher TPC values for all investigated rose species compared to aqueous extraction. TPC in ethanolic extracts varied from 255.9 mg to 766.0 mg GAE/100 g DW (Figure 1). Differences among the four investigated species were significant. Similarly to aqueous extraction, the highest TPC value was found in *R. spinosissima*, three fold higher than values of *R. gallica*, characterized by the lowest phenolic content. TPC levels in *R. canina* were significantly higher than those in *R. rugosa* and *R. gallica*. Significant differences between collecting sites were obtained only for *R. canina*: location 1 showed higher TPC values in ethanolic extracts than those of location 2.

3.2. Antioxidant Capacity

Antioxidant capacity was measured using FRAP assay, values for water and ethanolic extracts are represented in Figure 2. The FRAP values, expressed as ascorbic acid equivalents per g DW, varied from 123.8 mmol to 314.4 mmol in water extracts. The highest FRAP values were noted for *R. spinosissima*, followed by *R. canina*, then *R. rugosa*, while the lowest values were detected in *R. gallica*. Differences among the species were found to be statistically significant. FRAP in water extracts was only influenced by the growing site in the case of *R. canina*.

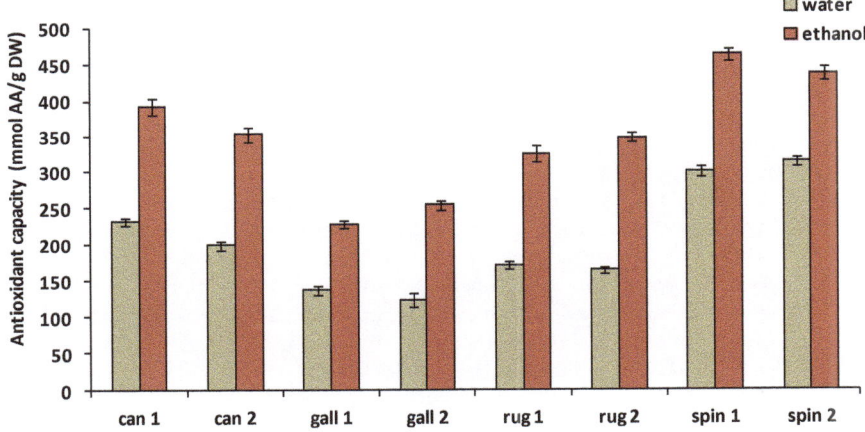

Figure 2. Antioxidant capacity (FRAP) of water and ethanolic extracts of *R. canina* (can), *R. gallica* (gall), *R. rugosa* (rug) and *R. spinosissima* (spin); means ± SD; 1 = location 1 (Gödöllő), 2 = location 2 (Szeged). AA: ascorbic acid.

Ethanolic extracts showed significantly higher antioxidant capacities than water extracts in all four *Rosa* species (Figure 2). FRAP values of ethanolic extracts of rosehips ranged from 228.2 mmol to 464.8 mmol AA/g DW. The highest antioxidant capacity was detected for *R. spinosissima*, two-fold higher than data obtained for *R. gallica*, representing the lowest values. FRAP values measured in ethanolic extracts of *R. canina* and *R. rugosa* were significantly lower than those of *R. spinosissima*, whereas no significant difference between *R. canina* and *R. rugosa* was detected. Ethanolic extracts of *R. spinosissima* and *R. canina* had significantly higher antioxidant properties in samples originating from Gödöllő (location 1) than those from Szeged (location 2). However, in the case of *R. gallica* and *R. rugosa*, location 2 was characterized by higher FRAP values than location 1.

4. Discussion

In the present study, total phenol content of water and ethanolic extracts from rosehips of different species were evaluated. Comparing the two extraction methods, ethanolic extracts showed significantly higher TPC values than water extracts in all cases. Detected ranges of TPC are in agreement with some earlier studies, although with slight quantitative differences. For *R. canina*, Roman et al. [41] found a TPC range from 326 mg to 575 mg GAE/100 g DW, Yoo et al. [42] measured 818 mg GAE/100 g DW in water extracts, while Fattahi et al. [43] measured 180–225 mg GAE/100 g DW, Yilmaz and

Ercisli [44] 102 mg GAE/100 g DW, and Barros et al. [45] 149.35 mg GAE/g extract in methanolic extracts. On the other hand, values over ten-fold higher than our findings were reported by Ercisli [12] (9600 mg GAE/100 g DW) and Demir et al. [14] (3108 mg GAE/100 g DW) in water extracts, and by Nadpal et al. [25] (6100 mg GAE/100 g DW in water, 5030 mg GAE/100 g DW in methanolic extract) for the same species. Najda and Buczkowska [26] obtained very low TPC levels: 215.14 mg GAE/100 g fresh weight for *R. rugosa*, and 121.38 mg GAE/100 g fresh weight for *R. spinosissima*. Much higher TPC was noted by Demir et al. [14] for *R. gallica* (3151 mg GAE/100 g DW) than measured in the present study.

Both extraction methods revealed significant differences in total phenolic content among the investigated species. The concentration of TPC was obtained in a decreasing order of *R. spinosissima* > *R. canina* > *R. rugosa* > *R. gallica*. In this study, *R. spinosissima* was responsible for the highest TPC value compared to the other three species. Fattahi et al. [43] evaluated similar values for *R. spinosissima* and *R. canina*, while Najda and Buczkowska [26] found significantly lower TPC level for *R. spinosissima* than for *R. rugosa*. Demir et al. [14] reported no differences between TPC content of *R. canina* and *R. gallica*.

Rosehips of four *Rosa* species were collected at the same time at two locations. Growing site had no determining effect on TPC and in the case of phenolic content it only significantly affected the results of *R. canina*, but not the other three investigated species.

Total antioxidant capacity was evaluated by using FRAP assay, both in water and ethanolic extracts. The obtained ranges of FRAP values proved to be similar to those found by Gao et al. [46], Demir et al. [14], Taneva et al. [47] and Nadpal et al. [25], but much higher than those reported by Koca et al. [48]. Other antioxidant capacity determination methods than FRAP are also frequently used in rosehip experiments. Barros et al. [45] and Tumbas et al. [9] used DPPH (1,1-diphenyl-2-picrylhydrazyl) radical scavenging activity, while Montazeri et al. [49] applied DPPH and ABTS (2,2′-azinobis-3-ethylbenzothiazoline-6-sulfonic acid) to characterize antioxidant properties of *R. canina*. Fattahi et al. [43] determined the antioxidant capacity of *R. canina* and *R. spinosissima* by DPPH assay and hydrogen peroxide (H_2O_2) radical scavenging assay. Franco et al. [50] and Olech et al. [51] investigated rosehip antioxidants using DPPH for *R. rubiginosa* and for *R. rugosa*, respectively, while Najda and Buczkowska [26] gained extracts with DPPH for *R. californica*, *R. damascena*, *R. rugosa* and *R. villosa*.

It is worth underlining the effect of different solvents on total phenol content and antioxidant activity. In this study, ethanolic extracts had markedly higher antioxidant capacities than those of water extracts. Therefore ethanol is a more effective solvent for extraction of antioxidant compounds of *Rosa* species. This result is in agreement with the findings of Taneva et al. [47] and Franco et al. [50]. Ilbay et al. [52] found methanol extraction three-fold more effective than water extraction. However, Olech et al. [51] reported that *R. rugosa* ethanol extract had an antioxidant activity similar to that of water extract. Nadpal et al. [25] found that methanol is a more effective solvent for the extraction of phenolic compounds than water in the case of *R. canina* but obtained just the opposite for *R. arvensis*. Higher phenolic levels and antioxidant capacity were found in methanolic and/or ethanolic extracts of other plant species compared to water extracts by some authors [53–56]. Therefore in recent scientific studies, alcoholic extraction is more frequently used than water extraction to determine antioxidant properties of different plant materials [57–60].

High variability was found in FRAP values among the four species. *R. spinosissima* was responsible for much higher antioxidant activity than the other species. FRAP values were detected, similarly to TPC, in a decreasing order of *R. spinosissima* > *R. canina* > *R. rugosa* > *R. gallica*. Our data showed that *R. spinosissima* exhibited the greatest total phenolic content and total antioxidant capacity among the four studied *Rosa* species. This result indicates that *R. spinosissima* can be used as a reliable source of natural antioxidants. Based on the findings, this species is highly recommended as a breeding material for medicinal purposes. In the past, several *R. spinosissima* varieties were cultivated, mainly in Europe. However, today only few remained, so this species became an underexploited genetic resource [32].

Investigation of various *Rosa* species for their antioxidant properties may draw more attention to their potential as a functional food or food additive.

Antioxidant capacity was affected by the growing location of the rosehip: FRAP values obtained in ethanolic extracts were significantly different in samples from the two sites in the case of all the investigated species. FRAP values of water extracts differed markedly only for *R. canina*. This result suggests that the antioxidant activity of *R. canina* is strongly dependent on environmental factors. As shown in Figure 2, antioxidant capacity of ethanolic extracts of *R. canina* and *R. spinosissima* was higher in samples from location 1, however, the opposite was found for *R. gallica* and *R. rugosa*. These differences indicate that the growing site influences the antioxidant properties depending on the species. In our case, location 2 is characterized by slightly higher temperatures and more sunshine hours in the vegetation period than location 1. These climatic conditions seem to favor the forming of antioxidant components in the case of *R. gallica* and *R. rugosa*.

As the results of this study demonstrate, antioxidant activity of different *Rosa* species is recommended to be analyzed more comprehensively. Furthermore, differences in the antioxidant properties among samples of the same species from different locations underline the importance of further investigations under different environmental conditions. The results also revealed that different solvents and extraction methods should also be examined as they play an important role in biological activity. The concentration of extracted bioactive ingredients greatly influences the medicinal effects of the rosehip.

Author Contributions: Conceptualization, N.K. and A.O.; Methodology, É.S.-B.; Validation, É.S.-B. and N.K.; Formal Analysis, A.O.; Investigation, N.K.; Resources, É.S.-B.; Data Curation, A.O.; Writing-Original Draft Preparation, N.K.; Writing-Review & Editing, A.O.; Visualization, N.K.; Supervision, É.S.-B.

Funding: This research received no external funding.

Conflicts of Interest: The authors declare no conflict of interest.

References

1. Bruneau, A.; Starr, J.R.; Joly, S. Phylogenetic relationships in the genus Rosa: New evidence from chloroplast DNA sequences and an appraisal of current knowledge. *Syst. Bot.* **2007**, *32*, 366–378. [CrossRef]
2. The Plant List. Available online: http://www.theplantlist.org/tpl1.1/search?q=rosa (accessed on 28 June 2018).
3. Brown, D. *New Encyclopedia of Herbs & Their Uses*, 1st ed.; Dorling Kindersley: London, UK. 2002; pp. 346–347, ISBN 0-7513-3386-7.
4. Cunja, V.; Mikulic-Petkovsek, M.; Stampar, F.; Schmitzer, V. Compound identification of selected rose species and cultivars: An insight to petal and leaf phenolic profiles. *J. Am. Soc. Hort. Sci.* **2014**, *139*, 157–166.
5. Orhan, D.D.; Hartevioğlu, A.; Küpeli, E.; Yesilada, E.J. In vivo anti-inflammatory and antinociceptive activity of the crude extract and fractions from *Rosa canina* L. fruits. *J. Ethnopharmacol.* **2007**, *112*, 394–400. [CrossRef] [PubMed]
6. Barros, L.; Carvalho, A.M.; Morais, J.S.; Ferreira, I.C.F.R. Strawberry-tree, blackthorn and rose fruits: Detailed characterisation in nutrients and phytochemicals with antioxidant properties. *Food Chem.* **2010**, *120*, 247–254. [CrossRef]
7. Willich, S.N.; Rossnagel, K.; Roll, S.; Wagner, A.; Mune, O.; Erlendson, J.; Kharazmi, A.; Sörensen, H.; Winther, K. Rose hip herbal remedy in patients with rheumatoid arthritis—A randomized controlled trial. *Phytomedicine* **2010**, *17*, 87–93. [CrossRef] [PubMed]
8. Mármol, I.; Sánchez-de-Diego, C.; Jiménez-Moreno, N.; Ancín-Azpilicueta, C.; Rodríguez-Yold, M.J. Therapeutic Applications of Rose Hips from Different Rosa Species. *Int. J. Mol. Sci.* **2017**, *18*, 1137. [CrossRef] [PubMed]
9. Tumbas, V.T.; Canadanovic-Brunet, J.M.; Cetojevic-Simin, D.D.; Cetkovic, G.S.; Ethilas, S.M.; Gille, L. Effect of rosehip (*Rosa canina* L.) phytochemicals on stable free radicals and human cancer cells. *J. Sci. Food Agric.* **2012**, *92*, 1273–1281. [CrossRef] [PubMed]

10. Patel, S. Rose hips as complementary and alternative medicine: Overview of the present status and prospects. *Mediterr. J. Nutr. Metab.* **2013**, *6*, 89. [CrossRef]
11. Fan, C.; Pacier, C.; Martirosyan, D.M. Rose hip (*Rosa canina* L.): A functional food perspective. *Funct. Foods Health Dis.* **2014**, *4*, 493–509.
12. Ercisli, S. Chemical composition of fruits in some rose (*Rosa* spp.) species. *Food Chem.* **2007**, *104*, 1379–1384. [CrossRef]
13. Adamczak, A.; Buchwald, W.; Zielinski, J.; Mielcarek, S. Flavonoid and organic acid content in rose hips (Rosa L., sect. Caninae dc. Em. Christ.). *Acta Biol. Cracov. Bot.* **2012**, *54*, 105–112. [CrossRef]
14. Demir, N.; Yildiz, O.; Alpaslan, M.; Hayaloglu, A. Evaluation of volatiles, phenolic compounds and antioxidant activities of rose hip (*Rosa* L.) fruits in Turkey. *LWT Food Sci. Technol.* **2014**, *57*, 126–133. [CrossRef]
15. Machmudah, S.; Kawahito, Y.; Sasaki, M.; Goto, M. Process optimization and extraction rate analysis of carotenoids extraction from rosehip fruit using supercritical CO_2. *J. Supercrit. Fluids* **2008**, *44*, 308–314. [CrossRef]
16. Nowak, R. Chemical composition of hips essential oils of some *Rosa* L. species. *Z. Naturforsch.* **2005**, *60c*, 369–378. [CrossRef]
17. Adamczak, A.; Grys, A.; Buchwald, W.; Zieliński, J. Content of oil and main fatty acids in hips of rose species native in Poland. *Dendrobiology* **2011**, *66*, 55–62.
18. Sharma, B.; Singh, B.; Dhyani, D.; Verma, P.K.; Karthigeyan, S. Fatty acid composition of wild growing rose species. *J. Med. Plants Res.* **2012**, *6*, 1046–1049. [CrossRef]
19. Wenzig, E.; Widowitz, U.; Kunert, O.; Chrubasik, S.; Bucar, F.; Knauder, E.; Bauer, R. Phytochemical composition and in vitro pharmacological activity of two rose hip (*Rosa canina* L.) preparations. *Phytomedicine* **2008**, *15*, 826–835. [CrossRef] [PubMed]
20. Ogah, O.; Watkins, C.S.; Ubi, B.E.; Oraguzie, N.C. Phenolic compounds in Rosaceae fruit and nut crops. *J. Agric. Food Chem.* **2014**, *62*, 9369–9386. [CrossRef] [PubMed]
21. Hosni, K.; Chrif, R.; Zahed, N.; Abid, I.; Medfei, W.; Sebei, H.; Brahim, N.B. Fatty acid and phenolic constituents of leaves, flowers and fruits of tunisian dog rose (*Rosa canina* L.). *Riv. Ital. Sostanze Gr.* **2010**, *87*, 117–123.
22. Türkben, C.; Uylaşer, V.; İncedayı, B.; Çelikkol, I. Effects of different maturity periods and processes on nutritional components of rose hip (*Rosa canina* L.). *J. Food Agric. Environ.* **2010**, *8*, 26–30.
23. Olsson, M.E.; Gustavsson, K.E.; Andersson, S.; Nilsson, A.; Duan, R.D. Inhibition of cancer cell proliferation in vitro by fruit and berry extracts and correlations with antioxidant levels. *J. Agric. Food Chem.* **2004**, *52*, 7264–7271. [CrossRef] [PubMed]
24. Elmastas, M.; Demir, A.; Genc, N.; Dölek, Ü.; Günes, M. Changes in flavonoid and phenolic acid contents in some Rosa species during ripening. *Food Chem.* **2017**, *235*, 154–159. [CrossRef] [PubMed]
25. Nadpal, J.D.; Lesjak, M.M.; Šibul, F.S.; Anackov, G.T.; Cetojevic´-Simin, D.D.; Mimica-Dukic, N.M.; Beara, I.N. Comparative study of biological activities and phytochemical composition of two rose hips and their preserves: *Rosa canina* L. and *Rosa arvensis* Huds. *Food Chem.* **2016**, *192*, 907–914. [CrossRef] [PubMed]
26. Najda, A.; Buczkowska, H. Morphological and chemical characteristics of fruits of selected *Rosa* sp. *Mod. Phytomorph.* **2013**, *3*, 99–103. [CrossRef]
27. Jiménez, S.; Jiménez-Moreno, N.; Luquin, A.; Laguna, M.; Rodríguez-Yoldi, M.J.; Ancín-Azpilicueta, C. Chemical composition of rosehips from different Rosa species: An alternative source of antioxidants for the food industry. *Food Add. Cont. A* **2017**, *34*, 1121–1130. [CrossRef] [PubMed]
28. Bäumler, S. Heilpflanzen. In *Praxis heute*, 2nd ed.; Urban & Fischer Verlag: München, Germany, 2012; pp. 261–262, ISBN 978-3-437-57272-2. (In German)
29. USDA (United States Department of Agriculture), Natural Resources Conservation Service. *Rosa canina* L. Dog Rose. In *The PLANTS Database*; National Plant Data Team: Greensboro, NC, USA. Available online: https://plants.usda.gov/plantguide/pdf/pg_roca3.pdf (accessed on 20 June 2018).
30. European Medicines Agency. Rosa Flower. EMA/237220/2017. Available online: http://www.ema.europa.eu/docs/en_GB/document_library/Herbal_-_Summary_of_assessment_report_for_the_public/2017/07/WC500230910.pdf (accessed on 20 June 2018).

31. USDA (United States Department of Agriculture), Natural Resources Conservation Service. *Rosa rugosa* Thunb. Rugosa Rose. In *The PLANTS Database*; National Plant Data Team: Greensboro, NC, USA. Available online: https://plants.usda.gov/factsheet/pdf/fs_roru.pdf (accessed on 20 June 2018).
32. Boyd, P.D.A. Scots Roses and Related Cultivars of *Rosa spinosissima*—A Review. In Proceedings of the ISHS Acta Horticulturae 1064 VI International Symposium on Rose Research and Cultivation, Hannover, Germany, 25 January 2015.
33. Magalhaes, L.M.; Segundo, M.A.; Reis, S.; Lima, J.L.F.C. Methodological aspects about in vitro evaluation of antioxidant properties. *Anal. Chim. Acta* **2008**, *613*, 1–19. [CrossRef] [PubMed]
34. Gündüz, K.; Özdemir, E. The effects of genotype and growing conditions on antioxidant capacity, phenolic compounds, organic acid and individual sugars of strawberry. *Food Chem.* **2014**, *155*, 298–303. [CrossRef] [PubMed]
35. Scalzo, J.; Politi, A.; Pellegrini, N.; Mezzetti, B.; Battino, M. Plant genotype affects total antioxidant capacity and phenolic contents in fruit. *Nutrition* **2005**, *21*, 207–213. [CrossRef] [PubMed]
36. Lima, V.L.A.G.; Mélo, E.A.; Maciel, M.I.S.; Prazeres, F.G.; Musser, R.S.; Lima, D.A.E.S. Total phenolic and carotenoid contents in acerola genotypes harvested at three ripening stages. *Food Chem.* **2005**, *90*, 565–568. [CrossRef]
37. Mphahlele, R.R.; Stander, M.A.; Fawole, O.A.; Opara, U.L. Effect of fruit maturity and growing location on the postharvest contents of flavonoids, phenolic acids, vitamin C and antioxidant activity of pomegranate juice (cv. Wonderful). *J. Sci. Food Agric.* **2016**, *96*, 1002–1009. [CrossRef] [PubMed]
38. Béla, L. *Pharmacopoea Hungarica*, 8th ed.; Medicina Kiadó: Budapest, Hungary, 2004; p. 1432.
39. Singleton, V.L.; Rossi, J.A. Colorimetry of total phenolics with phosphomolybdic phosphotungstic acid reagents. *Am. J. Enol. Vitic.* **1965**, *16*, 144–158.
40. Benzie, I.F.F.; Strain, J.J. Ferric reducing ability of plasma (FRAP) as a measure of antioxidant power: The FRAP assay. *Anal. Biochem.* **1996**, *1*, 70–76. [CrossRef] [PubMed]
41. Roman, I.; Stănilă, A.; Stănilă, S. Bioactive compounds and antioxidant activity of *Rosa canina* L. biotypes from spontaneous flora of Transylvania. *Chem. Cent. J.* **2013**, *7*, 73. [CrossRef] [PubMed]
42. Yoo, K.M.; Lee, C.H.; Lee, H.; Moon, B.; Lee, C.Y. Relative antioxidant and cytoprotective activities of common herbs. *Food Chem.* **2008**, *106*, 929–936. [CrossRef]
43. Fattahi, S.; Jamei, R.; Sarghein, S.H. Antioxidant and antiradicalic activity of *Rosa canina* and *Rosa pimpinellifolia* fruits from West Azerbaijan. *Iran. J. Plant Physiol.* **2012**, *2*, 523–529.
44. Yilmaz, S.O.; Ercisli, S. Antibacterial and antioxidant activity of fruits of some rose species from Turkey. *Rom. Biotechnol. Lett.* **2011**, *16*, 6407–6411.
45. Barros, L.; Carvalho, A.M.; Ferreira, I.C.F.R. Exotic fruits as a source of important phytochemicals: Improving the traditional use of *Rosa canina* fruits in Portugal. *Food Res. Int.* **2011**, *44*, 2233–2236. [CrossRef]
46. Gao, X.; Björk, L.; Trajkovski, V.; Uggla, M. Evaluation of antioxidant activities of rosehip ethanol extracts in different test systems. *J. Sci. Food Agric.* **2000**, *80*, 2021–2027. [CrossRef]
47. Taneva, I.; Petkova, N.; Dimov, I.; Ivanov, I.; Denev, P. Characterization of rose hip (*Rosa canina* L.) fruits extracts and evaluation of their in vitro antioxidant activity. *J. Pharmacogn. Phytochem.* **2016**, *5*, 35–38.
48. Koca, I.; Ustun, N.S.; Koyuncu, T. Effect of drying conditions on antioxidant properties of rosehip fruits (*Rosa canina* sp.). *Asian J. Chem.* **2009**, *21*, 1061–1068.
49. Montazeri, N.; Baher, E.; Mirzajani, F.; Barami, Z.; Yousefian, S. Phytochemical contents and biological activities of *Rosa canina* fruit from Iran. *J. Med. Plants Res.* **2011**, *5*, 4584–4589.
50. Franco, D.; Pinelo, M.; Sineiro, J.; Núñez, M.J. Processing of *Rosa rubiginosa*: Extraction of oil and antioxidant substances. *Bioresour. Technol.* **2007**, *98*, 3506–3512. [CrossRef] [PubMed]
51. Olech, M.; Nowak, R.; Los, R.; Rzymowska, J.; Malm, A.; Chrusciel, K. Biological activity and composition of teas and tinctures prepared from *Rosa rugosa* Thunb. *Cent. Eur. J. Biol.* **2012**, *7*, 172–182. [CrossRef]
52. İlbay, Z.; Şahin, S.; Kırbaşlar, S.I. Investigation of polyphenolic content of rose hip (*Rosa canina* L.) tea extracts: A comparative study. *Foods* **2013**, *2*, 43–52. [CrossRef] [PubMed]
53. Do, Q.D.; Angkawijaya, A.E.; Tran-Nguyen, P.L.; Huynh, L.H.; Soetaredjo, F.E.; Ismadji, S.; Ju, Y.H. Effect of extraction solvent on total phenol content, total flavonoid content, and antioxidant activity of *Limnophila aromatica*. *J. Food Drug Anal.* **2014**, *22*, 296–302. [CrossRef] [PubMed]
54. Koczka, N.; Móczár, Z.; Stefanovits-Bányai, É.; Ombódi, A. Differences in antioxidant properties of ginkgo leaves collected from male and female trees. *Acta Pharm.* **2015**, *65*, 99–104. [CrossRef] [PubMed]

55. Butsat, S.; Siriamornpun, S. Effect of solvent types and extraction times on phenolic and flavonoid contents and antioxidant activity in leaf extracts of *Amomum chinense* C. *Int. Food Res. J.* **2016**, *23*, 180–187.
56. Ghasemzadeh, A.; Jaafar, H.Z.E.; Juraimi, A.S.; Tayebi-Meigooni, A. Comparative evaluation of different extraction techniques and solvents for the assay of phytochemicals and antioxidant activity of Hashemi rice bran. *Molecules* **2015**, *20*, 10822–10838. [CrossRef] [PubMed]
57. Tuyen, P.T.; Xuan, T.D.; Khang, D.T.; Ahmad, A.; Quan, N.V.; Tu Anh, T.T.; Anh, L.H.; Minh, T.N. Phenolic compositions and antioxidant properties in bark, flower, inner skin, kernel and leaf extracts of *Castanea crenata* Sieb. et Zucc. *Antioxidants* **2017**, *6*, 31. [CrossRef] [PubMed]
58. Navarro-Hoyos, M.; Lebrón-Aguilar, R.; Quintanilla-López, J.E.; Cueva, C.; Hevia, D.; Quesada, S.; Azofeifa, G.; Moreno-Arribas, M.V.; Monagas, M.; Bartolomé, B. Proanthocyanidin characterization and bioactivity of extracts from different parts of *Uncaria tomentosa* L. (cat's claw). *Antioxidants* **2017**, *6*, 12. [CrossRef] [PubMed]
59. Wright, R.J.; Lee, K.S.; Hyacinth, H.I.; Hibbert, J.M.; Reid, M.E.; Wheatley, A.O.; Asemota, H.N. An investigation of the antioxidant capacity in extracts from *Moringa oleifera* plants grown in Jamaica. *Plants* **2017**, *6*, 48. [CrossRef] [PubMed]
60. Khang, D.T.; Dung, T.N.; Elzaawely, A.A.; Xuan, T.D. Phenolic profiles and antioxidant activity of germinated legumes. *Foods* **2016**, *5*, 27. [CrossRef] [PubMed]

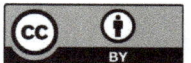

© 2018 by the authors. Licensee MDPI, Basel, Switzerland. This article is an open access article distributed under the terms and conditions of the Creative Commons Attribution (CC BY) license (http://creativecommons.org/licenses/by/4.0/).

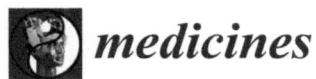

Article

An Investigation of Potential Sources of Nutraceuticals from the Niger Delta Areas, Nigeria for Attenuating Oxidative Stress

Lucky Legbosi Nwidu [1,2,*], Philip Cheriose Nzien Alikwe [3], Ekramy Elmorsy [2,4] and Wayne Grant Carter [2]

[1] Department of Experimental Pharmacology and Toxicology, Faculty of Pharmaceutical Sciences, University of Port Harcourt, Port Harcourt PMB 5323, Rivers State, Nigeria
[2] School of Medicine, University of Nottingham, Royal Derby Hospital Centre, Derby DE22 3DT, UK; ekramy_elmorsy@yahoo.com (E.E.); wayne.carter@nottingham.ac.uk (W.G.C.)
[3] Department of Animal Science, Niger Delta University, Wilberforce Island, Yenegoa PMB 071, Bayelsa State, Nigeria; bushdoctor2013@gmail.com
[4] Department of Forensic Medicine and Clinical Toxicology, Faculty of Medicine, Mansoura University, Mansoura 35516, Egypt
* Correspondence: menelucky@yahoo.com; Tel.: +234-803341-7432

Received: 18 December 2018; Accepted: 15 January 2019; Published: 20 January 2019

Abstract: Background: Diets rich in fruits, vegetables, and medicinal plants possess antioxidants potentially capable of mitigating cellular oxidative stress. This study investigated the antioxidant, anti-acetylcholinesterase (AChE), and total phenolic and flavonoids contents (TPC/TFC) of dietary sources traditionally used for memory enhancing in Niger Delta, Nigeria. **Methods:** *Dacroydes edulis* methanolic seed extract (DEMSE), *Cola lepidota* methanolic seed extract (CLMSE), *Terminalia catappa* methanolic seed extract (TeCMSE), *Tricosanthes cucumerina* methanolic seed extract (TrCMSE), *Tetrapleura tetraptera* methanolic seed extract (TTMSE), and defatted *Moringa oleifera* methanolic seed extract (DMOMSE); *Dennettia tripetala* methanolic fruit extract (DTMFE), *Artocarpus communis* methanolic fruit extract (ACMFE), *Gnetum africana* methanolic leaf extract (GAMLE), *Musa paradisiaca* methanolic stembark extract (MPMSE), and *Mangifera indica* methanolic stembark extract (MIMSE) were evaluated for free radical scavenging antioxidant ability using 2,2-Diphenyl-1-picrylhydrazyl (DPPH), reducing power capacity (reduction of ferric iron to ferrous iron), AChE inhibitory potential by Ellman assay, and then TPC/TFC contents determined by estimating milli-equivalents of Gallic acid and Quercetin per gram, respectively. **Results:** The radical scavenging percentages were as follows: MIMSE (58%), MPMSE (50%), TrCMSE (42%), GAMLE (40%), CLMSE (40%), DMOMSE (38%), and DEMFE (37%) relative to β-tocopherol (98%). The highest iron reducing (antioxidant) capacity was by TrCMSE (52%), MIMSE (40%) and GAMLE (38%). Extracts of MIMSE, TrCMSE, DTMFE, TTMSE, and CLMSE exhibited concentration-dependent AChE inhibitory activity ($p < 0.05$–0.001). At a concentration of 200 µg/mL, the AChE inhibitory activity and IC_{50} (µg/mL) exhibited by the most potent extracts were: MIMSE ($\approx$50%/111.9), TrCMSE ($\approx$47%/201.2), DTMFE ($\approx$32%/529.9), TTMSE ($\approx$26%/495.4), and CLMSE ($\approx$25%/438.4). The highest TPC were from MIMSE (156.2), TrCMSE (132.65), GAMLE (123.26), and CLMSE (119.63) in mg gallic acid equivalents/g, and for TFC were: MISME (87.35), GAMLE (73.26), ACMFE (69.54), CLMSE (68.35), and TCMSE2 (64.34) mg quercetin equivalents/gram. **Conclusions:** The results suggest that certain inedible and edible foodstuffs, most notably MIMSE, MPMSE, TrCMSE, GAMLE, and CLMSE may be beneficial to ameliorate the potentially damaging effects of redox stress.

Keywords: acetylcholinesterase inhibitor; antioxidants; memory enhancers; nutraceuticals

1. Introduction

Oxidative stress is associated with a number of diseases and arises as a consequence of an imbalance between reactive oxygen species (ROS), reactive nitrogen species (RNS), and their dissipation via enzymatic and non-enzymatic mechanisms [1]. Many factors including UV-irradiation, industrial emissions, tobacco smoke, licit or illicit drug usage, heavy metal exposure, inorganic and organic contaminants, and xenobiotics are among the potential exogenous sources of ROS generation in regions such as the Niger Delta, Nigeria. Endogenous sources of ROS include those generated via normal cellular metabolism and via pathological means [2]. The chronic exposure to exogenous factors and/or activation of endogenous means can provoke oxidative insults that may activate stress response pathways including inflammation, cytokine secretion, and apoptosis that might contribute to wide range of pathophysiological events [1,3].

Nutraceuticals are used as dietary supplements, but also as auxiliaries for the perceived prevention and/or treatment of a variety of diseases and disorders. The role of consumption of nutraceuticals and their protective effects in mammals and humans against diseases such as neurodegeneration that includes an elevation of oxidative stress have been reviewed [4,5]. Natural antioxidants in foods may exhibit protective antioxidant effects and thereby aid in the reduction of premature mortality [6,7]. One such group of antioxidants is flavonoids, compounds that are ubiquitous in many edible plants [8]. Collectively, there are an extensive number of low molecular weight organic compounds, including polyphenols and flavonoids that have been termed secondary metabolites or phytochemicals that can be specific to each plant. These arrays of secondary metabolites can exhibit a wide spectrum of pharmacological effects including provision of cellular antioxidant activities capable of scavenging damaging free radicals. This endowed useful activity provides potential functional benefits to humans beyond basic nutrition, and could be exploited as commercial sources of nutraceutical formulations [9]. These potential health benefits provide an impetus for subjecting plant extracts and fractions for scrutiny to elucidate and quantify their respective antioxidant and other health benefiting abilities.

In the Niger Delta region of Nigeria residents may benefit from the wide patronage and chronic consumption of numerous endogenous edible seeds, fruits, nuts, pods, green leafy vegetables, herbs, spices, and crops. These are commonly consumed in either raw or in cooked forms in various cuisines. Many of these foodstuffs have yet to be evaluated for their ability to mitigate oxidative stress. Additionally, there is an association of oxidative stress and a cholinergic deficit with neurodegenerative diseases such as Alzheimer's disease and Parkinson's diseases [10–14]. Hence, the intake of appropriate foodstuffs able to combat this cellular damage and loss of neuronal functionality may limit the development or indeed propagation of neurodegenerative disease [15–18].

Therefore, this study investigated extracts of *Dacroydes edulis* methanolic seed extract (DEMSE), *Cola lepidota* methanolic seed extract (CLMSE), *Terminalia catappa* methanolic seed extract (TeCMSE), *Tricosanthes cucumerina* methanolic seed extract (TrCMSE), *Tetrapleura tetraptera* methanolic seed extract (TTMSE), defatted *Moringa oleifera* methanolic seed extract (DMOMSE); *Dennettia tripetala* methanolic fruit extract (DTMFE), *Artocarpus communis* methanolic fruit extract (ACMFE), *Gnetum africana* methanolic leaf extract (GAMLE), *Musa paradisiaca* methanolic stembark extract (MPMSE), and *Mangifera indica* methanolic stembark extract (MIMSE) for in vitro antioxidant and anti-acetylcholinesterase effects and associated polyphenolic and flavonoid contents.

Dacryodes edulis G. Don Lam (Burseraceae) is an edible pear native to the tropics. In the Niger Delta, the fruit is boiled or softened by exposure to heat and used to eat Zea mays (maize) or guinea corn. The pulp may also be boiled or roasted to form a kind of butter [19,20]. *D. edulis* leaf, fruit, and resin extracts have numerous pharmacological activities including antioxidant [21], anti-microbial [22], and anti-carcinogenic [23] properties.

Cola lepidota (Sterculiaceae) is popularly known as monkey cola. The plant is indigenous to tropical Africa and has its center of greatest diversity in West Africa [24]. The native peoples of southern Nigeria and the Cameron relish the fruits as a source of foodstuffs. Seeds of the monkey cola species are not edible, unlike the seeds of kola nut (*C. nitida*). *C. lepidota* is used in traditional medicine with functions that include its use as a stimulant, and to suppress sleep and for pulmonary problems and cancer-related ailments [25,26], with seed and fruit pulp extracts also displaying antioxidant activity [27]. Phytochemical analysis of the plant included detection of flavonoids [28].

Trichosanthes cucumerina Linn (Cucurbitaceae) is an annual, dioecious climber, widely distributed in Asian countries [29]. *T. cucumerina* fruit is consumed as a vegetable by rural dwellers, especially in the Western part of Africa. It is commonly called snake gourd, viper gourd, snake tomato, or long tomato [30]. The fruit is used as a cathartic, the seeds used for stomach disorders, anti-febrile and anti-helmintic activities and cardioprotective activities have also been reported [31].

Dennettia tripetala G. Baker (Annonaceae) is a fruit used as a spice and condiment in West Africa [32]. *D. tripetala* fruit is used in ethnomedicine to treat cold, fever, typhoid, cough, worm infestation, vomiting, stomach upset, and as an appetite enhancer [33]. Strong anti-nociceptive effects comparable to opioid agonists and non-steroidal anti-inflammatory drugs have been demonstrated [33]. Tannins, terpenoids, and other phytochemicals of *D. tripetala* are reported to be responsible for wide range of bioactivities [34].

Artocarpus comminis (Moraceae) is a flowering tree from the mulberry family. It is locally called breadfruit tree because of the "bread-like texture" of its edible fruits. *A. comminis* grown in the Niger Delta region is extensively used as both a food and traditional medicine. Studies have shown that *A. communis* possesses several bioactivities, such as antioxidant [35], anti-cancer [36,37], and anti-inflammatory activities [38,39]. Biologically active phytochemicals within *A. communis* include flavonoids, chalcones, and stilbenes [40].

Terminalia catappa Linn. (Combretaceae) is native to Southeast Asia. It is widely planted throughout the tropics and the Niger Delta region of Nigeria. *T. catappa* nut kernel can be eaten raw [41]. The ethnopharmacological properties of this plant have yet to be fully evaluated.

Moringa oleifera (Moringaceae), commonly known as horseradish tree or drumstick tree, is widely cultivated in Africa and other regions including South East Asia, and is considered a multi-purpose plant [42]. There are a broad number of bioactive agents present within the seeds, and for which seed extracts have been reported to exhibit neuroprotective effects [43–45].

Tetrapleura tetraptera (Mimosaceae), locally referred to as "Arindan" in Yoruba, is a flowering plant of the pea family native to West Africa. The dried fruit is used as a seasoning spice in the Southern part of Nigeria [46,47] and in the Niger Delta areas, the pod, fruit, and seeds are used as spices. A neuroprotective effect of *T. tetraptera* has been reported in scopolamine-induced amnesic rats [48].

Gnetum africanum (Gnetaceae) leaf, also known as wild spinach, is utilized as a food [49]. The vegetable is locally known under different nomenclature: sorgo (in Ogoni in Rivers state, Nigeria), afang (Ibibios in South-South, Nigeria), okazi (Igbo in South-East Nigeria), okok or eru (Cameroun), and fumbwa (Democratic Republic of Congo). Leaves are eaten as a vegetable raw or cooked and revered for their nutritional and therapeutic properties. The vegetable is domesticated for its economic potential, and useful component of dietary fibre, essential amino acids, vitamins, and minerals [50].

Musa paradisiaca (Musaceae), a banana plant, has a number of reported medicinal uses, for example banana seed mucilage has been applied as a treatment for catarrh and diarrhea [51]. There is also an extensive list of reported pharmacological activities including hepatoprotective effects [51].

Mangifera indica (Anacardiaceae) aqueous stem bark extract has been utilized as a remedy for diarrhea, fever, gastritis, and ulcers [52]. It has a number of biological activities, including the ability to act as an anti-cancer, and anti-bacterial agent [53].

Collectively, the plants described above were among the commonly edible and non-edible components of daily diets of Niger Deltans, hence an investigation of their relative antioxidant and anti-cholinesterase activities were undertaken.

2. Materials and Methods

2.1. Collection and Identification of Plant Materials

The seeds of *Dacroydes edulis*, *Cola lepidota*, *Tricosanthes cucumerina*, *Terminalia catappa*, *Tetrapleura tetraptera*, and defatted *Moringa oleifera* seed; fruits of *Dennettia tripetala*, *Artocarpus communis*, green leafy vegetable of *Gnetum africana*; stembark of *Musa paradisiaca* and *Mangifera indica* were collected from Niger Delta University Agricultural Extension farm, Amassoma, Yenegoa, Bayelsa State, Nigeria in March 2015 and authenticated by Mr. Philip Cheriose Nzien Alikwe, an Agriculturalist from the Department of Animal Science, Niger Delta University, Wilberforce Island, Bayelsa State, Nigeria. The voucher numbers (NDUH/P/71-81) were deposited in the University's herbarium, Niger Delta University, Nigeria. All of the samples were shade or air-dried for seven days and powdered using an electrical blender.

2.2. Preparation of Hydromethanolic Extracts

The seeds of *Dacroydes edulis*, *Cola lepidota*, *Tricosanthes cucumerina*, *Terminalia catappa*, *Tetrapleura tetraptera*, and defatted *Moringa oleifera* seed; fruits of *Dennettia tripetala*, *Artocarpus communis* and leafy vegetable of *Gnetum africanum*; stembark of *Musa paradisiaca* and *Mangifera indica* were powdered, and 10 g of each were macerated in 100 mL of 50% methanol for 72 h with vigorous hand agitation for one minute three times daily. Double layered gauze was used for filtration to obtain filtrates that were then reduced in volume at 40 °C on a water bath (Model TT6, Techmel and Techmel, Asaba, Nigeria) to obtain dried extracts. The extracts were weighed and the yield recovered (as a percentage) and recorded (Table 1). Extracts were stored in a refrigerator at 4 °C in an airtight container until used for experimental studies.

Table 1. Percentage yield, DPPH radical scavenging activity, AChE inhibitory potency, and total phenolic and flavonoid content for the evaluated food sources.

Extracts of Plants	Yield (%)	IC_{50} Concentrations (µg/mL)		Total Phenolic Content (mg GAE/g)	Total Flavonoid Content (mg QUER E/g)
		DPPH Radical Scavenging	AChE Inhibition		
Edible Food					
TeCMSE	7.1	302	834.5	28.45 ± 1.40	21.43 ± 0.98
TrCMSE	59.8	854	201.2	132.65 ± 0.85	64.34 ± 1.43
TTMSE	66.7	205	967.9	25.36 ± 0.87	17.35 ± 1.53
DTMFE	39.4	134	654.3	75.64 ± 1.87	41.24 ± 1.56
ACMFE	3.4	890	576.4	102.45 ± 1.43	69.54 ± 1.73
DEMSE	5.0	138	529.9	95.73 ± 3.62	53.35 ± 2.37
GAMLE	11.2	825	321.9	123.26 ± 2.73	73.26 ± 1.78
CLMSE	13.5	526	438.4	119.63 ± 3.24	68.35 ± 2.65
DMOMSE	21.3	145	657.1	65.15 ± 1.35	31.43 ± 0.83
Non-Edible					
MIMSE	2.1	321	111.9	156.2 ± 2.43	87.35 ± 1.57
MPMSE	7.8	106	619.8	85.36 ± 0.95	42.83 ± 1.24

TeCMSE, *Terminalia catappa* methanolic seed extract; TrCMSE, *Tricosanthes cucumerina* methanolic seed extract; TTMSE, *Tetrapleura tetraptera* methanolic seed extract; DTMFE, *Dennettia tripetala* methanolic fruit extract; ACMFE, *Artocarpus communis* methanolic fruit extract; DEMSE, *Dacroydes edulis* methanolic seed extract; GAMLE, *Gnetum africanum* methanolic leaf extract; CLMSE, *Cola lepidota* methanolic seed extract; DMOMSE, Defatted *Moringa oleifera* methanolic seed extract; MIMSE, *Mangifera indica* methanolic stembark extract; MPMSE, *Musa Parasidisiaca* methanolic stem-bark extract. GAE: gallic acid equivalents; QUER E: quercetin equivalents. Extract was evaluated at least in triplicate across concentration range, and an approximate IC_{50} calculated.

2.3. Chemicals

Acetylthiocholine iodide (ATCI), L-ascorbic acid, bovine serum albumin (BSA), 2, 2-Diphenyl-1-picrylhydrazyl (DPPH), 5,5-dithiobis [2-nitrobenzoic acid] (DTNB), Folin-Ciocalteu reagent, physostigmine, and β-tocopherol were all purchased from Sigma Aldrich (Poole, UK), as were all the other chemicals used unless stated otherwise.

2.4. Animals

Rat brain homogenates from male F344 strain rats (200–230 g) were utilized as source of mammalian AChE, as described in an earlier report [54]. Rats were maintained at a controlled temperature of 21 ± 1 °C and a cycle of 16 h light/8 h dark with food intake daily and water ad libitum. Approval for the use of animals was obtained from the University of Nottingham Local Ethical Review Committee (study reference CHE 10, project licence approval code: PPL: 40/2624, approval date 13 June 2005 and the study was executed in line with the Animals Scientific Procedures Act (UK) 1986.

2.5. 2,2-Diphenyl-1-Picrylhydrazyl (DPPH) Radical Scavenging Effect

Spectrophotometric assays that utilized DPPH radical scavenging were used to quantify antioxidant activity. DPPH has been utilized extensively as a stable organic radical to evaluate scavenging activities of plethora of natural compounds such as flavonoids, polyphenols, and crude plant extracts and fractions. Antioxidants scavenge DPPH radicals by donating an electron to form reduced DPPH changing the colour of the solution from purple to yellow, the level of which can be quantified by spectrophotometry. DPPH radical scavenging assays were performed according to the method of Nwidu et al. [54]. Stock solutions of the plant extracts (5 mg/mL) were diluted to final concentrations of 200, 100, 50, 25, 12.5, and 6.25 µg/mL in ethanol. Then, 160 µL of 0.1 mM DPPH in ethanol solution was added to 20 µL solutions of the extracts as well as a standard and 20 µL H_2O. For the standard, β-tocopherol was prepared at concentrations of 1.56, 0.78, 0.39, 0.195, and 0.0975 mg/mL. Assays were performed at 37 °C for 40 min in the dark, and thereafter the absorbance was read at 517 nm, as described in a previous report [54]. All reactions were performed in triplicates, from which an average was generated.

2.6. Reducing Power Capacity Assay

The reducing capacity (antioxidant ability) of the plant extract was also estimated based on its ability to reduce ferric ions (Fe^{3+}) to ferrous ions (Fe^{2+}). The plant extracts were assayed over the concentration ranged of 6.25–50 µg/mL. Four µL of 5 mg/mL of each plant extract was mixed with 400 µL of phosphate buffer (0.2 M dibasic sodium phosphate and 0.2 M monobasic sodium phosphate buffer adjusted to pH 7.4), 250 µL of 1% potassium ferricyanide was then added and the mixture incubated at 50 °C for 20 min. Then, 250 µL of 10% trichloroacetic acid was added, and after mixing, the solution was centrifuged at 3000 rpm for 10 min. One hundred µL from the supernatant was mixed with an equal volume of water, followed by 20 µL of freshly prepared ferric chloride solution. After mixing, the absorbance was measured at 700 nm in a microtiter plate reader, as previously reported [54]. Ascorbic acid was the reference substrate and the following concentration range was employed (0.3, 0.6, 0.9, 1.2, 1.5, and 3 mg/mL). All reactions were performed in triplicates, from which an average reading was generated.

2.7. Acetylcholinesterase Inhibition Assay

The assay for AChE inhibition was based upon the method of Ellman et al. [55], but modified for a 96-well microtiter plate format, as reported in Nwidu et al. [54]. In a microtiter plate, 40 µL of plant extract (at concentrations of 200, 20, 2, 0.2 and 0.02 µg/mL) was mixed with 35 µL of 50 mM Tris-HCl (pH 8.0) containing 0.1% BSA, 50 µL of 3 mM DTNB, and 50 µL of AChE. The AChE used was either from electric eel at 1 mg/mL (Sigma, Poole, UK) or that present within rat brain homogenate (prepared at 10% (w/v), according to the procedure of Carter et al. [56,57], which had been diluted 1:10 in 10 mM Tris-HCl pH 8.0 for assays. Plates were incubated at 37 °C for 5 min before the cholinesterase reaction initiated by the addition of 25 µL of 15 mM ATCI substrate, resulting in the production of 5-thio-2-nitrobenzoate anion that was read at 412 nm every 5 s for 10 min using a Spectramax microplate reader (Thermo Fisher, Stafford, UK). Eserine was employed at 0.02 µg/mL as a positive control for AChE inhibition. At this concentration (or above), eserine inhibits AChE to ≈100% [55]. All reactions were performed in triplicates, from which an average reading was generated.

2.8. Determination of Total Phenolic Content

A Folin-Ciocalteu Reagent (FCR) spectrophotometric method was used to quantify the total phenolic content in plant extracts, as described previously [54]. Twenty µL of each concentration of the plant extracts (ranging from 1–100 µg/mL) was added to 90 µL of water followed by addition of 30 µL of FCR, and samples were vigorously shaken within a microtiter plate reader. Within 30 s and a total assay time of eight minutes, 60 µL of 7.5% Na_2CO_3 solution was added to each microtiter well and then plates were incubated at 40 °C on a shaking incubator. The absorbance of the mixture was read after 40 min at 760 nm, as detailed in a previous report [56]. Gallic acid was used as the positive control substance. All reactions were performed in triplicates, from which an average reading was generated.

2.9. Determination of Total Flavonoid Content

Total flavonoid contents of the plant extracts were determined according to the method described by Nwidu et al. [54] using quercetin as a reference compound. Twenty microliter of plant extracts (5 mg/mL) were dissolved in ethanol and then mixed with 200 µL of 10% aluminum chloride solution and 1 M potassium acetate solution in microtiter plate wells. Samples were incubated for 30 min at room temperature, after which the absorbance of the solution was measured at 415 nm, as reported earlier [54]. Quercetin was used as the reference compound. All reactions were performed in triplicates, from which an average reading was generated.

2.10. Statistical Analysis

Results are expressed as the mean ± SD. IC_{50} values for each extract or fraction were calculated using non-linear regression analysis. A Spearman rank-order correlation coefficient was used to assess the relationship between total phenolic content, total flavonoid content, antioxidant content, and inhibition of AChE activity. Statistical analyses were performed using GraphPad Prism (Version 5.3) for Windows (GraphPad Software, Inc., San Diego, CA, USA, www.graphpad.com). A p value of <0.05 for results was considered to be statistically significant.

3. Results

3.1. DPPH Radical Scavenging Activity

Aqueous methanolic extracts of the inedible stem-bark, edible fruits, seeds and leaf extracts displayed DPPH radical scavenging activities in a concentrations-dependent manner as shown in Figure 1. From these analyses IC_{50} values for radical scavenging were calculated with results displayed in Table 1. When assessed at a concentration of 1000 µg/mL, the majority of aqueous methanolic extracts displayed significant (p < 0.05–0.001) DPPH radical scavenging effects, that ranged from ≈38–58% of that observed with Vitamin E (set at 100%). For the tested extracts, MIMSE (IC_{50} = 321 µg/mL) and MPMSE (IC_{50} = 106 µg/mL) demonstrated the highest percent inhibitions of 58% and 50%, respectively, and the latter extract was also the most potent (lowest IC_{50} value). Collectively, the descending order of DPPH radical scavenging activity was: MIMSE > MPMSE > TrCMSE > GAMLE > CLMSE > DMOMSE > DEMSE > DTMSE > ACMFE > TeCMSE > TTMSE with radical scavenging percentages of 58%, 50%, 42%, 40%, 40%, 38%, 37%, 21%, 20%, 19%, and 18%, respectively. The descending orders of potency of the extracts as radical scavengers as determined via IC_{50} values (µg/mL) were: MPMSE > DTMFE > DEMSE > DMOMSE > TTMSE > TeCMSE > MIMSE > CLMSE > GAMLE > TrCMSE > ACMFE (Table 1).

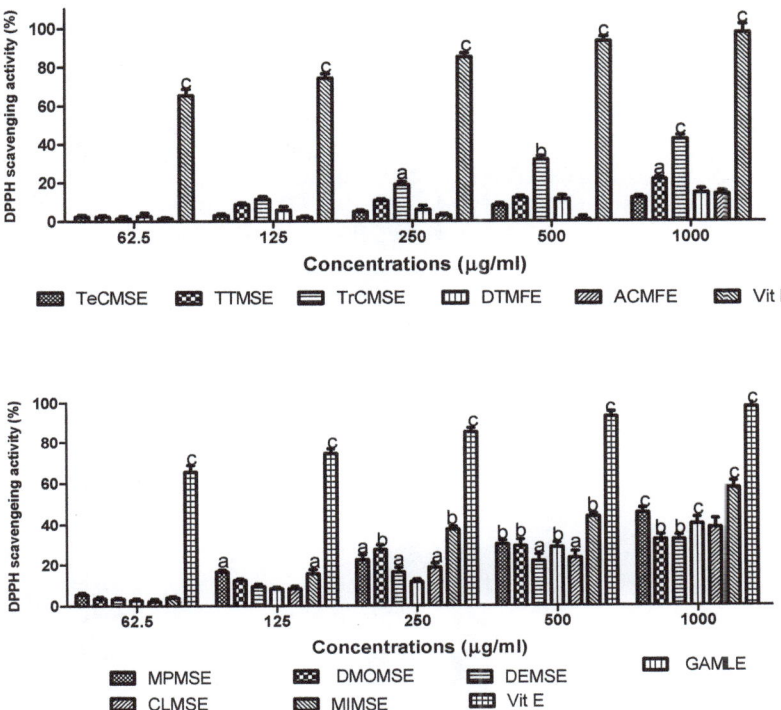

Figure 1. DPPH radical scavenging activity of plant extracts. Plant antioxidant activity was measured via percentage inhibition of radical scavenging of DPPH. Results are expressed as means ± SEM for three separate experiments at each concentration. TeCMSE, *Terminalia catappa* methanolic seed extract; TTMSE, *Tetrapleura tetraptera* methanolic seed extract; TrCMSE, *Tricosanthes cucumerina* methanolic seed extract; DTMFE, *Dennettia tripetala* methanolic fruit extract; ACMFE, *Artocarpus communis* methanolic fruit extract; MPMSE, *Musa parasidisiaca* methanolic stem-bark extract; DMOMSE, Defatted *Moringa oleifera* methanolic seed extract; DEMSE, *Dacroydes edulis* methanolic seed extract; GAMLE, *Gnetum africanum* methanolic leaf extract; CLMSE, *Cola lepidota* methanolic seed extract; MIMSE, *Mangifera indica* methanolic stem-bark extract; Vit E, Vitamin E (β-Tocopherol). Results are expressed as means ± SEM for three separate experiments at each concentration. For marked significance from controls, a: $p < 0.05$, b: $p < 0.01$, c: $p < 0.001$.

3.2. Reducing (Antioxidant) Capacity

An evaluation of the reducing capacity of the aqueous methanolic extracts from the edible and non-edible foods showed that these also displayed antioxidant abilities in a concentration-dependent manner (Figure 2).

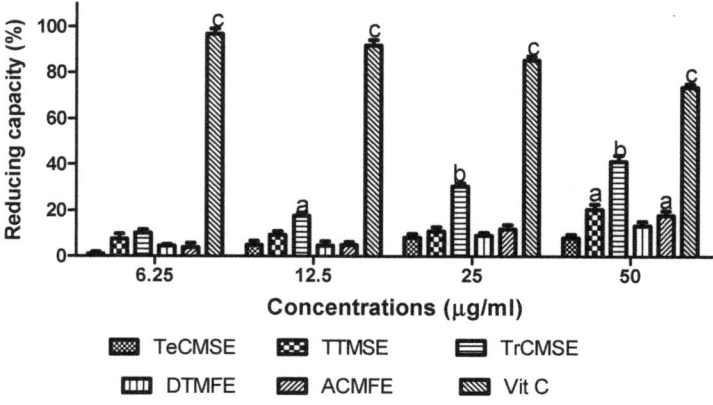

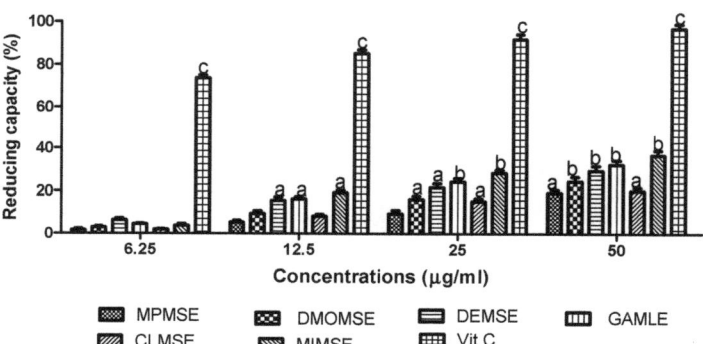

Figure 2. Reducing capacity of plant extracts. Plant reducing power was assessed via the ability to reduce ferric (Fe^{3+}) to ferrous (Fe^{2+}) iron. The percentage increase of reductive capacity with increasing plant extract concentration was determined. Vitamin C was used as a positive control. Results are expressed as means ± SEM for three separate experiments at each concentration. TeCMSE, *Terminalia catappa* methanolic seed extract; TTMSE, *Tetrapleura tetraptera* methanolic seed extract; TrCMSE, *Tricosanthes cucumerina* methanolic seed extract; DTMFE, *Dennettia tripetala* methanolic fruit extract; ACMFE, *Artocarpus communis* methanolic fruit extract; MPMSE, *Musa parasidisiaca* methanolic stem-bark extract; DMOMSE, Defatted *Moringa oleifera* methanolic seed extract; DEMSE, *Dacroydes edulis* methanolic seed extract; GAMLE, *Gnetum africanum* methanolic leaf extract; CLMSE, *Cola lepidota* methanolic seed extract; MIMSE, *Mangifera indica* methanolic stem-bark extract. Results are expressed as means ± SEM for three separate experiments at each concentration. For marked significance from controls, a: $p < 0.05$, b: $p < 0.01$, c: $p < 0.001$.

At a concentration of 50 µg/mL, all of the extracts demonstrated significant antioxidant effects except for TeCMSE and DTMFE when compared with Vitamin C (ascorbic acid). The highest antioxidant capacity was demonstrated by TCMSE2 (52%), MIMSE (40%) and then GAMLE (38%) relative to Vitamin C at 100%. The order of descending reducing capacity for the extracts was: TrCMSE > MIMSE > GAMLE > DEMSE > DMOMSE > ACMFE > CLMSE > MPMSE > DTMFE > TeCMSE.

3.3. Acetylcholinesterase Inhibitory Activity

Methanolic aqueous extracts of the inedible stem-bark, edible fruits, seeds, and leaf extracts of the evaluated plants displayed concentrations-dependent AChE inhibition, as shown in Figure 3.

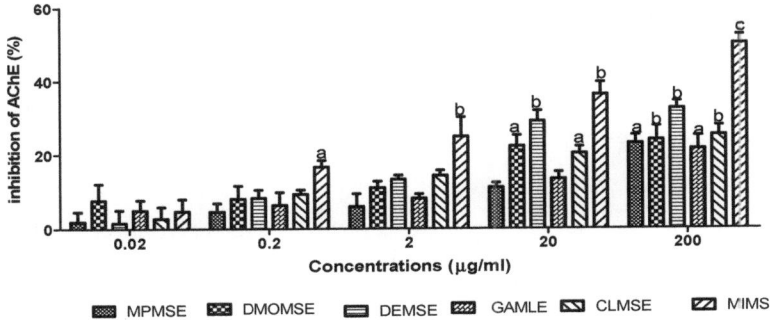

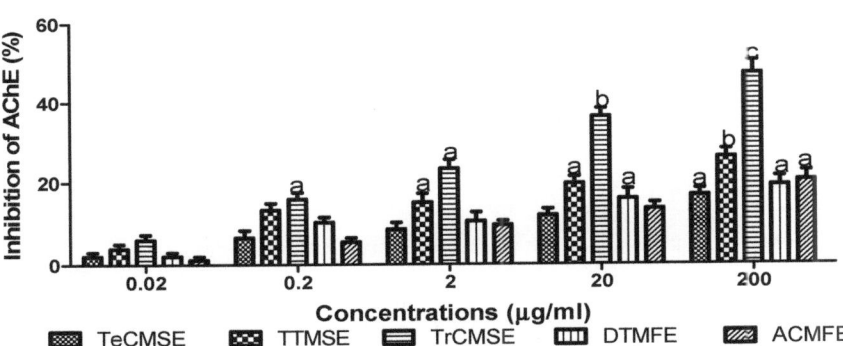

Figure 3. AChE inhibitory activity of plant extracts. Plant inhibition of AChE was measured using a modified Ellman assay, with percentage inhibition of AChE calculated relative to eserine. Results are expressed as means ± SEM for three separate experiments at each concentration. MPMSE, *Musa parasidisiaca* methanolic stem-bark extract; DMOMSE, Defatted *Moringa oleifera* methanolic seed extract; DEMSE, *Dacroydes edulis* methanolic seed extract; GAMLE, *Gnetum africanum* methanolic leaf extract; CLMSE, *Cola lepidota* methanolic seed extract; MIMSE, *Mangifera indica* methanolic stem-bark extract; TeCMSE, *Terminalia catappa* methanolic seed extract; TTMSE, *Tetrapleura tetraptera* methanolic seed extract; TrCMSE, *Tricosanthes cucumerina* methanolic seed extract; DTMFE, *Dennettia tripetala* methanolic fruit extract; ACMFE, *Artocarpus communis* methanolic fruit extract. Results are expressed as means ± SEM for three separate experiments at each concentration. For marked significance from controls, a: $p < 0.05$, b: $p < 0.01$, c: $p < 0.001$.

Across the investigated concentrations the level of AChE inhibition was used to generate IC_{50} concentrations (Table 1).

At the higher concentrations assayed, all evaluated extracts exhibited significant ($p < 0.001$) concentration dependent AChE inhibitory activity, with percentage AChE inhibitions at 200 µg/mL ranging from ≈17–50%. The descending order of AChE inhibitory activity for the extracts was MISME > TrCMSE > DEMSE > PPMS > TTMS > CLMSE > DMOMSE > MPMSE > GAMLE > ACMFE > TeCMSE.

The descending order of potency, as determined by IC_{50} values, were: MIMSE > TrCMSE > GAMLE > CLMSE > DEMSE > ACMFE > MPMSE > DTMSE > DMOMSE > TeCMSE > TTMSE.

3.4. Total Phenolic Content and Total Flavonoid Content

Total phenolic and total flavonoid contents were determined for each of the extracts and these have been included in Table 1. The relatively higher TPC levels (above 100 mg GAE/g) were observed for MISME, TrCMSE, GAMLE, CLMSE, and ACMFE at 156.2, 132.65, 123.26, 119.63, and 102.45 mg GAE/g, respectively. The relatively higher TFC levels (above 50 mg QUER/g) were recorded with MIMSE, GAMLE, ACMFE, CLMSE, TrCMSE, and DEMSE at 87.35, 73.26, 69.54, 68.35, 64.34, and 53.35 mg QUER/g, respectively.

3.5. Correlation between AChE Inhibition, Antioxidant Ability, and Total Phenolic and Flavonoid Contents

To consider if there was a relationship between AChE inhibition potency or DPPH radical scavenging potency and total phenolic or flavonoid content, Spearman rank correlations were calculated. The correlation coefficients (R-values) and significance of association (p-values) are shown in Table 2. The ability of extracts to inhibit AChE (measured as increasing IC_{50} values i.e., reduced potency) was significantly inversely correlated with increasing phenolic or increasing flavonoid content. Hence, extracts that displayed relatively high AChE inhibitory activity also retained relatively high phenolic or flavonoid content. By comparison, there was a positive but non-significant correlation between AChE inhibitory potency and either DPPH radical potency, or total phenolic or flavonoid content (Table 2).

Table 2. Correlation variables for AChE IC_{50}, DPPH radical scavenging IC_{50} and total phenolic and flavonoid content of the evaluated food sources.

Assessment	AChE Inhibition (IC_{50})	DPPH Radical Scavenging (IC_{50})
AChE inhibition (IC_{50})		R = 0.243 p = 0.42
DPPH Radical scavenging (IC_{50})	R = 0.243 p = 0.42	
Total phenolics	R = −0.972 p = 0.0001	R = 0.488 p = 0.127
Total flavonoids	R = −0.84 p = 0.0012	R = 0.392 p = 0.232

4. Discussion

Medicinal plants, spices, fruits, seeds, or vegetables provide an array of chemical entities with therapeutic potential. For example, medicinal plants may provide antioxidants in the form of flavonoids or polyphenols that are valuable assets for protection against oxidative stress and associated diseases. The public and scientific interest regarding the utilization of natural antioxidants continues to grow due to their potential or indeed perceived health-promoting effects.

Our analyses have shown *M. parasidisiaca* (106 µg/mL), *D. tripetala* (136 µg/mL), defatted *M. oleifera* (138 µg/mL), *T. tetraptera* (205 µg/mL), *T. catappa* (302 µg/mL) and *M. indica* (321 µg/mL) have highly active and significant DPPH (IC_{50}) radical scavenging abilities. Other independent studies have also reported antioxidant properties of *M. parasidisiaca* [58–60], *D. tripetala* [61] *M. oleifera* [62,63], *T. tetraptera* [64,65], *T. catappa* [66], *M. indica* [67,68], and *T. cucumenina* [69,70]. Additionally, the protective effect of a natural extract from the stem-bark of *M. indica* was able to counter age-associated oxidative stress in elderly humans, indicative of its potential to act as a nutraceutical in vivo [68]. The antioxidant effects of the fruit of *Artrocarpus communis* [71] and the leaves of *Dacroydes edulis* [72] have also been reported. Interestingly, fruit (*Dacroydes edulis*) and vegetable (*Gnetum africanum*) intake and an imbalance of oxidant/antioxidant status was reported to be associated with the development of diabetic retinopathy [72], with a recommendation that a diet rich in antioxidant supplements and tight glycemic control could postpone the onset of diabetic retinopathy [72].

The assessment of diets in a number of epidemiological studies and via quantitative evaluation have suggested that adherence to a Mediterranean-style diet and diets rich in fruits and vegetables may have protective benefits against age-related cognitive decline and neurodegenerative diseases [73–82]. This led us to consider the acetylcholinesterase inhibitory activity of these plants, since cholinesterase inhibitors are the mainstay of treatment for mild to moderate AD. An assessment of the potencies of a broad number of plant anticholinesterases inhibitors has been undertaken [83,84], with IC_{50} values ranging from 0.3 to 100.4 µg/mL. Hence, the plant extracts analyzed herein only displayed mild or moderate anti-AChE activities, with *M. indica* the most potent (IC_{50} of 111.9 µg/mL). Nevertheless, although only relatively weak cholinesterase inhibitors per se, chronic consumption of these foodstuffs might still provide provision of chemical entities able to ameliorate development or propagation of neurodegenerative disease. Indeed, an aqueous decoction of mango (*Mangifera indica* L.) stem bark has been developed on an industrial scale to be used as a nutritional supplement, cosmetic, and as a nutraceutical with neuroprotective effects [68,85,86]. Furthermore, neuroprotective effects of *Moringa oleifera* seed extract [52,53] and likewise *T. tetraptera* have also been demonstrated [48].

Our study also quantified the levels of phenolics and flavonoids, as these phytochemicals are widely distributed in the plant kingdom and possess antioxidant and anti-inflammatory activities [87]. Many of the active extracts investigated possessed high polyphenols and flavonoids content (Table 1) comparable to gallic acid and quercetin, respectively. Certain dietary phytochemicals, such as polyphenols have been reported to possess potential protection of cognitive function during aging [88] and may serve as natural neuroprotective agents [89–91]. In addition to their action as neuroprotective agents, flavonoids may also be efficacious candidates as potential pharmaceuticals or nutraceuticals for the treatment of AD [92]. Antioxidant activities of green tea phytochemicals and nutraceuticals such as curcumin, catechins, lycopene, resveratrol, piperine, and anthocyanins, have been reported using in vitro and in vivo models [93,94].

Of interest, there was a significant inverse correlation between the potency of AChE inhibition (IC_{50} values) and total phenolic or flavonoid contents. This suggests that the agent(s) responsible for the AChE inhibitory activity are resident within the phenolic and flavonoid compounds. By contrast, there was no significant correlation between the AChE inhibition potency and that for DPPH radical scavenging, suggesting that the agent(s) that provide AChE inhibition is different from that for radical scavenging. Likewise, there was no correlation between AChE inhibitory potency and antioxidant activity, or between antioxidant activity and TPC or TFC, hence the chemical agent(s) that provided antioxidant protection were not AChE inhibitors, or likely to be abundant polyphenols or flavonoids.

A clear limitation of our study is that we have only assessed in vitro properties of these plant parts and their respective polyphenol and flavonoid content. We are unable to directly comment on how much of these foodstuffs are typically eaten, and indeed this will vary extensively between peoples and their food preparation methods. However, irrespective of these limitations, it is provocative to propose that a suitable diet rich in certain phytochemicals may provide beneficial counter-measures against oxidative stress-induced damage and its impact upon disease pathogenesis and propagation.

Author Contributions: L.L.N. was involved with conception and design of the study, performed experiments, collection and assemblage of the data, drafting of the article and final approval of the article, provided administrative, technical and logistic support. P.C.N.A. provided the plant materials used for this investigation. E.E. performed experiments, analyzed and interpreted the data, and provided statistical expertise. W.G.C. participated in critical editing and revision of the article for important intellectual content; provision of laboratory space and funding.

Funding: This research received no external funding.

Acknowledgments: The authors are grateful to the University of Nottingham for the International Visiting Fellowship grants awarded to W.G.C. to support L.L.N. and E.E.

Conflicts of Interest: The authors confirm that there are no conflicts of interest connected with the publication of this manuscript. The funding sponsor had no role in the design of this study; in the collection, analyses, or interpretation of data; in the writing of the manuscript; or in the decision to publish the results in this journal.

References

1. Chen, Q.; Wang, Q.; Zhu, J.; Xiao, Q.; Zhang, L. Reactive oxygen species: Key regulators in vascular health and diseases. *Br. J. Pharmacol.* **2018**, *175*, 1279–1292. [CrossRef]
2. Birben, E.; Sahiner, U.M.; Sackesen, C.; Erzurum, S.; Kalayci, O. Oxidative stress and antioxidant defenses. *World Allergy Organ. J.* **2012**, *5*, 9–19. [CrossRef] [PubMed]
3. Espinosa-Diez, C.; Miguel, V.; Mennerich, D.; Kietzmann, T.; Sánchez-Pérez, P.; Cadenas, S.; Lamas, S. Antioxidant responses and cellular adjustments to oxidative stress. *Redox Biol.* **2015**, *6*, 183–197. [CrossRef] [PubMed]
4. Dadhania, V.P.; Trivedi, P.P.; Vikram, A.; Tripathi, D.N. Nutraceuticals against Neurodegeneration: A Mechanistic Insight. *Curr. Neuropharmacol.* **2016**, *14*, 627–640. [CrossRef] [PubMed]
5. Sadhukhan, P.; Saha, S.; Dutta, S.; Mahalanobish, S.; Sil, P.C. Nutraceuticals: An emerging therapeutic approach against the pathogenesis of Alzheimer's disease. *Pharmacol. Res.* **2018**, *129*, 100–114. [CrossRef]
6. Gupta, R.K.; Patel, A.K.; Shah, N.; Chaudhary, A.K.; Jha, U.K.; Yadav, U.C.; Gupta, P.K.; Pakuwal, U. Oxidative stress and antioxidants in disease and cancer: A review. *Asian Pac. J Cancer Prev.* **2014**, *15*, 4405–4409. [CrossRef] [PubMed]
7. Lobo, V.; Patil, A.; Phatak, A.; Chandra, N. Free radicals, antioxidants and functional foods: Impact on human health. *Pharmacogn. Rev.* **2010**, *4*, 118–126. [CrossRef] [PubMed]
8. Perez-Vizcaino, F.; Fraga, C.G. Research trends in flavonoids and health. *Arch. Biochem. Biophys.* **2018**, *646*, 107–112. [CrossRef]
9. Krzyzanowska, J.; Czubacka, A.; Oleszek, W. Dietary phytochemicals and human. *Adv. Exp. Med. Biol.* **2010**, *698*, 74–98.
10. Pratico, D.; Clark, C.M.; Liun, F.; Rokach, J.; Lee, V.Y.; Trojanowski, J.Q. Increase of brain oxidative stress in mild cognitive impairment: A possible predictor of Alzheimer disease. *Arch. Neurol.* **2002**, *59*, 972–976. [CrossRef]
11. Barnham, K.J.; Masters, C.L.; Bush, A.I. Neurodegenerative diseases and oxidative stress. *Nat. Rev. Drug Discov.* **2004**, *3*, 205–214. [CrossRef] [PubMed]
12. Keller, J.N.; Schmitt, F.A.; Scheff, S.W.; Ding, Q.; Chen, Q.; Butterfield, D.A.; Markesbery, W.R. Evidence of increased oxidative damage in subjects with mild cognitive impairment. *Neurology* **2005**, *64*, 1152–1156. [CrossRef] [PubMed]
13. Guidi, I.; Galimberti, D.; Lonati, S.; Novembrino, C.; Bamonti, F.; Tiriticco, M.; Fenoglio, C.; Venturelli, E.; Baron, P.; Bresolin, N.; et al. Oxidative imbalance in patients with mild cognitive impairment and Alzheimer's disease. *Neurobiol. Aging* **2006**, *27*, 262–269. [CrossRef] [PubMed]
14. Butterfield, D.A.; Boyd-Kimball, D. Oxidative Stress, Amyloid-β Peptide, and Altered Key Molecular Pathways in the Pathogenesis and Progression of Alzheimer's Disease. *J. Alzheimer Dis.* **2018**, *62*, 1345–1367. [CrossRef] [PubMed]
15. Da Costa, L.A.; Badawi, A.; El-Sohemy, A. Nutrigenetics and modulation of oxidative stress. *Ann. Nutr. Metab.* **2012**, *60*, 27–36. [CrossRef] [PubMed]
16. Thapa, A.; Carroll, N.J. Dietary Modulation of Oxidative Stress in Alzheimer's Disease. *Int. J. Mol. Sci.* **2017**, *18*, 1583. [CrossRef]
17. Ravi, S.K.; Narasingappa, R.B.; Vincent, B. Neuro-nutrients as anti-Alzheimer's disease agents: A critical review. *Crit. Rev. Food Sci. Nutr.* **2018**, *30*, 1–20. [CrossRef] [PubMed]
18. Lopes da Silva, S.; Vellas, B.; Elemans, S.; Luchsinger, J.; Kamphuis, P.; Yaffe, K.; Sijben, J.; Groenendijk, M.; Stijnen, T. Plasma nutrient status of patients with Alzheimer's disease: Systematic review and meta-analysis. *Alzheimer Dement.* **2014**, *10*, 485–502. [CrossRef]
19. Irvine, F.R. *Woody Plants of Ghana with Special Reference to Their Uses*; Oxford University Press: London, UK, 1961.
20. Leakay, R.R.B. Potential for Novel food products from Agroforestry Trees. A review. *Food Chem.* **1999**, *66*, 1–4. [CrossRef]

21. Erukainure, O.L.; Mopuri, R.; Oyebode, O.A.; Koorbanally, N.A.; Islam, M.S. *Dacryodes edulis* enhances antioxidant activities, suppresses DNA fragmentation in oxidative pancreatic and hepatic injuries; and inhibits carbohydrate digestive enzymes linked to type 2 diabetes. *Biomed. Pharmacother.* **2017**, *96*, 37–47. [CrossRef]
22. Tee, L.H.; Yang, B.; Nagendra, K.P.; Ramanan, R.N.; Sun, J.; Chan, E.S.; Tey, B.T.; Azlan, A.; Ismail, A.; Lau, C.Y.; et al. Nutritional compositions and bioactivities of Dacryodes species: A review. *Food Chem.* **2014**, *165*, 247–255. [CrossRef] [PubMed]
23. Atawodi, S.E. Nigerian foodstuffs with prostate cancer chemopreventive polyphenols. *Infect. Agent Cancer* **2011**, *6*, S9. [CrossRef] [PubMed]
24. Rusell, T.A. The *cola* of Nigeria and Cameroon. *Trop. Agric.* **1955**, *32*, 210–240.
25. Engel, N.; Opermann, C.; Falodun, A.; Udo, K. Proliferative effects of five traditional Nigerian medicinal plant extracts on human breast and bone cancer cell lines. *J. Ethnopharmacol.* **2011**, *137*, 1003–1010. [CrossRef]
26. Oghenerobo, V.I.; Falodun, A. Antioxidant activities of the leaf extract and fractions of *Cola lepidota*, K. Schum (Sterculiaceae). *Niger. J. Biotechnol.* **2013**, *25*, 31–36.
27. Essien, E.E.; Peter, N.S.; Akpan, S.M. Chemical Composition and Antioxidant Property of Two Species of Monkey Kola (*Cola rostrata* and *Cola lepidota*, K. Schum) Extracts. *Eur. J. Med. Plants* **2015**, *7*, 31–37. [CrossRef]
28. Ene-Obong, H.N.; Okudu, H.O.; Asumugha, U.V. Nutrient and phytochemical composition of two varieties of Monkey kola (*Cola parchycarpa and Cola lepidota*): An under utilised fruit. *Food Chem.* **2016**, *193*, 154–159. [CrossRef]
29. Jayaweera, D.M.A. *Medicinal Plants (Indigenous and Exotic) Used in Ceylon Part 2*; National Science Council of Sri Lanka: Colombo, Sri Lanka, 1980; pp. 162–163.
30. Sandhya, S.; Vinod, K.; Chandra, S.; Aradhana, R.; Vamshi, S. An Updated Review on *Trichosanthes cucumerina*, L. *Int. J. Pharm. Sci. Rev. Res.* **2010**, *1*, 56–58.
31. Shah, S.L.; Mali, V.R.; Zambare, G.N.; Bodhankar, S.L. Cardioprotective activity of methanol extract of fruit of *Trichosanthes cucumerina* on doxorubicin-induced cardiotoxicity in Wistar rats. *Toxicol. Int* **2012**, *19*, 167–172. [CrossRef]
32. Adjalian, E.; Sessou, P.; Fifa, TD.; Dangou, B.J.; Odjo, T.; Figueredo, G.; Noudogbessi, J.P.; Kossou, D.; Menut, C.; Sohounhloue, D. Chemical composition and bioefficacy of *Dennettia tripetala* and *Uvariodendron angustifolium* leaves essential oils against the angoumois grain moth, *Sitotroga cerealella*. *Int. J. Biosci.* **2014**, *5*, 161–172.
33. Oyemitan, I.A.; Iwalewa, E.O.; Akanmu, M.A.; Olugbade, T.A. Antinociceptive and anti-inflammatory effects of essential oil of *Dennettia tripetala*, G. Baker in rodents. *Afr. J. Tradit. Complement.* **2008**, *5*, 355–362. [CrossRef]
34. Lewis, K.; Ausubel, F.M. Prospects for plant-derived anti-bacterial. *Nat. Biotechnol.* **2006**, *24*, 1504–1507. [CrossRef] [PubMed]
35. Lee, C.W.; Ko, H.H.; Lin, C.C.; Chai, C.Y.; Chen, W.T.; Yen, F.L. Effect of *Artocarpus communis* Extract on UVB Irradiation-Induced Oxidative Stress and Inflammation in Hairless Mice. *Int. J. Mol. Sci.* **2013**, *14*, 3860–3873. [CrossRef] [PubMed]
36. Arung, E.T.; Wicaksono, B.D.; Handoko, Y.A.; Kusuma, I.W.; Shizu, K.; Yulia, D.; Sandra, F. Cytotoxic effect of artocarpin on T47D cells. *J. Nat. Med.* **2010**, *64*, 423–429. [CrossRef]
37. Tzeng, C.W.; Tzeng, W.S.; Lin, L.T.; Lee, C.W.; Yen, F.L.; Lin, C.C. *Artocarpus communis* induces Autophagic Instead of Apoptotic Cell Death in Human Hepatocellular Carcinoma Cells. *Phytomedicine* **2015**, *23*, 528–540. [CrossRef]
38. Lin, J.A.; Fang, S.C.; Wu, C.H.; Huang, S.M.; Yen, G.C. Anti-inflammatory effect of the 5,7,4'-trihydroxy-6-geranylflavanone isolated from the fruit of *Artocarpus communis* in S100B-induced human monocytes. *J. Agric. Food Chem.* **2011**, *59*, 105–111. [CrossRef] [PubMed]
39. Hsu, C.L.; Chang, F.R.; Tseng, P.Y.; Chen, Y.F.; El-Shazly, M.; Du, Y.C.; Fang, S.C. Geranyl flavonoid derivatives from the fresh leaves of *Artocarpus communis* and their anti-inflammatory activity. *Planta Med.* **2012**, *78*, 995–1001. [CrossRef]
40. Han, A.R.; Kang, YJ.; Windono, T.; Lee, S.K.; Seo, E.K. Prenylated flavonoids from the heartwood of *Artocarpus communis* with inhibitory activity on lipopolysaccharide-induced nitric oxide production. *J. Nat. Prod.* **2006**, *69*, 719–721. [CrossRef]

41. Anand, A.V.; Divya, N.; Kotti, P.P. An updated review of *Terminalia catappa*. *Pharmacog. Rev.* **2015**, *9*, 93–98. [CrossRef]
42. Singhal, A.K.; Naithani, V.; Bangar, O.P. Medicinal Plants with a Potential to Treat Alzheimer and Associated Symptoms. *Intern. J. Nutr. Pharmacol. Neurol. Dis.* **2012**, *2*, 84–91. [CrossRef]
43. Galuppo, M.; Giacoppo, S.; Iori, R.; De Nicola, G.R.; Milardi, D.; Bramanti, P.; Mazzon, E. 4(α-L-rhamnosyloxy)-benzyl isothiocyanate, a bioactive phytochemical that defends cerebral tissue and prevents severe damage induced by focal ischemia/reperfusion. *J. Biol. Regul. Homeost. Agents* **2015**, *29*, 343–356. [PubMed]
44. Jaafaru, M.S.; Nordin, N.; Shaari, K.; Rosli, R.; Abdull Razis, A.F. Isothiocyanate from *Moringa oleifera* seeds mitigates hydrogen peroxide-induced cytotoxicity and preserved morphological features of human neuronal cells. *PLoS ONE* **2018**, *13*, e0196403. [CrossRef] [PubMed]
45. Mensah, J.K.; Ikhajiagbe, B.; Edema, N.E.; Emokhor, J. Phytochemical, nutritional and antibacterial properties of dried leaf powder of *Moringa oleifera* (Lam.) from Edo Central Province Nigeria. *J. Nat. Prod. Plant Resour.* **2012**, *2*, 107–112.
46. Essien, E.U.; Izunwane, B.C.; Aremu, C.Y.; Eka, O.U. Significance for humans of the nutrient contents of the dry fruit of *Tetrapleura tetraptera*. *Food Hum. Nutr.* **1994**, *45*, 47–51. [CrossRef]
47. Aladesanmi, J.A. *Tetrapleura tetraptera*: Molluscicidal activity and chemical constituents. *Afr. J. Tradit. Complement. Altern. Med.* **2007**, *4*, 23–26. [CrossRef]
48. Odubanjo, V.O.; Ibukun, E.O.; Oboh, G.; Adefegha, S.A. Aqueous extracts of two tropical ethnobotanicals (*Tetrapleura tetraptera* and *Quassia undulata*) improved spatial and non-spatial working memories in scopolamine-induced amnesic rats: Influence of neuronal cholinergic and antioxidant systems. *Biomed. Pharmacother.* **2018**, *99*, 198–204. [CrossRef] [PubMed]
49. Ali, F.; Assanta, M.A.; Robert, C. *Gnetum africanum*: A wild food plant from the African forest with many nutritional and medicinal properties. *J. Med. Food* **2011**, *14*, 1289–1297. [CrossRef]
50. Alozie, Y.E.; Ene-Obong, H.N. Recipe standardization, nutrient composition and sensory evaluation of waterleaf (*Talinum triangulare*) and wild spinach (*Gnetum africanum*) soup "afang" commonly consumed in South-south Nigeria. *Food Chem.* **2018**, *238*, 65–72. [CrossRef]
51. Lavanya, K.; Abi Beaulah, G.; Vani, G. *Musa Parasidisiaca*—A review of phytochemistry and pharmacology. *World J. Pharm. Med. Res.* **2016**, *2*, 163–173.
52. Masibo, M.; He, Q. Mango Bioactive Compounds and Related Nutraceutical Properties—A Review. *Food Rev. Int.* **2009**, *25*, 346–370. [CrossRef]
53. Lauricella, M.; Emanuele, S.; Calvaruso, G.; Giuliano, M.; D'Anneo, A. Multifaceted Health Benefits of *Mangifera indica*, L. (Mango): The Inestimable Value of Orchards Recently Planted in Sicilian Rural Areas. *Nutrients* **2017**, *9*, 525. [CrossRef]
54. Nwidu, L.L.; Elmorsy, E.; Thornton, J.; Wijamunige, B.; Wijesekara, A.; Tarbox, R.; Warren, A.; Carter, W.G. Anti-acetylcholinesterase activity and antioxidant properties of extracts and fractions of *Carpolobia lutea*. *Pharm. Biol.* **2017**, *55*, 1875–1883. [CrossRef] [PubMed]
55. Ellman, G.L.; Courtney, K.D.; Andres, V.; Featherstone, R.M. A new and rapid colorimetric determination of acetylcholinesterase activity. *Biochem. Pharmacol.* **1961**, *7*, 88–95. [CrossRef]
56. Carter, W.G.; Tarhoni, M.; Rathbone, A.J.; Ray, D.E. Differential protein adduction by seven organophosphorus pesticides in both brain and thymus. *Hum. Exp. Toxicol.* **2007**, *26*, 347–353. [CrossRef] [PubMed]
57. Carter, W.G.; Tarhoni, M.H.; Ray, D.E. Analytical approaches to investigate protein-pesticide adducts. *J. Chromatogr. B* **2010**, *878*, 1312–1319. [CrossRef] [PubMed]
58. Vijayakumar, S.; Presannakumar, G.; Vijayalakshmi, N.R. Antioxidant activity of banana flavonoids. *Fitoterapia* **2008**, *79*, 279–282. [CrossRef] [PubMed]
59. Loganayaki, N.; Rajendrakumaran, D.; Manian, S. Antioxidant capacity and phenolic content of different solvent extracts from banana (*Musa paradisiaca*) and mustai (*Rivea hypocrateriformis*). *Food Sci. Biotechnol.* **2010**, *19*, 1251–1258. [CrossRef]
60. Panigrahi, P.N.; Dey, S.; Sahoo, M.; Dan, A. Antiurolithiatic and antioxidant efficacy of *Musa paradisiaca* pseudostem on ethylene glycol-induced nephrolithiasis in rat. *Indian J. Pharmacol.* **2017**, *49*, 77–83. [PubMed]

61. Okoh, S.O.; Iweriegbor, B.C.; Okoh, O.O.; Nwodo, U.U.I.; Okoh, A. Bactericidal and antioxidant properties of essential oils from the fruits *Dennettia tripetala* G. Baker. *BMC Complement. Altern. Med.* **2016**, *16*, 486. [CrossRef]
62. Randriamboavonjy, J.I.; Rio, M.; Pacaud, P.; Loirand, G.; Tesse, A. *Moringa oleifera* Seeds Attenuate Vascular Oxidative and Nitrosative Stresses in Spontaneously Hypertensive Rats. *Oxid. Med. Cell Longev.* **2017**, *2017*, 4129459. [CrossRef]
63. Lamou, B.; Taiwe, G.S.; Hamadou, A.; Abene; Houlray, J.; Atour, M.M.; Tan, P.V. Antioxidant and Antifatigue Properties of the Aqueous Extract of *Moringa oleifera* in Rats Subjected to Forced Swimming Endurance Test. *Oxid. Med. Cell Longev.* **2016**, *2016*, 3517824. [CrossRef] [PubMed]
64. Moukette, B.M.; Pieme, A.C.; Biapa, P.C.; Njimou, J.R.; Stoller, M.; Bravi, M.; Yonkeu, N.J. In Vitro Ion Chelating, Antioxidative Mechanism of Extracts from Fruits and Barks of *Tetrapleura tetraptera* and Their Protective Effects against Fenton Mediated Toxicity of Metal Ions on Liver Homogenates. *Evid. Based Complement. Altern. Med.* **2015**, *2015*, 423689. [CrossRef] [PubMed]
65. Ene-Obong, H.; Onuoha, N.; Aburime, L.; Mbah, O. Chemical composition and antioxidant activities of some indigenous spices consumed in Nigeria. *Food Chem.* **2018**, *238*, 58–64. [CrossRef] [PubMed]
66. Pandya, N.B.; Tigari, P.; Dupadahalli, K.; Kamurthy, H.; Nadendla, R.R. Antitumor and antioxidant status of *Terminalia catappa* against Ehrlich ascites carcinoma in Swiss albino mice. *Indian J. Pharmacol.* **2013**, *45*, 464–469.
67. Núñez-Sellés, A.J.; Vélez Castro, H.T.; Agüero-Agüero, J.; González-González, J.; Naddeo, F.; De Simone, F.; Rastrelli, L. Isolation and quantitative analysis of phenolic antioxidants, free sugars, and polyols from mango (*Mangifera indica* L.) stem bark aqueous decoction used in Cuba as a nutritional supplement. *J. Agric. Food Chem.* **2002**, *50*, 762–766. [CrossRef]
68. Pardo-Andreu, G.L.; Philip, S.J.; Riaño, A.; Sánchez, C.; Viada, C.; Núñez-Sellés, A.J.; Delgado, R. *Mangifera indica*, L. (Vimang) Protection against Serum Oxidative Stress in Elderly Humans. *Arch Med. Res.* **2006**, *37*, 158–164. [CrossRef] [PubMed]
69. Arawwawala, M.; Thabrew, I.; Arambewela, L. In vitro and in vivo evaluation of antioxidant activity of *Trichosanthes cucumerina* aerial parts. *Acta Biol. Hung.* **2011**, *62*, 235–243. [CrossRef] [PubMed]
70. Bamidele, O.P.; Fasogbon, M.B. Chemical and antioxidant properties of snake tomato (*Trichosanthes cucumerina*) juice and Pineapple (*Ananas comosus*) juice blends and their changes during storage. *Food Chem.* **2017**, *220*, 184–189. [CrossRef]
71. Lee, C.W.; Ko, H.H.; Lin, C.C.; Chai, C.Y.; Chen, W.T.; Yen, F.L. Artocarpin attenuates ultraviolet B-induced skin damage in hairless mice by antioxidant and anti-inflammatory effect. *Food Chem. Toxicol.* **2013**, *60*, 123–129. [CrossRef]
72. Moise, M.M.; Benjamin, L.M.; Etienne, M.; Thierry, G.; Ndembe Dalida, K.; Doris, T.M.; Samy, W.M. Intake of *Gnetum africanum* and *Dacryodes edulis*, imbalance of oxidant/antioxidant status and prevalence of diabetic retinopathy in central Africans. *PLoS ONE* **2012**, *7*, e49411. [CrossRef]
73. Martinez-Lapiscina, E.H.; Clavero, P.; Toledo, E.; Estruch, R.; Salas-Salvado, J.; San Julian, B.; Sanchez-Tainta, A.; Ros, E.; Valls-Pedret, C.; Martinez-Gonzalez, M.Á. Mediterranean diet improves cognition: The PREDIMED-NAVARRA randomised trial. *J. Neurol. Neurosurg. Psychiatry* **2013**, *84*, 1318–1325. [CrossRef] [PubMed]
74. Jin, Y.; Oh, K.; Oh, S.I.; Baek, H.; Kim, S.H.; Park, Y. Dietary intake of fruits and beta-carotene is negatively associated with amyotrophic lateral sclerosis risk in Koreans: A case-control study. *Nutr. Neurosci.* **2014**, *17*, 104–108. [CrossRef]
75. Hardman, R.J.; Kennedy, G.; Macpherson, H.; Scholey, A.B.; Pipingas, A. Adherence to a Mediterranean-style diet and effects on cognition in adults: A qualitative evaluation and systematic review of longitudinal and prospective trials. *Front. Nutr.* **2016**, *3*, 22. [CrossRef] [PubMed]
76. Dai, Q.; Borenstein, A.R.; Wu, Y.; Jackson, J.C.; Larson, E.B. Fruit and vegetable juices and Alzheimer's disease: The Kame Project. *Am. J. Med.* **2006**, *119*, 751–759. [CrossRef] [PubMed]
77. Fischer, K.; Melo van Lent, D.; Wolfsgruber, S.; Weinhold, L.; Kleineidam, L.; Bickel, H.; Scherer, M.; Eisele, M.; van den Bussche, H.; Wiese, B.; et al. Prospective Associations between Single Foods, Alzheimer's Dementia and Memory Decline in the Elderly. *Nutrients* **2018**, *10*, 852. [CrossRef] [PubMed]

78. Arnim, C.A.; Herbolsheimer, F.; Nikolaus, T.; Peter, R.; Biesalski, H.K.; Ludolph, A.C.; Riepe, M.; Nagel, G.; ActiFE Ulm Study Group. Dietary antioxidants and dementia in a population-based case-control study among older people in South Germany. *J. Alzheimer Dis.* **2012**, *31*, 717–724. [CrossRef]
79. Dardiotis, E.; Kosmidis, M.H.; Yannakoulia, M.; Hadjigeorgiou, G.M.; Scarmeas, N. The Hellenic Longitudinal Investigation of Aging and Diet (HELIAD): Rationale, study design, and cohort description. *Neuroepidemiology* **2014**, *43*, 9–14. [CrossRef]
80. De Rest, O.; Wang, Y.; Barnes, L.L.; Tangney, C.; Bennett, D.A.; Morris, M.C. APOE ε4 and the associations of seafood and long-chain omega-3 fatty acids with cognitive decline. *Neurology* **2016**, *86*, 2063–2070. [CrossRef]
81. Loughrey, D.G.; Lavecchia, S.; Brennan, S.; Lawlor, B.A.; Kelly, M.E. The Impact of the Mediterranean Diet on the Cognitive Functioning of Healthy Older Adults: A Systematic Review and Meta-Analysis. *Adv. Nutr. Bethesda* **2017**, *8*, 571–586.
82. Gardener, H.; Caunca, M.R. Mediterranean Diet in Preventing Neurodegenerative Diseases. *Curr. Nutr. Rep.* **2018**, *7*, 10–20. [CrossRef]
83. Murray, A.P.; Faraoni, M.B.; Castro, M.J.; Alza, N.P.; Cavallaro, V. Natural AChE inhibitors from plants and their contribution to Alzheimer's disease therapy. *Curr. Neuropharmacol.* **2013**, *11*, 388–413. [CrossRef] [PubMed]
84. Dos Santos, T.C.; Gomes, T.M.; Pinto, B.A.S.; Camara, A.L.; Paes, A.M.A. Naturally occurring anticholinesterases inhibitors and their potential use for Alzheimer's disease therapy. *Front. Pharmacol.* **2018**, *9*, 1192. [CrossRef]
85. Kawpoomhae, K.; Sukma, M.; Ngawhirunpat, T.; Opanasopit, P.; Sripattanaporn, A. Antioxidant and neuroprotective effects of standardized extracts of *Mangifera indica* leaf. *J. Pharm. Sci.* **2010**, *34*, 32–43.
86. Infante-Garcia, C.; Ramos-Rodriguez, J.J.; Delgado-Olmos, I.; Gamero-Carrasco, C.; Fernandez-Ponce, M.T.; Casas, L.; Mantell, C.; Garcia-Alloza, M. Long-Term Mangiferin Extract Treatment Improves Central Pathology and Cognitive Deficits in APP/PS1 Mice. *Mol. Neurobiol.* **2017**, *54*, 4696–4704. [CrossRef] [PubMed]
87. Biesalski, H.K. Polyphenols and inflammation: Basic interactions. *Curr. Opin. Clin. Nutr. Metab. Care* **2007**, *10*, 724–728. [CrossRef]
88. Thangthaeng, N.; Poulose, S.M.; Miller, M.G.; Shukitt-Hale, B. Preserving brain function in aging: The anti-glycative potential of berry fruit. *Neuromol. Med.* **2016**, *18*, 465–473. [CrossRef]
89. Ataie, A.; Shadifar, M.; Ataee, R. Polyphenolic antioxidants and neuronal regeneration. *Basic Clin. Neurosci.* **2016**, *7*, 81–90. [CrossRef]
90. Almeida, S.; Alves, M.G.; Sousa, M.; Oliveira, P.F.; Silva, B.M. Are Polyphenols Strong Dietary Agents Against Neurotoxicity and Neurodegeneration? *Neurotox. Res.* **2016**, *30*, 345–366. [CrossRef]
91. Ruan, Q.; Ruan, J.; Zhang, W.; Qian, F.; Yu, Z. Targeting NAD$^+$ degradation: The therapeutic potential of flavonoids for Alzheimer's disease and cognitive frailty. *Pharmacol. Res.* **2018**, *128*, 345–358. [CrossRef]
92. Darvesh, A.S.; Carroll, R.T.; Bishayee, A.; Geldenhuys, W.J.; Van der Schyf, C.J. Oxidative stress and Alzheimer's disease: Dietary polyphenols as potential therapeutic agents. *Expert Rev. Neurother.* **2010**, *10*, 729–745. [CrossRef]
93. Arab, H.; Mahjoub, S.; Hajian-Tilaki, K.; Moghadasi, M. The effect of green tea consumption on oxidative stress markers and cognitive function in patients with Alzheimer's disease: A prospective intervention study. *Caspian J. Int. Med.* **2016**, *7*, 188–194.
94. Rice-Evans, C.; Miller, N.; Paganga, G. Antioxidant properties of phenolic compounds. *Trends Plant Sci.* **1997**, *2*, 152–159. [CrossRef]

© 2019 by the authors. Licensee MDPI, Basel, Switzerland. This article is an open access article distributed under the terms and conditions of the Creative Commons Attribution (CC BY) license (http://creativecommons.org/licenses/by/4.0/).

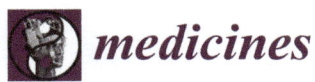

Article

Antioxidant and Anti-Inflammatory Activities of Fractions from *Bidens engleri* O.E. Schulz (Asteraceae) and *Boerhavia erecta* L. (Nyctaginaceae)

Moussa COMPAORE [1,2,*], Sahabi BAKASSO [3], Roland Nâg Tiero MEDA [4] and Odile Germaine NACOULMA [1]

1. Laboratory of Applied Biochemistry and Chemistry, University Ouaga I JKZ, Ouagadougou 03 BP 7021, Burkina Faso; odilenacoulma@yahoo.com
2. Culture Platform of Cell and Tissue (PCCT) U.F.R/S.V.T., University Ouaga I JKZ, Ouagadougou 09 BP 1001, Burkina Faso
3. Laboratory of Natural Products and Organic Synthesis, Department of Chemistry, Faculty of Science and Technology Abdou Moumouni University of Niamey, Niamey BP 10662, Niger; b_sahabi2000@yahoo.fr
4. Laboratory for Research and Education in Animal Health and Biotechnology, University Nazi Boni of Bobo-Dioulasso, Bobo-Dioulasso 01 BP 1091, Burkina Faso; meda_roland@yahoo.fr
* Correspondence: mcompaore_3@yahoo.fr or moussa.compaore@univ-ouaga.bf; Tel.: +226-700-647-42

Received: 25 May 2018; Accepted: 7 June 2018; Published: 12 June 2018

Abstract: Background: According to recent studies, reactive oxygen is the leader of human metabolic disease development. The use of natural antioxidants is the best way to stop or prevent this problem. Therefore, the aim of this study was to evaluate the antioxidant and anti-inflammatory activities and to determine the polyphenolic contents of the *Bidens engleri* and *Boerhavia erecta* fractions. **Methods:** Plant fractions were obtained using Soxhlet procedures with hexane, dichloromethane, acetonitrile, ethyl acetate, methanol, and butanol solvent, successively. The different fractions were compared according to their antioxidant, anti-inflammatory activities, total phenolic, and total flavonoid contents. The phenolic contribution to the biological activity was evaluated. **Result:** The *Bidens engleri* and *Boerhavia erecta* fractions showed the highest antioxidant abilities, notably the polar fractions, which inhibited significantly the radical 2,2-diphenyl-1-picrylhydrazyl (DPPH) and 2,2-O-azinobis(3-ethylbenzoline-6-sulphonate) (ABTS). The butanol fraction from *Bidens engleri* and methanol fraction from *Boerhavia erecta* have presented the best iron (III) reduction power with 211.68 and 198.55 mgAAE/g, respectively. Butanol and acetonitrile were the best solvents for extracting phenolic compounds from *Bidens engleri* and *Boerhavia erecta*, respectively. In contrast, dichloromethane was the best solvent for extracting a flavonoid from two plants with anti-COX-2 and anti-LOX-15 active compounds. The phenolic compound contributed significantly to antioxidant activity ($r > 0.80$). **Conclusion:** The *Bidens engleri* and *Boerhavia erecta* fractions possessed a potential antioxidant for fighting oxidative stress and helping to prevent diabetes, hypertension, and cardiovascular diseases. The uses of this plant could be promoted in Burkina Faso.

Keywords: antioxidants; cyclooxygenase; lipoxygenase; phenolic; flavonoid; traditional medicine

1. Introduction

Oxidative stress is an inevitable consequence of life in an oxygen-rich atmosphere. The environment is filled with a lot of reactive oxygen species (ROS) and reactive nitrogen species (RNS). In recent data, it was demonstrated that ROS and RNS played an important role in human disease development [1]. In Burkina Faso, some recent studies have shown some alarming data concerning the prevalence of metabolic diseases [2]. The oxidative stress plays a direct or indirect role in the pathophysiology of diseases, such as cancer, diabetes, and cardiovascular diseases [3,4]. However, the intake of natural antioxidants has been reported to reduce the risk of cancer, cardiovascular diseases, diabetes, and other diseases that are associated with aging [5,6].

Plants, fruits, vegetables, and medicinal herbs possess a wide variety of free radical scavenging biomolecules, such as phenolic compounds, flavonoids, vitamins, terpenoids, and some other endogenous phytometabolites, which are rich in antioxidant capacity [7–9]. *Bidens engleri* and *Boerhavia erecta* were some well-known medicinal plants in the Central Plateau, because they were used in the treatment of diabetes mellitus, hypertension, and old wounds [10]. According to Nacoulma's investigations, the traditional healers and herbalists used *Bidens engleri* and *Boerhavia erecta* in combination, for treating diabetes in Burkina Faso [10]. The same information was found in Cote d'Ivoire by ethnobotanical investigations [11].

The previous data demonstrated the antioxidant and anti-diabetic activities of *Boerhavia erecta* in India were associated with some polyphenolic compounds, such as phenolics and flavonoids [12,13]. Some antioxidant compounds, such as (+)-catechin (−)-epicatechin, quercetin, isorhamnetin, rutin, narcissin, isoquercitrin, and isorhamnetin 3-*O*-β-D-glucopyranoside, as well as other metabolites, were isolated from *B. erecta* leaves extract [14,15]. According to the medicinal importance of *B. engleri* and *B. erecta* in Burkina Faso, the present study aimed to highlight the potential of this plant by determining the antioxidant and anti-inflammatory activities, and the polyphenolic content of six organic fractions for identifying the type of metabolites that were responsible for biological activity.

2. Materials and Methods

2.1. Plant Material

Whole plants of *Bidens engleri* and *Boerhavia erecta* were taken from the Gampela region, which was situated in the mid-east of Kadiogo (central region), during the rainy season (August–September 2012). The sample was dried in the laboratory under ventilation. The sample was certified by Professor Jeanne MILLOGO, a botanist from the Laboratory of Plant Biology and Ecology (University of Ouagadougou). The herbaria were saved in the University Herbarium with numbers MC_501 and MC_502 for *Bidens engleri* and *Boerhavia erecta*, respectively.

2.2. Reagents and Solvents

The Folin–Ciocalteu reagent, sodium phosphate mono- and di-basics, sodium tetraborate, potassium persulfate, aluminum trichloride, trolox, 2,2-diphenyl-1-picrylhydrazyl (DPPH), 2,2-*O*-azinobis(3-ethylbenzoline-6-sulphonate) (ABTS), gallic acid, and trichloro acetic acid (TCA) were purchased from Sigma-Aldrich (Berlin, Germany). The sodium carbonate, potassium hexacyanoferrate, ascorbic acid, and ferric chloride were from Prolabo (Paris, France). The colorimetric COX (ovine) inhibitor screening assay kit, 15-lipoxygenase (soybean P1), linoleic, and arachidonic acids were purchased from Sigma-Aldrich, (New York, NY, USA).

2.3. Extraction Procedures

Of the sample, 20 g were successively extracted using hexane, dichloromethane, acetonitrile, ethyl acetate, methanol, and butanol in a Soxhlet system. The solvent was removed in a rotary evaporator system.

2.4. Antioxidant Effects Evaluation

2.4.1. Radical DPPH Inhibition Determination

The fractions' capacities to inhibit radical DPPH were evaluated according to the method that was presented by Compaoré et al. [16]. In a 96 micro-well plate, 200 µL of DPPH (20 mg/L) and 100 µL of fraction were incubated in the dark for 10 min, and the absorbencies were read at 517 nm using a spectrophotometer (BioTek Instruments, New York, NY, USA). Quercetin was used to generate a standard curve ($y = -27.94 + 8.15$, $r^2 = 0.99$, $p < 0.0001$). The results were expressed in milligram Quercetin equivalent per gram (mgQE/g).

2.4.2. Trolox Equivalent Antioxidant Capacity Assay

The method that was described by Compaoré et al. was used to evaluate the sample scavenging ABTS ability [16]. To 200 µL of diluted ABTS solution, 50 µL of fraction or trolox was added, with incubation in the dark for 5 min. The absorbance was read at 734 nm, with a microplate reader (BioTek Instruments, New York, NY, USA). Trolox was used to generate the standard curve ($y = -72.38x + 54.57$, $r^2 = 0.99$, $p < 0.001$) and the results were expressed in millimole Trolox equivalent per gram (mMTE/g).

2.4.3. Ferric (Fe III) Reducing Antioxidant Power (FRAP) Assay

The reducing power of the extracts was determined according to the method that was presented by Compaoré et al. [16]. The data were transformed to mg of ascorbic acid per gram of fraction (mgAAE/g), because the standard curve was obtained with ascorbic acid ($y = 105.9x$, $r^2 = 0.99$, $p < 0.0001$). The iron (III) reducing activity of each sample was obtained from two of the three independent determinations.

2.5. Anti-Inflammatory Tests

2.5.1. COX-1 and COX-2 Inhibition Assay

The inhibition of COXs was performed using a commercially available colorimetric COX (ovine) inhibitor screening assay kit (Cayman Chemical Company, New York, NY, USA). All of the inhibitors were dissolved in an appropriate solvent. The COX activity was evaluated using N,N,N′N′-tetramethyl-*p*-phenylenediamine (TMPD) as a co-substrate, with arachidonic acid. The TMPD oxidation was monitored spectrophotometrically at 590 nm (BioTek Instruments, New York, NY, USA). The inhibition percentage that was induced by 100 µg/mL of the sample was calculated.

2.5.2. Lipoxygenase 15 Inhibition Assay

The assay was performed according to the previous procedure that was presented by Compaoré et al. [17]. The incubation mixture consisted of the sample solution (100 µg/mL) in an appropriate solvent and 200 µL of the enzyme solution (167 U/mL) in a boric acid buffer (0.2 M, pH 9). After the incubation at room temperature for 5 min, the reaction was started by adding 250 µL of linoleic acid solution (250 mM in buffer). The conversion of linoleic acid to 13-hydroperoxylinoleic acid was recorded by measuring the samples' absorbencies at 234 nm, during 3 min, and against the appropriate blank solutions, without extracts. The inhibition percentage was calculated.

2.6. Polyphenolic Amount Quantification

2.6.1. Phenolic Content Determination

The total phenolic content was evaluated using a Folin–Ciocalteu colometric assay, as described by Compaoré et al. [16]. The sample was mixed with Folin-Ciocalteu Reagent (0.2N). After incubation in the dark, 100 µL of sodium carbonate was added. The absorbance (760 nm) was measured after a second incubation in the dark (2 h), using the Biotek equipment (BioTek Instruments, New York, NY, USA). Gallic acid was used to produce the standard curve ($y = 201x - 21.22$, $r^2 = 0.99$, $p < 0.0001$) and the results were expressed in mg gallic acid, equivalent per gram (mgGAE/g) of extract.

2.6.2. Total Flavonoid Content Evaluation

The total flavonoid content was determined according to the previous method that was described by Compaoré et al. [16]. Then, 100 µm of sample and 100 µL of $AlCl_3$ (2%) were mixed in 96 micro-wells and were incubated for 10 min. The absorbance was measured at 415 nm with a microplate reader

(BioTek Instruments, New York, NY, USA). Quercetin was used to generate the standard curve ($y = 39.8x - 3.5$, $r^2 = 0.99$, $p < 0.0001$) and the results were expressed at mg quercetin equivalent per gram (mgQE/g) of sample.

2.7. Statistical Analyses

Microsoft Excel was used to calculate the average and standard deviation of the repeated tests ($n = 2 \times 3$). GraphPad Prism 6.01 (San Diego, CA, USA, 2012) and Xlstat Pro 7.5 (Paris, France, 2005) were used to produce the standard curve and to measure the statistical significant results, respectively ($p < 5\%$).

3. Results and Discussion

3.1. Antioxidant Activities

The use of medicinal plants in Burkina Faso has been a current activity of the population [18]. However, the main role of the researchers was to promote the medicinal uses. The plant extracts' antioxidant potential is shown in Table 1. The radical DPPH scavenging effect was decreased from 63.94 mgQE/g to 2.25 mgQE/g, and the radical ABTS scavenging power was decreased from 22.86 mMTE/g to 7.16 mMTE/g. The hexane fractions presented radical ABTS scavenging activities contrary to the anti-DPPH radical effect. The butanol fraction from *Bidens engleri* demonstrated the best antiradical possibility, similar to the acetonitrile from *Boerhavia erecta*. The ability of the fractions to reduce iron (III) were increased from 10.20 mgAAE/g to 211.68 mgAAE/g. In general, the *B. erecta* sample presented some antioxidant activity that was superior to the *B. engleri* samples. This data demonstrated the importance of these plant samples in stress oxidative management. In the previous data, it was demonstrated that *B. erecta* possessed some antioxidant activity that was supported by the flavonoid compounds [14,19]. The anti-DPPH, anti-ABTS, and iron (III) reduction abilities were evaluated [13,20]. However, it was the first antioxidant activity data from *Bidens engleri*, according to our bibliographic survey. According to previous antioxidant activities of similar fractions from *Commifora africana* (A. Rich.) Engl. (Burseraceae) and *Loeseneriella africana* (Willd.) (Celastraceae), which were from the same region, the present plants possessed a lowest antioxidant power [16].

Table 1. Yield and antioxidant activity of fractions.

	Fractions	Yield * (mg/g)	DPPH (mgQE/g)	ABTS (mMTE/g)	FRAP (mgAAE/g)
B. engleri	Hexane fraction	15.94	Non-active	10.06 ± 1.33 [ef]	10.20 ± 0.61 [j]
	Dichloromethane fraction	12.11	2.25 ± 0.9 [f]	8.67 ± 2.06 [ef]	29.36 ± 0.75 [hi]
	Acetonitrile fraction	19.17	17.88 ± 0.91 [e]	11.42 ± 1.12 [def]	64.34 ± 0.92 [g]
	Ethyl acetate fraction	3.98	26.74 ± 1.84 [d]	11.88 ± 0.91 [cde]	74.61 ± 0.73 [f]
	Methanol fraction	137.84	37.67 ± 0.88 [c]	15.43 ± 1.04 [bcd]	97.14 ± 3.55 [e]
	Butanol fraction	1.23	51.88 ± 1.52 [b]	17.10 ± 0.54 [bcd]	211.68 ± 3.11 [a]
B. erecta	Hexane fraction	13.87	Non-active	7.16 ± 1.40 [f]	24.56 ± 1.54 [i]
	Dichloromethane fraction	6.03	5.80 ± 0.18 [f]	9.11 ± 0.96 [ef]	37.02 ± 2.40 [h]
	Acetonitrile fraction	20.79	64.14 ± 0.67 [a]	22.86 ± 1.30 [a]	174.16 ± 4.88 [c]
	Ethyl acetate fraction	3.07	55.28 ± 3.46 [b]	16.21 ± 1.75 [bc]	126.65 ± 2.44 [d]
	Methanol fraction	141.94	63.94 ± 0.78 [a]	21.57 ± 1.82 [a]	198.55 ± 4.54 [b]
	Butanol fraction	1.67	41.40 ± 0.90 [c]	14.86 ± 2.45 [bcd]	92.02 ± 3.69 [e]

Data in each column were statistically different letter ([a–j]) ($p < 0.05$) except data with same letters. The data were obtained in two independent triplate tests ($n = 2 \times 3$). Aterisk (*) indicated data that were obtained by one procedure extraction. DPPH: 2,2-diphenyl-1-picrylhydrazyl, ABTS—2,2-O-azinobis(3-ethylbenzoline-6-sulphonate); FRAP—ferric (Fe III) reducing antioxidant power. mgQE/g: milligram quercetin equivalent per gram, mMTE/g: millimole Trolox equivalent per gram, mgAAE/g: milligram ascorbic acid equivalent per gram.

3.2. Anti-Inflammatory Activity

Table 2 presents the data concerning the inhibition of prostaglandin production from COXs and LOX-15 regular activities. COX-2 was more sensitive than COX-1 and LOX-15, which were not sensitive to the *B. erecta* fractions. The percentage inhibition of COX-2 was from 23.65% to 64.72% at 100 µg/mL, as the final concentration of the fraction. The LOX-15 inhibition percentage was increased from 36.76 to 64.90%. The maximal inhibition of COX-1 was obtained with ethyl acetate (42.51%) from *B. engleri*. Interestingly, the dichloromethane fractions from *B. engleri* and *B. erecta* were the active fractions for COX-2 (64.72 ± 2.13%) and LOX-15 (62.55 ± 5.09%), respectively, according to the enzyme activity classification scale [21]. According to the previous data, *B. erecta* possessed some anti-inflammatory activity in vivo [22], but in the present study, the *B. erecta* fractions could not significantly inhibit the prostaglandin production from the COXs and LOX-15 activity. It was suggested that the enzyme inhibition was not the method of action of this anti-inflammatory effect. This was the first study of the evaluation of the COXs and LOX-15 inhibition power of two plants. These enzyme inhibition activities of the *B. engleri* fractions were very little compared with the *Commifora africana* and *Loeseneriella africana* fractions inhibition effect [16]. In contrast, the butanol and dichloromethane fractions from *B. engleri* presented some interesting inhibition activity of LOX-15, compared with the *Bauhinia rufescens* extract, Lam. (Caesalpiniaceae) [17].

Table 2. Anti-inflammatory activities of fractions.

	Fractions	COX-2 (%Inhibition)	COX-1 (%Inhibition)	LOX-15 (%Inhibition)
Bidens engleri	Hexane fraction	42.74 ± 6.23 [b]	Non active	Non active
	Dichloromethane fraction	64.72 ± 2.13 [a]	Non active	62.55 ± 5.09 [a]
	Acetonitrile fraction	31.17 ± 11.02 [bc]	8.90 ± 1.15 [c]	36.76 ± 3.59 [b]
	Ethyl acetate fraction	37.39 ± 5.67 [bc]	42.52 ± 0.90 [a]	64.90 ± 4.78 [a]
	Methanol fraction	32.31 ± 4.84 [bc]	1.46 ± 0.46 [d]	57.35 ± 0.01 [a]
	Butanol fraction	37.87 ± 2.41 [bc]	31.35 ± 2.30 [b]	60.83 ± 0.80 [a]
Boerhavia erecta	Hexane fraction	23.65 ± 2.55 [c]	Non active	Non active
	Dichloromethane fraction	36.05 ± 2.19 [bc]	Non active	Non active
	Acetonitrile fraction	31.10 ± 3.54 [bc]	Non active	Non active
	Ethyl acetate fraction	26.44 ± 3.29 [c]	Non active	Non active
	Methanol fraction	32.41 ± 3.08 [bc]	Non active	Non active
	Butanol fraction	31.97 ± 6.07 [bc]	Non active	Non active

Data in each column were statistically different letter ($p < 0.05$) except data with same letters ([a–j]). The data were obtained in triplicate tests ($n = 3$).

3.3. Total Phenolic and Total Flavonoid Contents

As the metabolites were the main contributor to the antioxidant and anti-inflammatory powers, the phenolic and flavonoid contents were evaluated [16,23]. The yield of extraction is shown in Table 1. The methanol was the best solvent for extracting some metabolites from two plants, with a yield that was superior to 100 mg/g. Figure 1 shows the amount of flavonoid and phenolic in all of the fractions from *B. erecta* and *B. engleri*. The phenolic content was decreased from 425.12 to 5.92 mgGAE/g, and the flavonoid amount was increased from 2.62 to 30.38 mgQE/g. A notable variable distribution of polyphenolic compounds was found in concordance with the solvent polarities. Notably, *B. engleri* contained some non-polar flavonoids in the major compound that were extracted in dichloromethane, in contrast to *B. erecta*, which presented some polar compounds that were extractible by acetonitrile, ethyl acetate, and methanol. In previous phytochemical investigations, the flavonoid and phenolic contents were evaluated in the extracts from *B. erecta*. It was found that the ethanol and phosphate buffer were able to extract the flavonoid and phenolic compounds [13,14]. The flavonoid and phenolic individual compounds, with a radical scavenging activity and iron (III) reduction ability, were previously detected in the *B. erecta* extracts [24–26]. It was quercetin and isorhamnetin and their glycosides, rutin, narcissin, isoquercitrin, and isorhamnetin 3-O-β-D-glucopyranoside, as well as the two flavan-3-ols, [(+)-catechin] and [(−)-epicatechin], that are well known antioxidant phytometabolites [24–26]. These compounds showed anti-COX and anti-LOX properties [27,28].

The correlation analysis showed that phenolic contributed significantly to the radical scavenging and iron (III) reduction. The contribution to the anti-DPPH, anti-ABTS, and iron (III) reduction were 0.91, 0.86, and 0.99, respectively ($p < 0.0001$). Similar findings were shown in a previous study [16,29,30]. Additionally, it was found in this study that there was an insignificant correlation between the COX-2 and phenolic compound, contrary to a previous study [16].

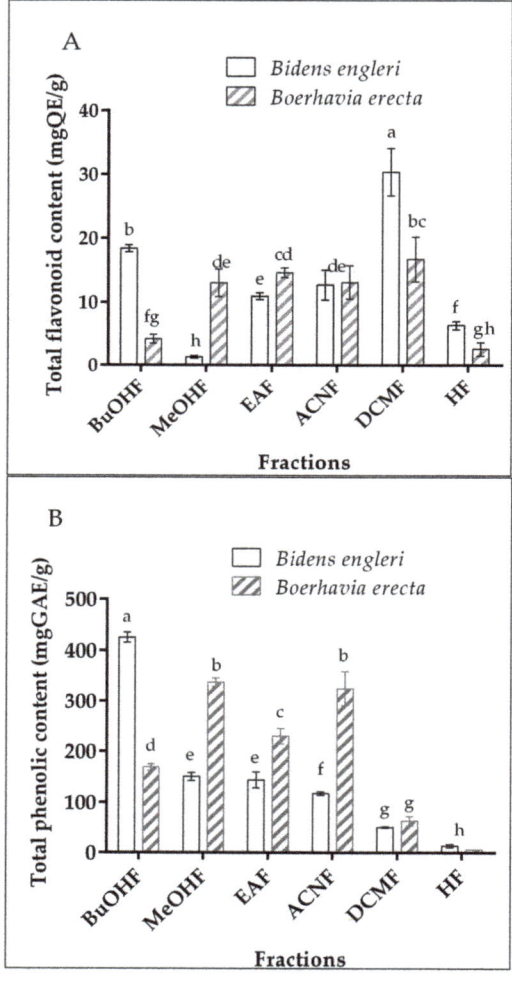

Figure 1. Polyphenolic content of fractions. A—total flavonoid contents; B—total phenolic contents. The data were obtained in two independent triplate tests ($n = 2 \times 3$). The data in each histogram were statistically different ($p < 0.05$), except for the data with the same letters (a–h). BuOHF: butanol Fraction, MeOHF: methanol fraction, EAF: ethyl acetate fraction, ACNF: acetonitrile fraction, DCMF: dichloromethane fraction, HF: hexane fraction, mgQE/g: milligram quercetin equivalent per gram, mgGAE milligram gallic acid equivalent per gram.

4. Conclusions

This study highlighted the antioxidant, anti-inflammatory, and the phytochemical potential of six fractions from *B. engleri* and *B. erecta*, well-known medicinal plants of Burkina Faso. Their utilization could be supported partially by antiradical scavenging and iron (III) reduction. According to the interesting biological activity of *B. engleri*, the next step would be to isolate the anti-radical flavonoid from butanol, ethyl acetate, and acetonitrile fractions, as well as the anti-COX-2 and anti-LOX-15 compounds from the dichloromethane in vitro model.

Author Contributions: M.C. corresponding author, sampling, conception of protocol, redaction of paper, and data analysis; R.N.T.M. conception of protocol, redaction, and correction; S.B. redaction and correction of the article; and O.G.N. laboratory headmaster, validation of plant list, and correction.

Funding: This research was funded by the International Foundation for Sciences grant number AF/20286.

Acknowledgments: Supported by International Foundation for Sciences (grant No. AF/20286). We also thanked Professor Jeanne MILLOGO for the botanical authentication of two plants.

Conflicts of Interest: The authors declare no conflicts of interest.

References

1. Rajendran, P.; Nandakumar, N.; Rengarajan, T.; Palaniswami, R.; Gnanadhas, E.N.; Lakshminarasaiah, U.; Gopas, J.; Nishigaki, I. Antioxidants and human diseases. *Clin. Chim. Acta* **2014**, *436*, 332–347. [CrossRef] [PubMed]
2. Sagna, Y.; Yanogo, D.A.R.; Tiéno, H.; Guira, O.; Bagbila, A. Nutritional Disorders & Therapy Obesity and Metabolic Syndrome in a Burkina Faso Urban Area: Prevalence, Associated Factors and Comorbidities. *J. Nutr. Disord. Ther.* **2014**, *4*, 2–7. [CrossRef]
3. Marie, D.; Ateba, G.; Felicité, K.D.; Fernando, K.L.; Chia, M.; Henry, L.N. Oxidative Stress in Patients with Chronic Inflammatory Diseases in a Tertiary Health Care Setting in Africa. *J. Autoimmun. Disord.* **2017**, *3*, 47.
4. Uttara, B.; Singh, A.V.; Zamboni, P.; Mahajan, R.T. Oxidative Stress and Neurodegenerative Diseases: A Review of Upstream and Downstream Antioxidant Therapeutic Options. *Curr. Neuropharmacol.* **2009**, *7*, 65–74. [CrossRef] [PubMed]
5. Ganjifrockwala, F.A.; Joseph, J.T.; George, G. Decreased total antioxidant levels and increased oxidative stress in South African type 2 diabetes mellitus patients Decreased total antioxidant levels and increased oxidative stress in South African type 2 diabetes mellitus patients. *J. Endocrinol. Metab. Diabetes S. Afr.* **2017**, *22*, 21–25. [CrossRef]
6. Cosme, F.; Pinto, T.; Vilela, A. Phenolic Compounds and Antioxidant Activity in Grape Juices: A Chemical and Sensory View. *Beverages* **2018**, *4*, 22. [CrossRef]
7. Gullo, G.; Dattola, A.; Liguori, G.; Vonella, V. Evaluation of fruit quality and antioxidant activity of kiwifruit during ripening and after storage. *J. Berry Res.* **2016**, *6*, 25–35. [CrossRef]
8. Pistollato, F.; Battino, M.; Cliniche, S.; Biochimica, S. Role of plant-based diets in the prevention and regression of metabolic syndrome and neurodegenerative diseases. *Trends Food Sci. Technol.* **2014**, *40*, 62–81. [CrossRef]
9. Zhang, Y.; Gan, R.; Li, S.; Zhou, Y.; Li, A.; Xu, D. Antioxidant Phytochemicals for the Prevention and Treatment of Chronic Diseases. *Molecules* **2015**, *20*, 21138–21156. [CrossRef] [PubMed]
10. Nacoulma, O.G. Plantes Médicinales et Pratiques Médicales Traditionnelles au Burkina Faso: Cas du Plateau Central. Ph.D. Thesis, University Ouagadougou, Ouagadougou, Burkina Faso, 1996; p. 303.
11. Konkon, N.G.; Ouatara, D.; Kpan, W.B.; Kouakou, T.H. Medicinal plants used for treatment of diabetes by traditional practitioners in the markets of Abidjan district in Côte d'Ivoire. *J. Med. Plants Stud.* **2017**, *5*, 39–48.
12. Nisha, M.; Vinod, B.N.; Sunil, C. Evaluation of *Boerhavia erecta* L. for potential antidiabetic and antihyperlipidemic activities in streptozotocin-induced diabetic Wistar rats. *Futur. J. Pharm. Sci.* **2018**, in press. [CrossRef]
13. Govindan, P.; Muthukrishnan, S. Evaluation of total phenolic content and free radical scavenging activity of *Boerhavia erecta*. *J. Acute Med.* **2013**, *3*, 103–109. [CrossRef]
14. Petrus, A.J.A.; Hemalatha, S.S.; Suguna, G. Isolation and Characterisation of the Antioxidant Phenolic Metabolites of *Boerhaavia erecta* L. leaves. *J. Pharm. Sci. Res.* **2012**, *4*, 1856–1861.

15. Nugraha, A.S.; Hilou, A.; Vandegraaff, N.; David, I.; Haritakun, R.; Keller, P.A. Bioactive glycosides from the African medicinal plant *Boerhavia erecta* L. *Nat. Prod. Res.* **2015**, *29*, 37–41. [CrossRef] [PubMed]
16. Compaoré, M.; Meda, R.N.-T.; Bakasso, S.; Vlase, L.; Kiendrebeogo, M. Antioxidative, anti-inflammatory potentials and phytochemical profile of *Commiphora africana* (A. Rich.) Engl. (Burseraceae) and *Loeseneriella africana* (Willd.) (Celastraceae) stem leaves extracts. *Asian Pac. J. Trop. Biomed.* **2016**, *6*, 665–670. [CrossRef]
17. Compaoré, M.; Lamien, C.E.; Vlase, L.; Kiendrébéogo, M.; Ionescu, C.; Nacoulma, O. Antioxidant, xanthine oxidase and lipoxygenase inhibitory activities and phenolics of *Bauhinia rufescens* Lam. (Caesalpiniaceae). *Nat. Prod. Res.* **2012**, *26*, 1069–1074. [CrossRef] [PubMed]
18. Zizka, A.; Thiombiano, A.; Dressler, S.; Nacoulma, B.M.; Ouédraogo, A.; Ouédraogo, I.; Ouédraogo, O.; Zizka, G.; Hahn, K.; Schmidt, M. Traditional plant use in Burkina Faso (West Africa): A national-scale analysis with focus on traditional medicine. *J. Ethnobiol. Ethnomed.* **2015**, *11*, 11–19. [CrossRef] [PubMed]
19. Rajeswari, P.; Krishnakumari, S. *Boerhaavia erecta*—A potential source for phytochemicals and antioxidants. *J. Pharm. Sci. Res.* **2010**, *2*, 728–733.
20. Shareef, M.I.; Gopinath, S.M.; Gupta, A.; Gupta, S. Antioxidant and Anticancer Study of *Boerhavia erecta*. *Int. J. Curr. Microbiol. Appl. Sci.* **2017**, *6*, 879–885.
21. Fawole, O.A.; Amoo, S.O.; Ndhlala, A.R.; Light, M.E.; Finnie, J.F.; Van Staden, J. Anti-inflammatory, anticholinesterase, antioxidant and phytochemical properties of medicinal plants used for pain-related ailments in South Africa. *J. Ethnopharmacol.* **2010**, *127*, 235–241. [CrossRef] [PubMed]
22. Muthumani, P.; Meera, R.; Devi, P.; Arabath, S.A.; Jeyasundari, K.; Babmanaban, R. Phytochemical investigation, diuretic and anti-inflammatory activity of root and stem extracts of *Boerhaavia erecta* Linn in experimental animals. *Int. J. Appl. Biol. Pharm. Technol.* **2010**, *1*, 1285–1292. [CrossRef]
23. Yi, Y.; Sun, J.; Xie, J.; Min, T.; Wang, L.-M.; Wang, H.-X. Phenolic Profiles and Antioxidant Activity of Lotus Root Varieties. *Molecules* **2016**, *21*, 863. [CrossRef] [PubMed]
24. Seyoum, A.; Asres, K.; El-Fiky, F.K. Structure–radical scavenging activity relationships of flavonoids. *Phytochemistry* **2006**, *67*, 2058–2070. [CrossRef] [PubMed]
25. Cai, Y.; Sun, M.; Xing, J.; Luo, Q.; Corke, H. Structure–radical scavenging activity relationships of phenolic compounds from traditional Chinese medicinal plants. *Life Sci.* **2006**, *78*, 2872–2888. [CrossRef] [PubMed]
26. Bubols, B.G.; da Rocha Vianna, D.; Medina-Remón, A.; von Poser, G.; Maria Lamuela-Raventos, R.; Lucia Eifler-Lima, V.; Cristina Garcia, S. The Antioxidant Activity of Coumarins and Flavonoids. *Mini-Rev. Med. Chem.* **2013**, *13*, 318–334. [CrossRef] [PubMed]
27. Sadik, C.D.; Sies, H.; Schewe, T. Inhibition of 15-lipoxygenases by flavonoids: Structure-activity relations and mode of action. *Biochem. Pharmacol.* **2003**, *65*, 773–781. [CrossRef]
28. Aravindaram, K.; Yang, N. Anti-Inflammatory Plant Natural Products for Cancer Therapy. *Planta Med.* **2010**, *76*, 1103–1117. [CrossRef] [PubMed]
29. Agregán, R.; Munekata, P.E.S.; Franco, D.; Carballo, J.; Barba, F.J.; Lorenzo, J.M. Antioxidant Potential of Extracts Obtained from Macro- (*Ascophyllum nodosum*, *Fucus vesiculosus* and *Bifurcaria bifurcata*) and Micro-Algae (*Chlorella vulgaris* and *Spirulina platensis*) Assisted by Ultrasound. *Medecines* **2018**, *5*, 33. [CrossRef] [PubMed]
30. Lamien-Meda, A.; Lamien, C.E.; Compaoré, M.M.Y.; Meda, R.N.; Kiendrebeogo, M.; Zeba, B.; Millogo, J.F.; Nacoulma, O.G. Polyphenol Content and Antioxidant Activity of Fourteen Wild Edible Fruits from Burkina Faso. *Molecules* **2008**, *13*, 581–594. [CrossRef] [PubMed]

© 2018 by the authors. Licensee MDPI, Basel, Switzerland. This article is an open access article distributed under the terms and conditions of the Creative Commons Attribution (CC BY) license (http://creativecommons.org/licenses/by/4.0/).

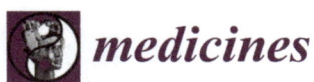 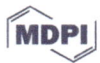

Article

Effect of Hochuekkito (Buzhongyiqitang) on Nasal Cavity Colonization of Methicillin-Resistant *Staphylococcus aureus* in Murine Model

Masaaki Minami [1,*], Toru Konishi [2] and Toshiaki Makino [2]

[1] Department of Bacteriology, Graduate School of Medical Sciences, Nagoya City University, 1 Kawasumi, Mizuho-ku, Nagoya 467-8601, Japan

[2] Department of Pharmacognosy, Graduate School of Pharmaceutical Sciences, Nagoya City University, 3-1 Tanabe-Dori, Mizuho-ku, Nagoya 467-8603, Japan; c142902@ed.nagoya-cu.ac.jp (T.K.); makino@phar.nagoya-cu.ac.jp (T.M.)

* Correspondence: minami@med.nagoya-cu.ac.jp; Tel.: +81-52-853-8166

Received: 29 June 2018; Accepted: 25 July 2018; Published: 1 August 2018

Abstract: Background: Methicillin-resistant *Staphylococcus aureus* (MRSA) infections are largely preceded by colonization with MRSA. Hochuekkito is the formula composing 10 herbal medicines in traditional Kampo medicine to treat infirmity and to stimulate immune functions. We evaluated the efficacy of hochuekkito extract (HET) against MRSA colonization using a nasal infection murine model. **Methods:** We evaluated the effects of HET as follows: (1) the growth inhibition by measuring turbidity of bacterial culture in vitro, (2) the nasal colonization of MRSA by measuring bacterial counts, and (3) the splenocyte proliferation in mice orally treated with HET by the ^{3}H-thymidine uptake assay. **Results:** HET significant inhibited the growth of MRSA. The colony forming unit (CFU) in the nasal fluid of HET-treated mice was significantly lower than that of HET-untreated mice. When each single crude drug—Astragali radix, Bupleuri radix, Zingiberis rhizoma, and Cimicifugae rhizome—was removed from hochuekkito formula, the effect of the formula significantly weakened. The uptake of ^{3}H-thymidine into murine splenocytes treated with HET was significantly higher than that from untreated mice. The effects of the modified formula described above were also significantly weaker than those of the original formula. **Conclusions:** Hochuekkito is effective for the treatment of MRSA nasal colonization in the murine model. We suggest HET as the therapeutic candidate for effective therapy on nasal cavity colonization of MRSA in humans.

Keywords: MRSA; Hochuekkito; Japanese traditional Kampo medicine; murine colonization model

1. Introduction

Staphylococcus aureus infection, such as surgical site infection, is a common hospital-associated infectious disease. It causes the extension of hospital stays and increases the costs of health-care [1]. The increasing rates of clinical isolates of *S. aureus* worldwide are methicillin-resistant [2]. The attributable mortality of *S. aureus* septicemia infection is about 20% for methicillin-sensitive strains and about 30% for methicillin-resistant *S. aureus* (MRSA) [3]. The development of new effective medication is desired for the improvement of morbidity and mortality regarding *S. aureus* infection.

Nasal colonization is an important risk factor for *S. aureus* infection. It is associated with up to 13-fold increased risk of *S. aureus* infection [4]. A study of nosocomial *S. aureus* bacteremia demonstrated nasal colonization on admission in most cases [5]. Nasal colonization is the predecessor to infection because the infecting strain was identical to the isolated colonizing strain before infection in four-fifths of *S. aureus* septicemia cases [6]. Decolonization therapy reduces the risk of healthcare-associated *S. aureus* infection in high-risk settings such as surgery, supporting the hypothesis that colonization leads to infection [7].

Traditional Chinese medicine (TCM) is one of the most popular alternative, complementary therapies worldwide [8]. In Japan, Kampo medicine, which is the traditional medicine developed from ancient Chinese medicine, is recognized as an effective alternative medicine against several diseases [9,10]. Hochuekkito (Buzhongyiqitang) is a formula in both traditional Japanese Kampo medicine and Chinese medicine. This formula comprises 10 crude drugs shown in Table 1. Hochuekkito extract (HET) has been used to treat severe infirmity such as weakness and loss of appetite of the elderly [11]. As HET is a popular alternative medicine in Japan, limited scientific evidence is available on the use of HET for the treatment of MRSA colonization [12,13]. Thus, the clarification of the precise mechanism of Hochuekkito efficacy against MRSA colonization has been desired.

In the present study, we evaluated the efficacy of HET against MRSA colonization using a nasal infection murine model. Furthermore, we also evaluated the efficacy of the constitutive crude drug of HET against MRSA and immunological activity of murine splenocytes from HET-treated mice.

Table 1. Composition of hochuekkito.

Name of Crude Drug	Origin	Daily Dose (g)
Astragali radix	The dried root of *Astragalus propinquus* Schischkin, Fabaceae	4.0
Ginseng radix	The dried root of *Panax ginseng* C.A. Mayer, Araliaceae	4.0
Atractylodes rhizome	The dried rhizome of *Atractylodes japonica* Koidzumi ex Kitamura, Asteraceae	4.0
Angelicae radix	The dried root of *Angelica acutiloba* (Siebold & Zucc.) Kitag., Apiaceae	4.0
Zizyphi fructus	The dried fruit of *Ziziphus jujuba* Miller, Rhamnaceae	3.0
Aurantii nobilis pericarpium	The dried ripe fruit skin of *Citrus reticulata* Blanco, Rutaceae	2.0
Bupleuri radix	The dried root of *Bupleurum falcatum* Linné, Apiaceae	2.0
Glycyrrhizae radix	The dried root and stolon of *Glycyrrhiza uralensis* Fisher, Fabaceae	1.5
Cimicifugae rhizome	The dried rhizome of *Actaea simplex* (DC.) Wormsk. ex Prantl, Ranunculaceae	1.0
Zingiberis rhizome	The dried rhizome of *Zingiber officinale* Roscoe, Zingiberaceae	0.5

Daily doses of crude drugs in hochuekkito are in Japanese Pharmacopoeia 17th Edition [14].

2. Materials and Methods

2.1. Bacterial Strains and Culture Condition

MRSA (ATCC_BAA-1556 (FPR3757)) (American Type Culture Collection, Rockville, MD, USA) was used in this study. After overnight pre-incubation on TSAII sheep blood agar (Nihon Becton Dickinson, Tokyo, Japan), a fresh colony of bacteria was cultured for 16 h at 37 °C. The bacteria were harvested by centrifugation and re-suspended in sterile Luria–Bertani (LB) medium (Becton Dickinson, Franklin Lakes, NJ, USA). Bacterial density was determined by measuring the absorbance at 600 nm (A600). The bacterial suspension was then diluted with LB to 10^6 CFU (colony forming unit)/mL using a standard growth curve to relate measured A600 to bacterial concentration. The bacteria were cultured at 37 °C and A600 was measured at every 2 h.

2.2. Crude Drugs and Exteact Preparation

Astragali radix (lot number, 6C30M), 4.0 g of Ginseng radix (5D25), 4.0 g of Atractylodes rhizome (3J07M), 3.0 g of Angelicae radix (5G06M), 2.0 g of Zizyphi fructus (5G07M), 2.0 g of Aurantii nobilis pericarpium (6B16M), 2.0 g of Bupleuri radix (6C15M), 1.5 g of Glycyrrhizae radix (6B22), 1.0 g of Cimicifugae rhizome (0F28M), and 0.5 g of Zingiberis rhizome (5G07M). These cut crude drugs were purchased from Daiko Shoyaku (Nagoya, Japan) and standardized by Japanese Pharmacopoeia 17th Edition [14]. Voucher specimens of each single crude drug were deposited in the Department of Pharmacognosy, Graduate School of Pharmaceutical Sciences, Nagoya City University. The mixture of the above crude drugs was boiled in 20-times weight of water for 30 min, and filtered. The decoction was lyophilized to yield powdered extract (HET, the ratio of the extract yielded was 36%). A fingerprint pattern of this HET was created as follows. HET (50 mg) was suspended with MeOH (1 mL) and sonicated for 30 min. The supernatant (30 μL) was injected to HPLC with the following conditions: system, Shimadzu LC-10A$_{VP}$ (Kyoto, Japan); column, TSK-GEL ODS-80$_{TS}$ (4.6 × 250 mm, Tosoh, Tokyo,

Japan); mobile phase, 0.05 M AcOH–AcONH$_4$ buffer (pH 3.6)/CH$_3$CN 90:10 (0 min)–45:55 (40 min), linear gradient; flow rate, 1.0 mL/min; column temperature, 40 °C; and detection, 200–400 nm by a photodiode array detector. Some peaks were identified by the retention times and UV spectra of the standard compounds. The fingerprint chromatogram of HET extract is shown in Figure 1. HET was suspended in distilled water to prepare the stock solution at a concentration of 0.1 g/mL, and kept at −20 °C until use. From the 10 crude drugs of hochuekkito formula, each single crude drug was removed to make 10 kinds of modified hochuekkito formula containing 9 crude drugs. The extracts of the modified formula were prepared in the same way.

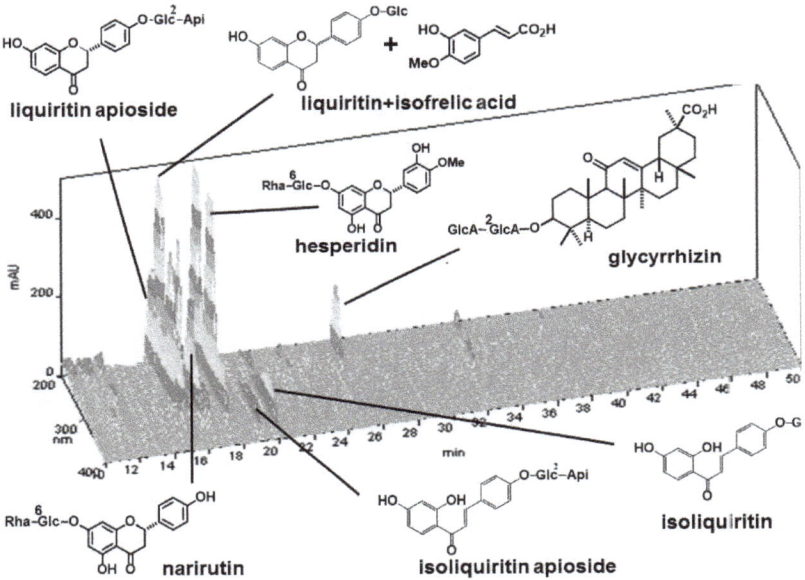

Figure 1. HPLC fingerprint of hochuekkito extract (HET). Compounds were identified by comparison of the retention times of the UV spectra with those of standard compounds.

2.3. Murine Model of Bacterial Nasal Infection

This study was approved by the Animal Experiment Committee of Graduated School of Medical Sciences of Nagoya City University in accordance with the guidelines of the Japanese Council on Animal Care. Ethical approval code: H28M-05. Date of approval: 2 March 2016. Mice were purchased from Japan SLC (Hamamatsu, Japan). The ability of the colonized effect of MRSA in mice after nasal inoculation was assessed using a previous procedure [15]. In brief, bacteria were harvested after 16 h of growth on TSAII sheep blood agar, and were mixed in 1 mL of phosphate buffered saline (PBS, pH 7.2, 0.15 M), then centrifuged at 2000× g for 2 min. The pellets were diluted in 100 µL PBS to 1×10^7 CFU, and then inoculated into both nostrils of inbred six-week-old female Balb/c mice using a micropipette. The number of CFU inoculated was verified for each experiment by plating the bacteria on TSAII sheep blood agar and counting CFU. Mice were observed daily. In the HET-treated group, mice were administered with HET (0.85, 1.7, or 3.4 g/kg body weight/day body weight, which were equivalent to 5, 10, and 20 times the dosage of humans, respectively) on days −1, 0, 1, 2, and 3 after the bacterial inoculation (Figure 2). The mice in the control group were given PBS without infection.

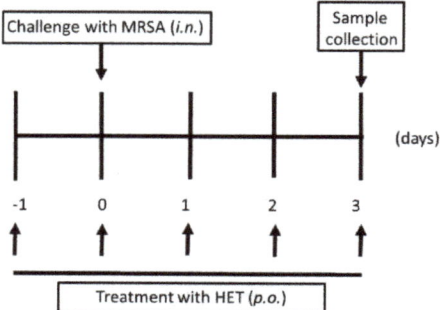

Figure 2. Protocols for murine experiments of methicillin-resistant *Staphylococcus aureus* (MRSA) colonized model. In the infected group, 1×10^7 colony forming unit (CFU) bacteria were injected into both nostrils of mice using a 29 gauge needle at day 0. In the hochuekkito extract (HET)-treated group, mice were administrated with HET *p.o.*

2.4. Nasal Lavage Cultures

The procedure of nasal cultures was described elsewhere [16]. In brief, the mice were sacrificed by CO_2 inhalation. After that, the external noses, oral cavity, and head were disinfected with a moist alcohol swab and allowed to dry. Nasal lavage was performed with 200 µL of PBS. The recovered fluid was then serially diluted, and 10 µL of each dilution was plated onto TSAII sheep blood agar plates. The plates were incubated for 24 h, and then colonies of bacteria were counted. The results were quantified as the number of CFU/mL.

2.5. Determination of Splenocyte Proliferative Response

The oral administration protocol for this assay was done in almost the same manner for bacterial nasal infection, except for no-infection with MRSA. After the mice were sacrificed by CO_2 inhalation, the spleen was removed aseptically, and splenocytes were filtered and cultured in RPMI 1640 (Wako Pure Chemical Industry, Osaka, Japan) containing 5% fetal calf serum (FBS, Sigma-Aldrich, St. Louis, MO, USA). At 20 h prior to the culmination of the splenocyte culture, ^{3}H-thymidine (2.0 Ci/mmol; PerkinElmer, Waltham, MA, USA) was added into the medium, and the cells were further incubated for 4 h. Then, the cells were adsorbed on 0.45-µm membrane filters, washed with distilled water, and then dried. The filters were transferred to vials filled with liquid scintillator cocktail (Ultima Gold, Perkin Elmer, Inc., Waltham, MA, USA), and the radioactivity was measured by using a liquid scintillation counter (LSC-6100, Hitachi Aloka Medical, Tokyo, Japan). The results are given as disintegrations per minute (DPM).

2.6. Statistical Analysis

All statistical analyses were conducted using Tukey/Bonferroni's multiple comparison test for differences among multiple groups (EZR version 1.36, http://www.jichi.ac.jp/saitama-sct/SaitamaHP.files/statmedEN.html). Values less than 0.01 indicated statistical significance.

3. Results

3.1. Bacterial Growth Inhibitory Effect

First of all, we tried to evaluate whether or not HET could inhibit the growth of MRSA. MRSA was grown in LB medium with or without HET, and the inhibitory ability of bacterial growth was assessed.

As expected, HET (10 mg/mL) significantly inhibited the growth of MRSA ($p < 0.01$). We confirmed that this inhibitory ability was in dose- and time-dependent manners (Figure 3).

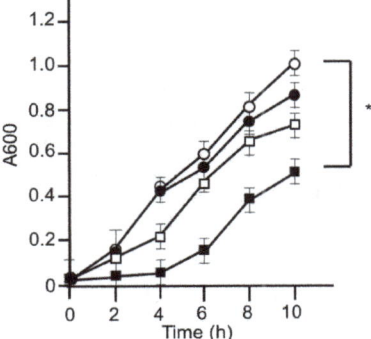

Figure 3. Bacterial growth inhibitory effect of hochuekkito extract (HET). MRSA was cultured on Luria–Bertani (LB) medium with or without HET for 10 h. The bacterial growth was evaluated by measuring absorbance at 600 nm. Open circle, closed circle, open square, and closed square exhibited HET 0, 0.1, 1, and 10 mg/mL, respectively. Data shown represent the mean ± S.D. ($n = 6$). ** $p < 0.01$ by Tukey/Bonferroni's multiple comparison test.

3.2. Murine Nasal Infection Model

Next, we tried to assess whether HET would provide in vivo effects against MRSA. Four days after nostril infection of MRSA, we evaluated the bacterial colony counts in murine nose. The CFUs of HET-treated murine nasal lavage were lower than those of HET-untreated mice in dose-dependent manners, and the group treated with 3.4 g/kg/day exhibited statistical significance ($p < 0.01$) (Figure 4). In order to find the active components in the hochuekkito formula, we prepared the extracts of the modified formulas, which contain nine crude drugs. The extracts of modified hochuekkito formulas—that is, Astragali radix, Bupleuri radix, Zingiberis rhizoma, or Cimicifugae rhizome—exhibited significantly lower activities than HET, respectively ($p < 0.01$) (Figure 5).

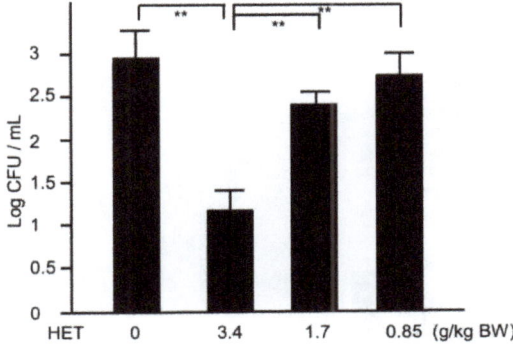

Figure 4. The colonies of MRSA in hochuekkito extract (HET)-treated and untreated murine nasal lavage. The nasal fluids were inoculated on TSAII sheep blood agar and incubated for 24 h. Comparisons of colony count between HET-treated and untreated mice were performed. Data represent the mean ± S.D. ($n = 6$). ** $p < 0.01$ by Tukey/Bonferroni's multiple comparison test.

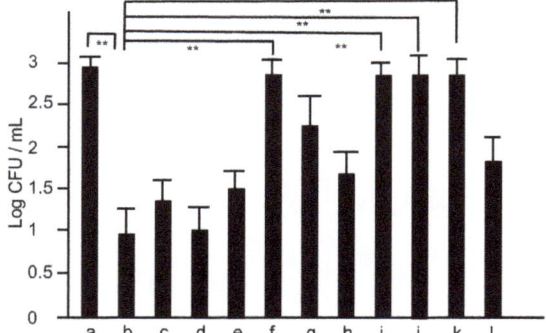

Figure 5. The colonies of MRSA of nasal lavage collected from mice treated with the extracts of modified hochuekkito formulas. The nasal fluids were inoculated on TSAII sheep blood agar and incubated for 24 h. a: untreated, b: hochuekkito extract (HET)-treated, c: aurantii nobilis pericarpium-removed HET, d: zizyphi fructus-removed HET, e: angelicae radix-removed HET, f: zingiberis rhizome-removed HET, g: Atractylodes rhizome-removed HET, h: Ginseng radix-removed HET, i: astragali radix-removed HET, j: bupleuri radix-removed HET, k: cimicifugae rhizome-removed HET, l: glycyrrhizae radix-removed HET, respectively. Dosage of HET was 3.4 g/kg/day, and those of the extracts of other modified hochueekito formulas were equivalent to this dosage. Data represent the mean ± S.D. ($n = 6$). ** $p < 0.01$ by Tukey/Bonferroni's multiple comparison test.

3.3. Splenocyte Proliferative Activity in HET-Treated Mice

We also studied the activity of splenocyte in mice treated with HET, because splenocytes play major roles in murine bacterial infection models. To determine whether or not the activity of the splenocytes collected from HET-treated mice was elevated, we performed ^{3}H-thymidine uptake analysis. As shown in Figure 6, the uptake of ^{3}H-thymidine into splenocytes collected from mice orally treated with HET was significantly ($p < 0.01$) higher than that from untreated mice in dose-dependent manners. The extracts of modified hochuekkito formulas—that is, Astragali radix, Bupleuri radix, Zingiberis rhizoma, or Cimicifugae rhizome—exhibited significantly lower ^{3}H-thymidine uptake compared with HET ($p < 0.01$) (Figure 7).

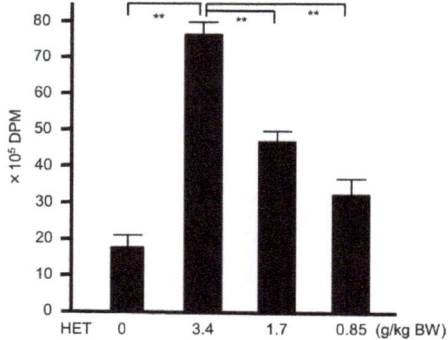

Figure 6. ^{3}H-thymidine-uptake assay in hochuekkito extract (HET)-treated and untreated murine splenocyte. Six-week-old female Balb/c mice were administrated with HET for four days, and the splenocyte were collected. Data represent the mean ± S.D. ($n = 6$). ** $p < 0.01$ by Tukey's/Bonferroni multiple comparison test. DPM—disintegrations per minute.

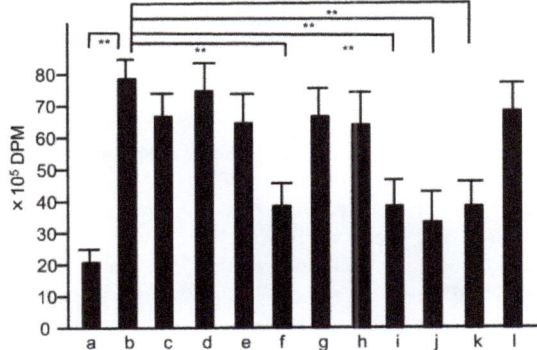

Figure 7. ^{3}H-thymidine-uptake assay of the splenocytes collected from mice treated with the extracts of modified hochuekkito formulas. Six-week-old female Balb/c mice were administrated with hochuekkito extract (HET) for four days, and splenocytes were collected. Symbols of a–l and the dosages of the samples were as same as those shown in Figure 5. Data represent the mean ± S.D. ($n = 6$). ** $p < 0.01$ by Tukey/Bonferroni's multiple comparison test.

4. Discussion

In this study, we tried to clarify that HET would be effective for the eradication in the MRSA-colonized murine model. Our results showed that the turbidity of the bacteria increases over time at the start and that the turbidity decreases compared with the control when HET is added, so this is the growth suppressing effect. After MRSA nasal infection, HET-treated mice showed a reduction of MRSA colonization in murine nose and the upregulation of murine splenocyte activity. Furthermore, we demonstrated that four crude drug components of HET—Astragali radix, Bupleuri radix, Zingiberis rhizoma, and Cimicifugae rhizome—affected the eradication of MRSA. Our results suggest that HET can play a crucial part in protection against MRSA colonization in the mouse model.

Several studies of HET on microbial infections have been investigated. In a small-scale clinical trial about MRSA infection, eradication of MRSA was successful when HET was administered to five MRSA carriers' patients [12]. Another study showed that when HET was administered to 34 asymptomatic patients from which MRSA was isolated from urine, MRSA was not isolated from urine in 12 patients, and 10 patients decreased the bacterial volume to less than 1/100 [13]. Other human clinical trials in lung *Mycobacterium avium* complex patients with HET for six months resulted in weight gain and increased serum albumin value without a tendency for infectious disease to exacerbate on chest radiograph [17]. Even in healthy elderly humans, natural killer (NK) cell activity increased at 30 days and 120 days after administration of HET. The serum interferone (IFN)-γ activity also increased [18]. A clinical large-scale trial to confirm the effect of HET on MRSA carriage of human nasal cavity is desired from the investigation of the effect of HET on these bacterial colonizations and chronic infections for humans and our experimental results.

Non-human experimental studies also revealed the efficacy of HET against bacterial infection. When *Listeria monocytogenes* was infected intraperitoneally in mice, HET showed an increase in polynuclear leukocytes and macrophages in the spleen. HET also confirmed renewal of phagocytic capacity of *L. monocytogenes* in intraperitoneal macrophages [19]. In a mouse infected with *L. monocytogenes*, HET showed a decrease in bacterial quantities in Peyer's patches, lymph nodes, and liver. HET showed increased phagocytosis of liver macrophages against bacteria. It also showed an increase in IFN-γ producing cells in intraepithelial lymphocytes [20]. When HET was administered in *L. monocytogenes* infected infant mice, the amount of *L. monocytogenes* in the liver and spleen decreased. Activation of IFN-γ producing CD4 T cells enhanced IFN-γ activity. The ability of macrophages to present antigen by MHC class II expression is enhanced [21]. In vitro experiments inhibited the growth of *Helicobacter pylori* at a concentration of HET 2.5 mg/mL. In addition, the amounts of bacteria in the stomach were decreased in mice by oral administration of HET in an in vivo experiment. Furthermore, the expression of IFN-γ in the gastric mucosa was elevated [22]. As our bacterial growth study showed that HET suppressed the MRSA in a dose-dependent manner, HET may have a bacterial inhibitory effect regardless of bacterial species. By infecting mice with *Brucella abortus*, causing a chronic fatigue syndrome, the combined effect of HET and IFN-γ increased the activity of thymic NK cells [23]. HET treatment increased the expression of human monocyte-like THP-1 cells on the cell surface of toll-like receptor (TLR) 4, resulting in an increase in receptors responsive to gram-negative bacteria. From this result, it is also considered to activate the protective effect against pathogenic bacteria [24].

Several reports about viral infection also showed that HET was effective for respiratory viral infection via immunomodulation system such as cytokines. As the nasal cavity belongs to respiratory organs, the anti-infective effect against respiratory infections may give some hint to the eradication of nasal colonization. HET administration resulted in improvement of survival rate and survival time with the mouse influenza virus infection. We also found suppression of viral load in bronchoalveolar lavage fluid (BALF) [25]. An increase in lung interleukin (IL)-1β and tumor necrosis factor-α was observed in combination with HET and osetamivir for influenza A virus-infected mice. In addition, hyperactivity of mouse alveolar macrophages was also observed [26]. In the mouse influenza virus infection model, virus titres decreased in BALF with HET administration. HET also stimulated not only the release of type 1 IFN in the lung, but also the anti-inflammatory response derived from granulocyte macrophage colony-stimulating factor. Furthermore, the defensin expression of the antimicrobial peptide was also increased [27]. When mice were infected with rhinovirus, it was thought that HET inhibited intracellular migration of rhinovirus by decreased expression of intercellular adhesion molecule-1 of airway epithelial cells. It also inhibited IL-1β, IL-6, and IL-8 secretion from respiratory epithelial cells. In our results, glycyrrhizae radix that contains glycyrrhizin was not prominent in the effect of HET, but it is reported that glycyrrhizin reduced viral antibody titter [28].

Splenocytes are the major immunomodulation system against bacterial infection [29]. Several crude drug are known to promote immunostimulation of spleen cells. Atractylodes rhizome extract promotes T cell activity by expressing CD28 of T cells in spleen [30]. It also promotes secretion of IL-2, 6, 10, and T cell differentiation via phosphorylation of extracellular signal-regulated kinases [31]. In addition, it reduces the IFN-γ secretion from T cells in helper T (Th) 1 cells and promotes the IL-4 secretion in Th2 cells [32]. Zingiberis rhizoma extract stimulates CD8+ T cells of splenocytes [33,34]. In addition, it is involved in the TLR2/NF-κB pathway by suppressing the expression of TLR2/NF-κB p65 in lung tissue with mouse pneumococcal infection [35]. Bupleuri radix extract reduces the Th1 subunit and increases the Th2 subunit of peripheral blood [36]. It also has B cell mitogenic activity in spleen cells [37]. Moreover, it also has antimicrobial and antiviral action [38]. Our findings also suggested that these constitutional crude drugs of HET were involved in the activation of spleen cells.

Furthermore, three kinds of active crude drugs, Bupleuri radix, Cimicifugae rhizoma, and Zingiberis rhizome, in hochuekkito belong to superfices-syndrome relieving drugs in Kampo medicinal theory, which means that it excludes the *evils* of the inner surface of the body. This traditional medicinal theory may explain that these three crude drugs have the effect of nasal infection of bacteria.

5. Conclusions

In summary, HET is significantly effective for the treatment of nasal cavity colonization of MRSA in the murine model. We suggest HET as the therapeutic candidate for effective therapy on nasal cavity colonization of MRSA in humans.

Author Contributions: M.M., T.K. and T.M. conceived and designed the experiments; M.M. and T.K. performed the experiments and analyzed the data; M.M. and T.M. wrote the paper.

Funding: This work was supported by Grants-in-Aid for Scientific Research (JSPS KAKENHI) grant number JP16K09251, and the Research Foundation for Oriental Medicine.

Acknowledgments: We thank Masashi Ishihara, and Miwako Fujimura for excellent support through this investigation.

Conflicts of Interest: All authors have no conflicts of interest.

References

1. Wisplinghoff, H.; Bischoff, T.; Tallent, S.M.; Seifert, H.; Wenzel, R.P.; Edmond, M.B. Nosocomial bloodstream infections in US hospitals: Analysis of 24,179 cases from a prospective nationwide surveillance study. *Clin. Infect. Dis.* **2004**, *39*, 309–317. [CrossRef] [PubMed]
2. Klevens, R.M.; Edwards, J.; Tenover, F.C.; McDonald, L.C.; Horan, T.; Gaynes, R. Changes in the epidemiology of methicillin-resistant *Staphylococcus aureus* in intensive care units in US hospitals, 1992–2003. *Clin. Infect. Dis.* **2006**, *42*, 389–391. [CrossRef] [PubMed]
3. Cosgrove, S.E.; Sakoulas, G.; Perencevich, E.N.; Schwaber, M.J.; Karchmer, A.W.; Carmeli, Y. Comparison of mortality associated with methicillin-resistant and methicillin-susceptible *Staphylococcus aureus* bacteremia: A meta-analysis. *Clin. Infect. Dis.* **2003**, *36*, 53–59. [CrossRef] [PubMed]
4. Keene, A.; Vavagiakis, P.; Lee, M.H.; Finnerty, K.; Nicolls, D.; Cespedes, C.; Quagliarello, B.; Chiasson, M.A.; Chong, D.; Lowy, F.D. *Staphylococcus aureus* colonization and the risk of infection in critically ill patients. *Infect. Control Hosp. Epidemiol.* **2005**, *26*, 622–628. [CrossRef] [PubMed]
5. Wertheim, H.F.; Vos, M.; Ott, A.; van Belkum, A.; Voss, A.; Kluytmans, J.A.; van Keulen, P.H.; Vandenbroucke-Grauls, C.M.; Meester, M.H.; Verbrugh, H.A. Risk and outcome of nosocomial *Staphylococcus aureus* bacteraemia in nasal carriers versus non-carriers. *Lancet* **2004**, *364*, 703–705. [CrossRef]
6. Wertheim, H.F.; Melles, D.C.; Vos, M.C.; van Leeuwen, W.; van Belkum, A.; Verbrugh, H.A.; Nouwen, J.L. The role of nasal carriage in *Staphylococcus aureus* infections. *Lancet Infect. Dis.* **2005**, *5*, 751–762. [CrossRef]
7. Bode, L.G.; Kluytmans, J.A.; Wertheim, H.F.; Bogaers, D.; Vandenbroucke-Grauls, C.M.; Roosendaal, R.; Troelstra, A.; Box, A.T.; Voss, A.; van der Tweel, I.; et al. Preventing surgical-site infections in nasal carriers of *Staphylococcus aureus*. *N. Engl. J. Med.* **2010**, *362*, 9–17. [CrossRef] [PubMed]
8. Park, H.L.; Lee, H.S.; Shin, B.C.; Liu, J.P.; Shang, Q.; Yamashita, H.; Lim, B. Traditional medicine in China, Korea, and Japan: A brief introduction and comparison. *Evid. Based Complement. Alternat. Med.* **2012**, *2012*, 429103. [CrossRef] [PubMed]
9. Uezono, Y.; Miyano, K.; Sudo, Y.; Suzuki, M.; Shiraishi, S.; Terawaki, K. A review of traditional Japanese medicines and their potential mechanism of action. *Curr. Pharm. Des.* **2012**, *18*, 4839–4853. [CrossRef] [PubMed]
10. Motoo, Y.; Seki, T.; Tsutani, K. Traditional Japanese medicine, Kampo: Its history and current status. *Chin. J. Integr. Med.* **2011**, *17*, 85–87. [CrossRef] [PubMed]
11. Satoh, N.; Sakai, S.; Kogure, T.; Tahara, E.; Origasa, H.; Shimada, Y.; Kohoda, K.; Okubo, T.; Terasawa, K. A randomized double blind placebo-controlled clinical trial of Hochuekkito, a traditional herbal medicine, in the treatment of elderly patients with weakness N of one and responder restricted design. *Phytomedicine* **2005**, *12*, 549–554. [CrossRef] [PubMed]
12. Itoh, T.; Itoh, H.; Kikuchi, T. Five cases of MRSA-infected patients with cerebrovascular disorder and in a bedridden condition, for whom bu-zhong-yi-qi-tang (hochu-ekki-to) was useful. *Am. J. Chin. Med.* **2000**, *28*, 401–408. [CrossRef] [PubMed]
13. Nishida, S. Effect of Hochu-ekki-to on asymptomatic MRSA bacteriuria. *J. Infect. Chemother.* **2003**, *9*, 58–61. [CrossRef] [PubMed]
14. Pharmaceutical and Medical Device Regulatory Science Society of Japan. *Japanese Pharmacopoeia*, 17th ed.; Jiho: Tokyo, Japan, 2016.
15. Minami, M.; Konishi, T.; Takase, H.; Jiang, Z.; Arai, T.; Makino, T. Effect of Shin'iseihaito (Xinyiqingfeitang) on acute *Streptococcus pneumoniae* murine sinusitis via macrophage activation. *Evid. Based Complement. Alternat. Med.* **2017**, *2017*, 4293291. [CrossRef] [PubMed]
16. Minami, M.; Konishi, T.; Takase, H.; Makino, T. Comparison between the effects of oral and intramuscular administration of shin'iseihaito (xinyiqingfeitang) in a *Streptococcus pyogenes*-induced murine sinusitis model. *Evid. Based Complement. Alternat. Med.* **2018**, *2018*, 8901215. [CrossRef] [PubMed]

17. Enomoto, Y.; Hagiwara, E.; Komatsu, S.; Nishihira, R.; Baba, T.; Kitamura, H.; Sekine, A.; Nakazawa, A.; Ogura, T. Pilot quasi-randomized controlled study of herbal medicine Hochuekkito as an adjunct to conventional treatment for progressed pulmonary *Mycobacterium avium complex* disease. *PLoS ONE* **2014**, *9*, e104411. [CrossRef] [PubMed]
18. Kuroiwa, A.; Liou, S.; Yan, H.; Eshita, A.; Naitoh, S.; Nagayama, A. Effect of a traditional Japanese herbal medicine, hochu-ekki-to (Bu-Zhong-Yi-Qi Tang), on immunity in elderly persons. *Int. Immunopharmacol.* **2004**, *4*, 317–324. [CrossRef] [PubMed]
19. Li, X.Y.; Takimoto, H.; Miura, S.; Yoshikai, Y.; Matsuzaki, G.; Nomoto, K. Effect of a traditional Chinese medicine, bu-zhong-yi-qi-tang (Japanese name: Hochu-ekki-to) on the protection against *Listeria monocytogenes* infection in mice. *Immunopharmacol. Immunotoxicol.* **1992**, *14*, 383–402. [CrossRef] [PubMed]
20. Yamaoka, Y.; Kawakita, T.; Kishihara, K.; Nomoto, K. Effect of a traditional Chinese medicine, Bu-zhong-yi-qi-tang on the protection against an oral infection with *Listeria monocytogenes*. *Immunopharmacology* **1998**, *39*, 215–223. [CrossRef]
21. Yamaoka, Y.; Kawakita, T.; Nomoto, K. Protective effect of a traditional Japanese medicine Hochu-ekki-to (Chinese name: Bu-zhong-yi-qi-tang), on the susceptibility against *Listeria monocytogenes* in infant mice. *Int. Immunopharmacol.* **2001**, *1*, 1669–1677. [CrossRef]
22. Yan, X.; Kita, M.; Minami, M.; Yamamoto, T.; Kuriyama, H.; Ohno, T.; Iwakura, Y.; Imanishi, J. Antibacterial effect of Kampo herbal formulation Hochu-ekki-to (Bu-Zhong-Yi-Qi-Tang) on *Helicobacter pylori* infection in mice. *Microbiol. Immunol.* **2002**, *46*, 475–482. [CrossRef] [PubMed]
23. Chen, R.; Moriya, J.; Luo, X.; Yamakawa, J.; Takahashi, T.; Sasaki, K.; Yoshizaki, F. Hochu-ekki-to combined with interferon-gamma moderately enhances daily activity of chronic fatigue syndrome mice by increasing NK cell activity, but not neuroprotection. *Immunopharmacol. Immunotoxicol.* **2009**, *31*, 238–245. [CrossRef] [PubMed]
24. Mita, Y.; Dobashi, K.; Shimizu, Y.; Nakazawa, T.; Mori, M. Surface expression of toll-like receptor 4 on THP-1 cells is modulated by Bu-Zhong-Yi-Qi-Tang and Shi-Quan-Da-Bu-Tang. *Methods Find. Exp. Clin. Pharmacol.* **2002**, *24*, 67–70. [CrossRef] [PubMed]
25. Mori, K.; Kido, T.; Daikuhara, H.; Sakakibara, I.; Sakata, T.; Shimizu, K.; Amagaya, S.; Sasaki, H.; Komatsu, Y. Effect of Hochu-ekki-to (TJ-41), a Japanese herbal medicine, on the survival of mice infected with influenza virus. *Antivir. Res.* **1999**, *44*, 103–111. [CrossRef]
26. Ohgitani, E.; Kita, M.; Mazda, O.; Imanishi, J. Combined administration of oseltamivir and hochu-ekki-to (TJ-41) dramatically decreases the viral load in lungs of senescence-accelerated mice during influenza virus infection. *Arch. Virol.* **2014**, *159*, 267–275. [CrossRef] [PubMed]
27. Dan, K.; Akiyoshi, H.; Munakata, K.; Hasegawa, H.; Watanabe, K. A Kampo (traditional Japanese herbal) medicine, Hochuekkito, pretreatment in mice prevented influenza virus replication accompanied with GM-CSF expression and increase in several defensin mRNA levels. *Pharmacology* **2013**, *91*, 314–321. [CrossRef] [PubMed]
28. Yamaya, M.; Sasaki, T.; Yasuda, H.; Inoue, D.; Suzuki, T.; Asada, M.; Yoshida, M.; Seki, T.; Iwasaki, K.; Nishimura, H.; et al. Hochu-ekki-to inhibits rhinovirus infection in human tracheal epithelial cells. *Br. J. Pharmacol.* **2007**, *150*, 702–710. [CrossRef] [PubMed]
29. Tarantino, G.; Scalera, A.; Finelli, C. Liver-spleen axis: Intersection between immunity, infections and metabolism. *World J. Gastroenterol.* **2013**, *19*, 3534–3542. [CrossRef] [PubMed]
30. Clements, J.R.; Monaghan, P.L.; Beitz, A.J. An ultrastructural description of glutamate-like immunoreactivity in the rat cerebellar cortex. *Brain Res.* **1987**, *421*, 343–348. [CrossRef]
31. Gao, Q.T.; Cheung, J.K.; Li, J.; Jiang, Z.Y.; Chu, G.K.; Duan, R.; Cheung, A.W.; Zhao, K.J.; Choi, R.C.; Dong, T.T.; et al. A Chinese herbal decoction, Danggui Buxue Tang, activates extracellular signal-regulated kinase in cultured T-lymphocytes. *FEBS Lett.* **2007**, *581*, 5087–5093. [CrossRef] [PubMed]
32. Kang, H.; Ahn, K.S.; Cho, C.; Bae, H.S. Immunomodulatory effect of Astragali Radix extract on murine TH1/TH2 cell lineage development. *Biol. Pharm. Bull.* **2004**, *27*, 1946–1950. [CrossRef] [PubMed]
33. Ikemoto, K.; Utsunomiya, T.; Ball, M.A.; Kobayashi, M.; Pollard, R.B.; Suzuki, F. Protective effect of shigyaku-to, a traditional Chinese herbal medicine, on the infection of herpes simplex virus type 1 (HSV-1) in mice. *Experientia* **1994**, *50*, 456–460. [CrossRef] [PubMed]
34. Suzuki, F.; Kobayashi, M.; Komatsu, Y.; Kato, A.; Pollard, R.B. Keishi-ka-kei-to, a traditional Chinese herbal medicine, inhibits pulmonary metastasis of B16 melanoma. *Anticancer Res.* **1997**, *17*, 873–878. [PubMed]

35. Yang, P.; Jin, S.A.; Che, L.J.; He, S.M.; Yuan, Y. Study on effect of four traditional Chinese medicines distributed along lung meridian on TLR2 and NF-κB expressions in mice with lung heat syndrome. *China J. Chin. Mater. Medica* **2014**, *39*, 3359–3362.
36. Zhang, Q.; Li, T.; Xu, Y.G.; Yang, X.H. Effect of Chinese herbs used in treating multiple sclerosis on T subsets using association rules. *Chin. J. Integr. Tradit. West. Med.* **2016**, *36*, 425–429.
37. Oka, H.; Ohno, N.; Iwanaga, S.; Izumi, S.; Kawakita, T.; Nomoto, K.; Yadomae, T. Characterization of mitogenic substances in the hot water extracts of bupleuri radix. *Biol. Pharm. Bull.* **1995**, *18*, 757–765. [CrossRef] [PubMed]
38. Yang, F.; Dong, X.; Yin, X.; Wang, W.; You, L.; Ni, J. Radix Bupleuri: A review of traditional uses, botany, phytochemistry, pharmacology, and toxicology. *BioMed Res. Int.* **2017**, *2017*, 7597596. [CrossRef] [PubMed]

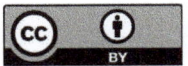

© 2018 by the authors. Licensee MDPI, Basel, Switzerland. This article is an open access article distributed under the terms and conditions of the Creative Commons Attribution (CC BY) license (http://creativecommons.org/licenses/by/4.0/).

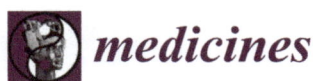

Article

Optimisation of the Microwave-Assisted Ethanol Extraction of Saponins from Gac (*Momordica cochinchinensis* Spreng.) Seeds

Anh V. Le [1,2,*], Sophie E. Parks [1,3], Minh H. Nguyen [1,4] and Paul D. Roach [1]

1. School of Environmental and Life Sciences, University of Newcastle, Ourimbah, NSW 2258, Australia; sophie.parks@dpi.nsw.gov.au (S.E.P.); Minh.Nguyen@newcastle.edu.au (M.H.N.); Paul.Roach@newcastle.edu.au (P.D.R.)
2. Faculty of Bio-Food Technology and Environment, University of Technology (HUTECH), HCMC 700000, Vietnam
3. Central Coast Primary Industries Centre, NSW Department of Primary Industries, Ourimbah, NSW 2258, Australia
4. School of Science and Health, Western Sydney University, Penrith, NSW 2751, Australia
* Correspondence: vananh.le@uon.edu.au

Received: 6 June 2018; Accepted: 1 July 2018; Published: 3 July 2018

Abstract: Background: Gac (*Momordica cochinchinensis* Spreng.) seeds contain saponins that are reportedly medicinal. It was hypothesised that the extraction of saponins from powdered Gac seed kernels could be optimised using microwave-assisted extraction (MAE) with ethanol as the extraction solvent. The aim was to determine an appropriate ethanol concentration, ratio of solvent to seed powder and microwave power and time for extraction. Whether or not defatting the Gac seed powder had an impact on the extraction of saponins, was also determined. **Methods**: Ethanol concentrations ranged from 60–100% were used to compare total saponins content (TSC) extracted from full-fat and defatted Gac seeds. Ratios of solvent to Gac seeds ranged from 10 to 100 mL g^{-1} and microwave conditions ranged from 1–4 cycles at power levels ranged from 360–720 W, were examined successively to evaluate their efficiency in extracting saponins from full-fat Gac seeds. **Results**: A four-fold higher of TSC was obtained in extracts from full-fat Gac seed powder than from defatted powder (100 vs. 26 mg aescin equivalents (AE) per gram of Gac seeds). The optimal parameters for the extraction of saponins were a ratio of 30 mL of 100% absolute ethanol per g of full-fat Gac seed powder with the microwave set at 360 W for three irradiation cycles of 10 s power ON and 15 s power OFF per cycle. **Conclusions**: Gac seed saponins could be efficiently extracted using MAE. Full-fat powder of the seed kernels is recommended to be used for a better yield of saponins. The optimised MAE conditions are recommended for the extraction of enriched saponins from Gac seeds for potential application in the nutraceutical and pharmaceutical industries.

Keywords: Gac seeds; *Momordica cochinchinensis*; saponins; microwave-assisted extraction; optimization

1. Introduction

Momordica cochinchinensis Spreng. is a perennial climber, which belongs to the Cucurbitaceae family. It ranges from China to the Moluccas and has been used in food and traditional medicine in East and Southeast Asia [1]. The most important part of the mature fruit is the red flesh surrounding the seeds, called the aril, which is used as a colorant in rice or as a material for further processing into functional food ingredients. The seeds are not eaten and they are removed from the aril and are mostly considered waste [2]. However, in traditional medicine, Gac seeds are alleged to have a wide array of therapeutic effects for a wide variety of conditions, including fluxes, liver and spleen disorders, hemorrhoids, wounds, bruises, inflammation, swelling and infections [1,3]. Modern science has reported biological activities for Gac seed extracts, including being a gastroprotective agent [4,5] and accelerating the healing of gastric ulcers in rats [6], and possessing antitumour [7], anticancer [8] and anti-inflammatory [9,10] activities.

Gac seed saponins have been reported to be critical constituents in Gac seed extracts, which were responsible for their medicinal properties [9,11]. These constituents of Gac seeds have been investigated by several investigators: two saponins, referred to as momordica saponin I and II, have been isolated and characterised [12], in which momordica saponin I is a major gastroprotective ingredient [5]. Another saponin, karounidiol, a compound possessing cytotoxic activity against human cancer cell lines [13], has been reported to be present in Gac seeds [14]. The potential valuable pharmaceutical properties of the Gac seed saponins warrants investigating how they are best extracted from the seeds i.e., which extraction technique(s) will maximise the yield of saponins.

The conventional extraction technique, in which the solid material is suspended in extraction solvent with no assistance for breaking the cell structure of the solid material, is often associated with a long heating time, which risks the degradation of bioactive compounds. This has led to the proposed use of advanced techniques such as microwave-assisted extraction (MAE) and ultrasonic-assisted extraction (UAE) that are efficient in terms of extraction time and solvent consumption. Microwave heating or ultrasonic cavitation is able to disrupt the plant cell structure via an increase in the internal pressure of the cell and thereby, release the bioactive compounds [15,16]. However, in a comparative study being carried out by the same authors [17], it was found that while the MAE significantly improved Gac seed saponin extraction in comparison to the conventional method, UAE did not. MAE, therefore, is the technique which needs to be further optimised. The MAE method is likely to be effective for the extraction of saponins from the Gac seeds, as it has been reported that microwave assistance significantly improved the recovery of saponins from a wide range of plant sources such as *Phyllanthus amarus* [18], yellow horn [19], *Ganoderma atrum* [20], chick pea [21] and ginseng [22], among others.

The choice of the extraction solvent is also important. Low alcohols such as methanol and ethanol have usually been used as effective solvents for the extraction of saponins from plant materials. However, according to the US Food and Drug Administration [23], methanol belongs to the Class 2 solvents, which should be limited in pharmaceutical products because of their inherent toxicity. Ethanol, on the other hand, belongs to the Class 3 solvents [23], which are less toxic and of lower risk to human health and therefore, should be used instead of methanol for the extraction of plant bioactive compounds. Moreover, ethanol in form of wines has been traditionally used for maceration of Gac seeds, therefore, it is reasonable to investigate the efficiency of this solvent for modern extraction methods. In addition, ethanol is also an excellent microwave absorbing solvent and has been used to advantage in MAE [16].

When it comes to extraction of saponins from seeds, defatting is often carried out before the saponins are extracted [24]. Although the defatting might make it simpler for the saponin extraction in terms of technique, and does not greatly affect the saponin yield for some type of seeds, it can cause a great loss of saponin for others.

Therefore, in this study, the extraction of saponins from powdered Gac seed kernels was optimised using MAE with ethanol as the extraction solvent. The aim was to determine an appropriate ethanol concentration, ratio of solvent to seed powder and microwave power and time for saponin extraction. Whether or not defatting the Gac seed powder had an impact on the extraction of saponins, was also determined.

2. Materials and Methods

2.1. Materials

2.1.1. Solvents, Reagents and Chemicals

Absolute ethanol ($\geq$99.8%), methanol and chemicals including vanillin, sulphuric acid, and potassium persulfate were products of Merck (Bayswater, VIC, Australia) and 2,4,6-tris(2-pyridyl)-*s*-triazine; ($\pm$)-6-hydroxy-2,5,7,8-tetramethylchromane-2carboxylic acid (trolox), aescin, 2,2-diphenyl-1-picrylhydrazyl (DPPH), 2,2'-Azino-bis(3ethylbenzothiazoline-6-sulfonic acid) diammonium salt (ABTS) were products of Sigma-Aldrich Co. (Castle Hill, NSW, Australia).

2.1.2. Gac Seed Kernel Powder

Gac seeds, were collected from 450 kg of fresh Gac fruit, from accession VS7 as classified by Wimalasiri, Piva, Urban and Huynh [25]. These fruits were bought at Gac fruit farms in Dong Nai province, Ho Chi Minh city, Vietnam (Latitude: 10.757410; Longitude: 106.673439). After their separation from the fresh fruit, the seeds were vacuum dried at 40 °C for 24 h to reduce moisture and increase the crispness of the shell to facilitate shell removal. The dried seeds were de-coated to obtain the kernels, which were then packaged in vacuum-sealed aluminum bags and stored at -18 °C prior to use.

2.1.3. Preparation of Gac Seed Kernel Powder

The Gac seed kernels were ground in an electric grinder (100 g ST-02A Mulry Disintegrator), to produce powder, which could pass through a sieve of 1.4 mm. The powder was then freeze-dried using a Dynavac FD3 freeze dryer (Sydney, NSW, Australia) for 48 h at -45 °C under vacuum at a pressure loading of 10^{-2} mbar (1 Pa) to reduce the moisture content to 1.21 ± 0.02%, as determined using a MOC63u moisture analyser (Shimazdu, Kyoto, Japan). This Gac seed kernel powder was referred to as 'full-fat powder' and was stored in vacuum-sealed polyethylene bags under vacuum at -20 °C until used.

2.1.4. Preparation of Defatted Gac Seed Kernel Powder

To prepare defatted Gac seed kernel powder, the freeze-dried kernel powder was extracted three times for thirty minutes with hexane (1:5 w/v) on a magnetic stirrer at room temperature. Each time, the resulting slurry was suction-filtered and the final residue was air-dried for 12 h and stored in a desiccator at ambient temperature until used. This Gac seed kernel powder was referred to as 'defatted powder'.

2.2. Methods

The experimental design for the study is shown in Figure 1.

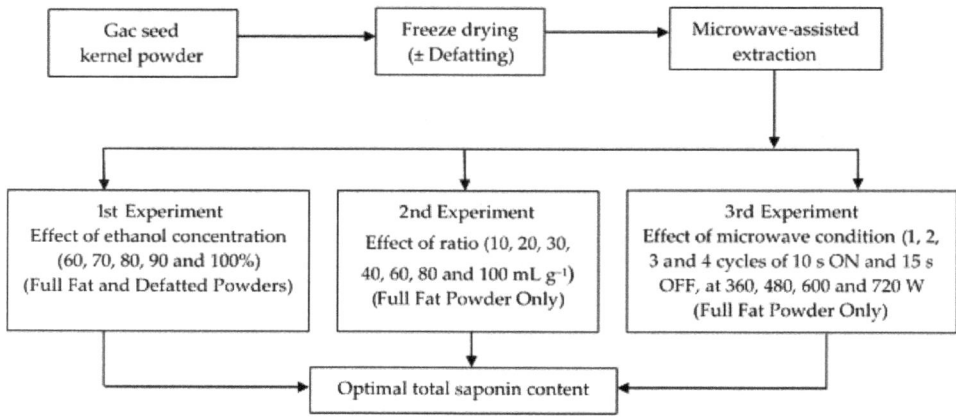

Figure 1. Experimental design for optimisation of saponin yield from Gac seeds.

2.2.1. Microwave Assisted Extraction (MAE)

The MAE was performed using a R395YS Sharp Carousel microwave oven (Sharp Corporation, Bangkok, Thailand) bought from a local Target store (Tuggerah, NSW, Australia). Gac seed kernel powder was mixed with ethanol of various concentrations with water in a 100 mL conical flask. The suspension was left pre-leaching for 30 min at ambient temperature before microwave treatment was applied for varying number of cycles, which consisted of 10 s power ON and 15 s power OFF per cycle. The temperature of the suspension was recorded at the end of the MAE process.

2.2.2. Extraction of Saponins from Full-Fat and Defatted Gac Seed Kernel Powders

Prior to weighing for extraction, the moisture content of the powder samples was measured using a MOC63u moisture analyser (Shimazdu, Kyoto, Japan), which was used in the determination of saponin yield.

The effect of the ethanol concentration was investigated for the MAE of saponins from both the full-fat and the defatted powders. The concentration of ethanol was varied (60%, 70%, 80%, 90% and 100%) but the solvent to powder ratio and the microwaving conditions were kept constant at 30 mL g^{-1} and 600 W for four cycles, respectively (1st experiment in Figure 1). After finishing the extractions, the suspensions were rapidly cooled to $\leq$20 °C in an ice water bath and filtered through a 0.45 µm membrane filter. The clear extracts were collected and kept at -20 °C for analysis within a week.

2.2.3. Extraction of Saponins from the Full-Fat Seed Kernel Powder

The full-fat powder was selected for the following two experiments since it resulted in a higher extraction of saponins for all the concentrations of ethanol; and 100% absolute ethanol was chosen because it resulted in the highest extraction of saponins from the full-fat powder.

Two experiments (Figure 1) were done using the full-fat powder and 100% ethanol as the extraction solvent to determine the effect of three individual parameters, (i) the ratio of solvent to powder (10, 20, 30, 40, 60, 80 and 100 mL g^{-1}) (Figure 1, 2nd Experiment), (ii) microwave radiation power (360, 480, 600, 720 and 840 W) and (iii) microwave irradiation time (1, 2, 3 and four cycles) (Figure 1, 3rd Experiment), on the recovery of saponins from the Gac seed kernel powder was investigated. When one parameter was examined, the other was maintained constant; for the 2nd experiment (Figure 1), the microwave conditions were 600 W with four cycles and for the 3rd experiment, the ratio of ethanol to powder was 30 mL g^{-1}. After finishing the extractions, the suspensions were rapidly cooled to

≤20 °C in an ice water bath and filtered through a 0.45 μm membrane filter. The clear extracts were collected and kept at −20 °C for less than a week before analysis.

2.2.4. Verifying Optimal Conditions for Gac Seed Saponin Extraction

From the findings in the 3rd experiment, two possible optimal sets of microwave parameters were chosen for the extraction of saponins from the full-fat powder. Therefore, these two sets of microwave parameters were repeated to validate the findings. A control (no microwave) extract was also run with 100% ethanol and the optimal solvent to powder ratio but where the heat was provided using a water bath instead of the microwave oven. The water bath temperature was chosen to be 76 °C and the incubation was done for 100 s because it was the maximum temperature and incubation time achieved during the MAE using the two sets of microwave parameters. These three extracts were analysed for TSC and antioxidant capacity–measured with two assays, ABTS and DPPH. The energy consumption for these extracts was also estimated according to the Equation (1) as follows:

$$W_i = P_i \times t_i \tag{1}$$

where W_i is the consumed electrical energy for the extraction method (kWh), P_i is the electrical power supplied for the extraction method (kW) and t_i is the electricity consumption time for the extraction method (h).

2.3. Analytical Methods

2.3.1. Determination of Total Saponin Content (TSC)

Determination of the total saponin content was conducted using the colorimetric method of Hiai, Oura and Nakajima [26] with slight modifications. The principle of this method is the reaction of sulphuric acid-oxidised saponins with vanillin to produce a distinctive red-purple colour, which is measured at 560 nm using a spectrophotometer.

To 0.25 mL of the appropriately diluted Gac seed ethanol extract samples, 0.25 mL 8% vanillin in ethanol (w/v) was added followed by 2.5 mL of 72% H_2SO_4 (v/v). The test tube was vortexed, covered, incubated at 60 °C for 15 min and cooled to ambient temperature in an iced-water bucket for 2 min. With a reagent blank as reference, the absorbance was measured at 560 nm using a Carry 50 Bio spectrophotometer (Varian Pty. Ltd., Mulgrave, VIC, Australia).

A standard curve of aescin (100–1000 μg/mL) was constructed to determine the saponin concentrations. The results were expressed as mg aescin equivalents (AE) per gram dry weight of Gac seed kernel powder (mg AE g^{-1}).

2.3.2. Determination of Antioxidant Capacity

The antioxidant capacity was tested for the optimal and control extracts using two assays: ABTS and DPPH.

ABTS Assay

The ABTS assay [27] was used as described by Tan et al. [28] with slight modifications. Stock solutions of 7.4 mM ABTS and 2.6 mM potassium persulfate were prepared and kept at 4 °C until use. Fresh working solution was prepared for each assay by mixing the 2 stock solutions in equal quantities and incubating them for 15 h in the dark at ambient temperature. Then, 1 mL of the working solution was diluted with ~30 mL of methanol to obtain an absorbance of 1.1 ± 0.02 units at 734 nm. To 0.15 mL of each standard, blank and appropriately diluted extract sample, 2.85 mL of the working solution was added. The tubes were incubated for 2 h in the dark at ambient temperature and the absorption was measured at 734 nm using a Carry 50 Bio spectrophotometer (Varian Pty. Ltd., Mulgrave, VIC,

Australia). Trolox was used as the standard and the results were expressed as mg Trolox equivalents per gram dry weight of Gac seed kernel powder (mg TE g^{-1}).

DPPH Assay

The DPPH assay [29] was used as described by Tan et al. [28]. A stock solution of 0.6 M DPPH in methanol was prepared and kept at $-20\ °C$ until use. The working solution was prepared by mixing 10 mL of stock solution with ~45 mL of methanol to obtain an absorbance of 1.1 ± 0.02 units at 515 nm. To 0.15 mL of each standard, blank and appropriately diluted extract sample, 2.85 mL of the working solution was added. The tubes were allowed to stand for 3 h in the dark at ambient temperature and the absorption was measured at 515 nm using a Carry 50 Bio spectrophotometer (Varian Pty. Ltd., Mulgrave, VIC, Australia). Trolox was used as the standard and results were expressed as mg Trolox equivalents per gram of dry weight Gac seed kernel powder (mg TE g^{-1}).

2.4. Statistical Analyses

Experiments were performed in triplicate and values were expressed as means $\pm$ SD and were assessed for statistical significance using the one-way ANOVA and Tukey's *Post Hoc* Multiple Comparison test using the IBM SPSS Statistics 24 program (IBM Corp., Armonk, NY, USA). Correlation and regression analyses were done using Microsoft Excel 2016. Differences between means, correlations and regressions were considered statistically significant at $p < 0.05$.

3. Results

3.1. Effect of the Ethanol Concentration on the MAE of Saponins from Full-Fat and Defatted Gac Seed Kernel Powders

The full-fat and defatted Gac seed kernel powders were extracted using MAE with the ethanol concentration ranging from 60% to 100% (in water) in the extraction solvent. Figure 2 shows that at the lower ethanol concentrations, from 60% to 80%, there was no significant difference in the measured TSC for the full-fat powder. The measured TSC was higher with 90% ethanol and the highest (100.3 mg AE g^{-1}) with 100% ethanol as the extraction solvent. In contrast, changing the ethanol concentration from 60% to 100% did not increase the measured TSC of the defatted Gac seed kernel powder, which was lower than for the full-fat powder for all the ethanol concentrations. Therefore, the full-fat Gac seed kernel powder and 100% absolute ethanol, as the extraction solvent, gave the best MAE extraction of saponins and they were used in the subsequent experiments.

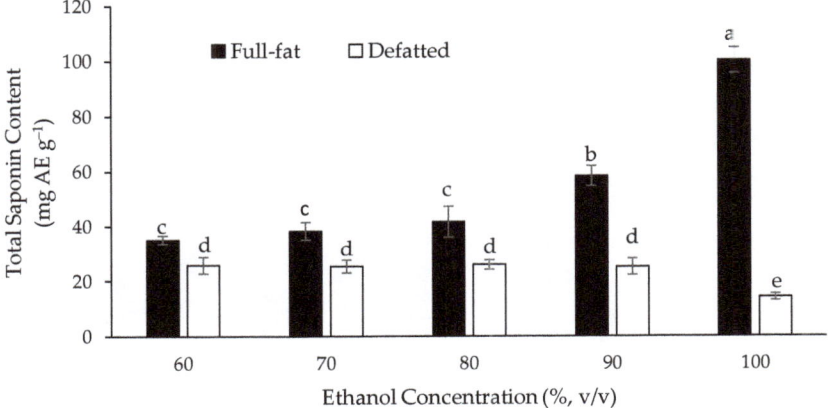

Figure 2. Effect of the ethanol concentration, in the extraction solvent used for microwave-assisted extraction (MAE), on the measured total saponin content (TSC) of the full-fat and defatted Gac seed kernel powders. The values are the means of three replicates for each extraction and columns not sharing the same superscript letter are significantly different at $p < 0.05$.

3.2. Effect of the Ethanol to Sample Ratio on the MAE of Saponins from the Full-Fat Gac Seed Kernel Powder

Seven ratios of 100% absolute ethanol to full-fat powder, from 10 to 100 mL g^{-1}, were investigated. Figure 3 shows that increasing the ratio from 10 to 30 mL g^{-1} had a significant effect on the measure TSC value after MAE, which increased by 30% from 70.4 to 100.8 mg AE g^{-1}. However, increasing the ratio from 30 to 100 mL g^{-1} resulted in less pronounced increases in the measured TSC. Therefore, although the measured TSC was slightly and significantly higher with the ratio of 100 mL g^{-1} compared to 30 mL g^{-1} (Figure 3), the ratio of ethanol to powder of 30 mL g^{-1} was deemed to be the better ratio, from the conservation of solvent perspective, and it was chosen for investigating the microwave parameters.

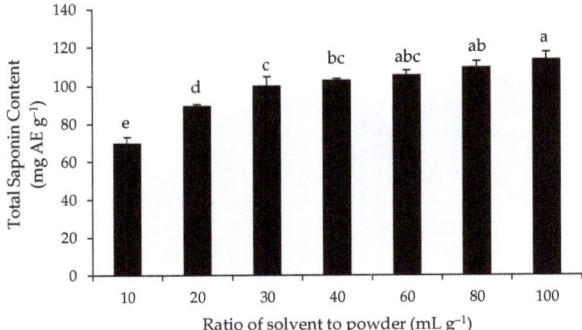

Figure 3. Effect of the ethanol to powder ratio on the TSC of the full-fat Gac seed kernel powder measured using MAE. The values are the means of three replicates for each extraction and columns not sharing the same superscript letter are significantly different at $p < 0.05$.

3.3. Effect of the Microwave Parameters on the MAE of Saponins from the Full-Fat Gac Seed Kernel Powder

Four levels of microwave power (360, 480, 600 and 720 W) were investigated and at every power level, the number of irradiation cycles was also varied (1, 2, 3 and four cycles). Each cycle consisted of 10 s power ON (irradiation) followed by 15 s power OFF (no irradiation). The full-fat powder was used and the ratio of 100% ethanol to powder was 30 mL g^{-1}. In general, Figure 4 shows that the measured TSC gradually increased as the power and irradiation time were increased for the MAE but that many of the values were not significantly different from each other. Notably, from 600 W to two cycles upwards (to the right in Figure 4), there was no significant increase in the measured TSC values. However, the two sets of parameters, which only shared the a superscript in Figure 4, 360 W and three cycles and 480 W and four cycles, were selected as possibly optimal for the MAE extraction of saponins from the full-fat Gac seed kernel powder.

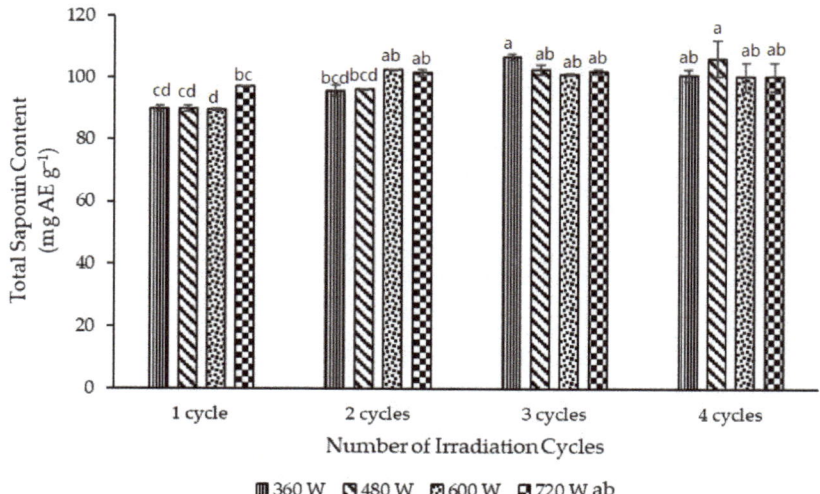

Figure 4. Effect of microwave power and irradiation time (cycles) on the TSC of the full-fat Gac seed kernel powder measured using MAE. The values are the means of three replicates for each extraction and columns not sharing the same superscript letter are significantly different at $p < 0.05$.

3.4. Correlations between the TSC and the MAE Temperature

The temperature of the extracts at the end of each MAE in Figure 4 was recorded using a digital thermometer. Their temperature ranged from 43.4 to 75.6 °C. Correlation analysis revealed that the measured TSC of the extracts was positively correlated with the temperature of the extraction mixture at the end of the MAE (Figure 5).

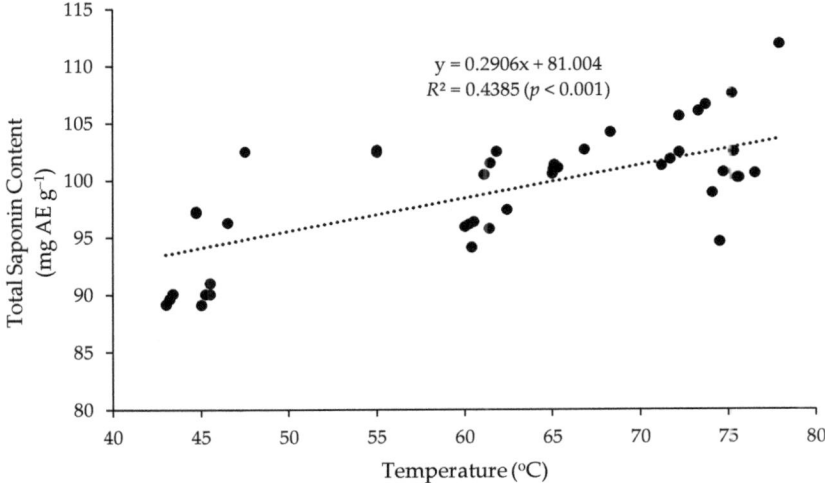

Figure 5. Correlation between the TSC and the temperature of the extract at the end of various MAE treatments. The black dots: TSC at different temperature of the extracts.

Table 1 shows that the temperature of the extracts at the end of the MAE was almost all due (92.5%) to the number of irradiation cycles (length of the microwave irradiation time) during the MAE; in contrast, there was no correlation between the temperature and the microwave power. Consisted with this, the measured TSC of the extracts was positively correlated with the number of microwave irradiation cycles but wasn't correlated with the power used during the MAE. Moreover, there was no interaction between the microwave power and the number of irradiation cycles.

Table 1. Correlations between the TSC and the MAE parameters.

	R^2 (p Value)			
	TSC	Number of Cycle	Power	Cycle and Power
Temperature	0.439 ($p < 0.001$)	0.925 ($p < 0.001$)	0.002 ($p > 0.5$)	0.926 ($p < 0.001$)
Number of cycle	0.362 ($p < 0.001$)	-	-	-
Power	0.000 ($p > 0.5$)	-	-	-
Cycle and Power	0.188 ($p > 0.1$)	-	-	-

3.5. Verification of the Optimal MAE Conditions for the Extraction of Saponins from Full-Fat Gac Seed Kernel Powder

Two possible optimal sets of microwave parameters (360 W and three cycles, 480 W and four cycles) were chosen for the extraction of saponins from the full-fat powder (Figure 4). Notably, the temperature measured at the end of the MAE using the two sets of microwave parameters (360 W and three cycles, 480 W and four cycles) was 72.2 ± 1.2 and 75.6 ± 1.9 °C, respectively, and they were not significantly different from each other.

These two sets of microwave parameters were repeated to validate the findings. A control (no microwave) set of extracts was also run with 100% ethanol and the optimal solvent to powder ratio where the temperature measured at the 480 W and four cycles MAE (76 °C) was provided using a water bath instead of the microwave oven. Also, the time used for the control extraction was chosen to be 100 s in order to match the length of time used for the 480 W and four cycles MAE.

These three sets of extracts were analysed for their saponin content and their ABTS and DPPH antioxidant activities. The results revealed that there was no difference among the three extracts in saponin content and antioxidant capacity (Table 2). However, the ABTS values were low and the DPPH assay did not detect any antioxidant activity for any of these extracts (Table 2).

Table 2. Saponin content, antioxidant activities and energy consumption of the optimal MAE and control extracts.

Extract	TSC (mg AE g^{-1})	ABTS (μmol TE g^{-1})	DPPH (μmol TE g^{-1})	Energy Consumption (kWh)
Optimal treatment 1 [†]	105.69 ± 2.40 [a]	1.47 ± 0.12 [a]	Undetected	0.003
Optimal treatment 2 [‡]	109.23 ± 2.69 [a]	1.80 ± 0.31 [a]	Undetected	0.005
Control (no microwave) [§]	109.64 ± 4.79 [a]	1.63 ± 0.10 [a]	Undetected	0.325

The results are mean values ± standard deviations (n = 3) and the values not sharing the same superscript letter in the same column, are significantly different at $p < 0.05$. [†] Ethanol + Full-fat powder (30 mL g^{-1}); MAE at 360 W, three cycles for 75 s. [‡] Ethanol + Full-fat powder (30 mL g^{-1}); MAE at 480 W, four cycles for 100 s. [§] Ethanol + Full-fat powder (30 mL g^{-1}); Shaking water bath at 76 °C for 100 s.

From the point of view of saving energy, the optimal treatment 1 MAE parameters (Table 2) of 360 W with three irradiation cycles of 10 s power ON and 15 s power OFF per cycle (total of 75 s), were the best microwave conditions for the extraction of saponins from full-fat Gac seed kernel powder (0.003 kWh). The conventional extraction for 100 s in a shaking water bath at the same temperature (76 °C) as at the end of the optimal treatment 2 MAE settings also gave the same results but this also required more energy than the optimal treatment 1 MAE parameters because of the energy needed (0.325 kWh) to bring the temperature of the 5 L water bath from 20 °C up to 76 °C.

4. Discussion and Conclusions

The full-fat Gac seed kernel powder was the more suitable material to use as defatting caused a considerable loss of saponins (~75%). The highest TSC of extracts were obtained with 100% absolute ethanol, a 30 mL g^{-1} ratio of ethanol to full-fat Gac seed kernel powder and several sets of MAE conditions. Furthermore, when two sets of the MAE parameters, which gave the highest measured TSC in the extracts, were re-tested, the two extracts had the same TSC. However, from the point of view of saving energy, the optimal 1 MAE parameters of 360 W with three irradiation cycles of 10 s power ON and 15 s power OFF per cycle (total of 75 s), were the best conditions for the extraction of saponins from the full-fat powder.

It was concluded that, to extract Gac seed saponins, it was better to use the full-fat seed kernel powder rather than kernel powder from which the fat had been extracted. The Gac seed saponins appeared to be mainly associated with the fat component of the seeds because they were largely lost during the defatting process with hexane. Undoubtedly, most of the Gac seed saponins (75%) were highly non-polar, which is consistent with a previous finding that saponins were found in the unsaponifiable matter from Gac seed oil [14]. The saponin content of the full-fat Gac seed kernels was also similar to that reported for other oily plant extracts, such as eucalyptus [30] and *Phyllanthus amarus* [31], and significantly higher than the non-oily extract from the flesh of bitter melon [28].

Absolute ethanol was found to be the best concentration of ethanol for extracting the saponins from the full-fat Gac seed kernel powder. This is also consistent with the Gac seed saponins being hydrophobic in nature and consistent with Gac seeds having a high fat content [32]. This result is also consistent with the earlier findings that Gac seed oil has a high content of unsaponifiable matter [33] and that this unsaponifiable material contains triterpenoid saponins [14]. It may be that more non-polar class 3 solvents, such as 1-propanol, isobutyl alcohol and n-butanol, could further improve the extraction of saponins from full-fat Gac seed kernels. However, because of the higher costs of these solvents, ethanol would be the solvent of choice for recovery of the Gac seed saponins on economic grounds.

The ratio of 30 mL ethanol per 1 g of Gac seed powder was the ratio of choice because, at this ratio, the saponin yield was improved significantly compared to the two lower ratios and there was not much improvement at the higher ratios. Although it varies for different plant materials, in the conventional extraction method, the higher the ratio of solvent volume to solid sample the better the extraction of compounds is. However, in the case of MAE, a higher solvent: sample ratio may not necessarily give a better yield due to non-uniform distribution and exposure to microwaves [16].

Varying the MAE parameters did not greatly affect the saponin extraction, mostly likely due to ethanol being a very good solvent [16] for the extraction of the Gac seed saponins and for increasing in temperature even under mild microwave conditions. When the optimal MAE conditions were compared with a control extraction (no microwave), it was found that the same level of saponin extraction was achieved irrespective of the heating source. However, from the point of view of saving energy, the optimal 1 MAE parameters were the best conditions for the extraction of saponins from full-fat Gac seed kernel powder. The energy saving characteristic of MAE has been confirmed in numerous reports [15]. This is due to the heat is generated inside the materials and then comes outwards, whereas in conventional heating the surface is heated first. Thus, the microwave heating is rapid and effective as heat is transferred directly to the material.

The antioxidant capacity of the Gac seed saponin extracts was low. This is possibly due to the more lipophilic nature of the Gac seed saponins, which is consistent with the findings that lipophilic compounds such as carotenoids, which do not show DPPH-radical scavenging activity [34], and tocopherols, which do not show much activity in the ABTS assay [35].

In conclusion, this study demonstrated that the extraction parameters play an important role in the extraction of saponins from Gac seeds. Accordingly, the MAE optimal parameters for the extraction of saponins were a ratio of 30 mL of 100% absolute ethanol per g of full-fat Gac seed kernel powder with the microwave set at 360 W for three irradiation cycles of 10 s power ON and 15 s power OFF per cycle. These parameters are recommended for the extraction of enriched saponins from Gac seeds for potential application in the nutraceutical and pharmaceutical industries.

Author Contributions: Conceptualization, A.V.L., M.H.N. and P.D.R.; Methodology, A.V.L.; Validation, A.V.L.; Formal Analysis, A.V.L.; Investigation, A.V.L.; Data Curation, A.V.L. and P.D.R.; Writing-Original Draft Preparation, A.V.L.; Writing-Review & Editing, P.D.R., M.H.N. and S.E.P.; Supervision, P.D.R., M.H.N. and S.E.P.

Funding: This research received no external funding.

Acknowledgments: A.V.L. acknowledges the University of Newcastle and VIED for their financial support.

Conflicts of Interest: The authors declare no conflict of interest.

References

1. Perry, L.M.M. *Medicinal Plants of East Southeast Asia: Attributed Properties and Uses*; MIT Press: Cambridge, MA, USA, 1980.
2. Chuyen, H.V.; Nguyen, M.H.; Roach, P.D.; Golding, J.B.; Parks, S.E. Gac fruit (*Momordica cochinchinensis* Spreng.): A rich source of bioactive compounds and its potential health benefits. *Int. J. Food Sci. Technol.* **2015**, *50*, 567–577. [CrossRef]
3. Yin, M.H.; Kang, D.G.; Choi, D.H.; Kwon, T.O.; Lee, H.S. Screening of vasorelaxant activity of some medicinal plants used in Oriental medicines. *J. Ethnopharmacol.* **2005**, *99*, 113–117. [CrossRef] [PubMed]
4. Kang, J.M.; Kim, N.; Kim, B.; Kim, J.-H.; Lee, B.-Y.; Park, J.H.; Lee, M.K.; Lee, H.S.; Jang, I.-J.; Kim, J.S. Gastroprotective action of *Cochinchina momordica* seed extract is mediated by activation of CGRP and inhibition of cPLA2/5-LOX pathway. *Dig. Dis. Sci.* **2009**, *54*, 2549–2560. [CrossRef] [PubMed]
5. Jung, K.; Chin, Y.-W.; Chung, Y.H.; Park, Y.H.; Yoo, H.; Min, D.S.; Lee, B.; Kim, J. Anti-gastritis and wound healing effects of *Momordicae semen* extract and its active component. *Immunopharmacol. Immunotoxicol.* **2013**, *35*, 126–132. [CrossRef] [PubMed]
6. Kang, J.M.; Kim, N.; Kim, B.; Kim, J.-H.; Lee, B.-Y.; Park, J.H.; Lee, M.K.; Lee, H.S.; Kim, J.S.; Jung, H.C. Enhancement of gastric ulcer healing and angiogenesis by *Cochinchina momordica* seed extract in rats. *J. Korean Med. Sci.* **2010**, *25*, 875–881. [CrossRef] [PubMed]

7. Tien, P.G.; Kayama, F.; Konishi, F.; Tamemoto, H.; Kasono, K.; Hung, N.T.K.; Kuroki, M.; Ishikawa, S.-E.; Van, C.N.; Kawakami, M. Inhibition of tumor growth and angiogenesis by water extract of Gac fruit (*Momordica cochinchinensis* Spreng.). *Int. J. Oncol.* **2005**, *26*, 881–889. [CrossRef] [PubMed]
8. Zheng, L.; Zhang, Y.-M.; Zhan, Y.-Z.; Liu, C.-X. *Momordica cochinchinensis* seed extracts suppress migration and invasion of human breast cancer ZR-75-30 cells via down-regulating MMP-2 and MMP-9. *Asian Pac. J. Cancer Prev.* **2014**, *15*, 1105–1110. [CrossRef] [PubMed]
9. Yu, J.S.; Kim, J.H.; Lee, S.; Jung, K.; Kim, K.H.; Cho, J.Y. Src/Syk-Targeted Anti-inflammatory actions of *Triterpenoidal saponins* from Gac (*Momordica cochinchinensis*) seeds. *Am. J. Chin. Med.* **2017**, *45*, 1–15. [CrossRef] [PubMed]
10. Jung, K.; Chin, Y.-W.; Yoon, K.D.; Chae, H.-S.; Kim, C.Y.; Yoo, H.; Kim, J. Anti-inflammatory properties of a triterpenoidal glycoside from *Momordica cochinchinensis* in LPS-stimulated macrophages. *Immunopharmacol. Immunotoxicol.* **2013**, *35*, 8–14. [CrossRef] [PubMed]
11. Yu, J.S.; Roh, H.-S.; Lee, S.; Jung, K.; Baek, K.-H.; Kim, K.H. Antiproliferative effect of *Momordica cochinchinensis* seeds on human lung cancer cells and isolation of the major constituents. *Rev. Bras. Farmacogn.* **2017**, *27*, 329–333. [CrossRef]
12. Masayo, I.; Hikaru, O.; Tatsuo, Y.; Masako, T.; Yoshie, R.; Shuji, H.; Kunihide, M.; Ryuichi, H. Studies on the constituents of *Momordica cochinchinensis* Spreng. I. Isolation and characterization of the seed saponins, Momordica saponins I and II. *Chem. Pharm. Bull.* **1985**, *33*, 464–478.
13. Akihisa, T.; Tokuda, H.; Ichiishi, E.; Mukainaka, T.; Toriumi, M.; Ukiya, M.; Yasukawa, K.; Nishino, H. Anti-tumor promoting effects of multiflorane-type triterpenoids and cytotoxic activity of karounidiol against human cancer cell lines. *Cancer Lett.* **2001**, *173*, 9–14. [CrossRef]
14. Kan, L.; Hu, Q.; Chao, Z.; Song, X.; Cao, X. Chemical constituents of unsaponifiable matter from seed oil of *Momordica cochinchinensis*. *China J. Chin. Mater. Med.* **2006**, *31*, 1441–1444.
15. Desai, P.J.; Parikh, P. Extraction of natural products using microwaves as a heat source. *Sep. Purif. Rev.* **2010**, *39*, 1–32. [CrossRef]
16. Tatke, P.; Jaiswal, Y. An overview of microwave assisted extraction and its applications in herbal drug research. *Res. J. Med. Plant* **2011**, *5*, 21–31. [CrossRef]
17. Le, A.V.; Roach, P.D.; Nguyen, M.H.; Parks, S.E. The microwave- and ultrasonic-assisted aqueous extraction of bioactive compounds from Gac (*Momordica cochinchinensis* S.) seeds. In Proceedings of the 4th World Congress on Medicinal Plants and Natural Products Research, Osaka, Japan, 8–9 August 2018.
18. Nguyen, V.T.; Bowyer, M.C.; Van Altena, I.A.; Scarlett, C.J. Microwave-assisted extraction as an advanced technique for optimization of saponin yield and antioxidant potential from *Phyllanthus amarus*. *Sep. Sci. Technol.* **2017**, *52*, 2721–2731. [CrossRef]
19. Li, J.; Zu, Y.-G.; Fu, Y.-J.; Yang, Y.-C.; Li, S.-M.; Li, Z.-N.; Wink, M. Optimization of microwave-assisted extraction of *Triterpene saponins* from defatted residue of yellow horn (*Xanthoceras sorbifolia* Bunge.) kernel and evaluation of its antioxidant activity. *Innov. Food Sci. Emerg. Technol.* **2010**, *11*, 637–643. [CrossRef]
20. Chen, Y.; Xie, M.-Y.; Gong, X.-F. Microwave-assisted extraction used for the isolation of total *Triterpenoid saponins* from *Ganoderma atrum*. *J. Food Eng.* **2007**, *81*, 162–170. [CrossRef]
21. Kerem, Z.; German-Shashoua, H.; Yarden, O. Microwave-assisted extraction of bioactive *saponins* from chickpea (*Cicer arietinum* L.). *J. Sci. Food Agric.* **2005**, *85*, 406–412. [CrossRef]
22. Kwon, J.-H.; Belanger, J.M.; Pare, J.J.; Yaylayan, V.A. Application of the microwave-assisted process (MAP™☆) to the fast extraction of ginseng *saponins*. *Food Res. Int.* **2003**, *36*, 491–498. [CrossRef]
23. Food and Drug Administration. Guidance for Industry: Q3C—Tables and List. In *USHaH Services*; Food and Drug Administration: Silver Spring, MD, USA, 2012.
24. Cheok, C.Y.; Salman, H.A.K.; Sulaiman, R. Extraction and quantification of *saponins*: A review. *Food Res. Int.* **2014**, *59*, 16–40. [CrossRef]
25. Wimalasiri, D.; Piva, T.; Urban, S.; Huynh, T. Morphological and genetic diversity of *Momordica cochinchinensis* (Cucurbitaceae) in Vietnam and Thailand. *Genet. Resour. Crop Evol.* **2016**, *63*, 19–33. [CrossRef]
26. Hiai, S.; Oura, H.; Nakajima, T. Color reaction of some *sapogenins* and *saponins* with vanillin and sulfuric acid. *Planta Med.* **1976**, *29*, 116–122. [CrossRef] [PubMed]
27. Re, R.; Pellegrini, N.; Proteggente, A.; Pannala, A.; Yang, M.; Rice-Evans, C. Antioxidant activity applying an improved ABTS radical *Cation decolorization* assay. *Free Radic. Biol. Med.* **1999**, *26*, 1231–1237. [CrossRef]

28. Tan Vuong, Q.V.; Stathopoulos, C.E.; Parks, S.E.; Roach, P.D. Optimized aqueous extraction of *saponins* from bitter melon for production of a saponin-enriched bitter melon powder. *J. Food Sci.* **2014**, *79*, E1372–E1381.
29. Blois, M.S. Antioxidant determinations by the use of a stable free radical. *Nature* **1958**, *131*, 1199. [CrossRef]
30. Bhuyan, D.J.; Vuong, Q.V.; Chalmers, A.C.; van Altena, I.A.; Bowyer, M.C.; Scarlett, C.J. Investigation of phytochemicals and antioxidant capacity of selected Eucalyptus species using conventional extraction. *Chem. Pap.* **2016**, *70*, 567–575. [CrossRef]
31. Pham, H.N.T.; Bowyer, M.C.; van Altena, I.A.; Scarlett, C.J. Influence of solvents and novel extraction methods on bioactive compounds and antioxidant capacity of *Phyllanthus amarus*. *Chem. Pap.* **2016**, *70*, 556–566.
32. Ishida, B.K.; Turner, C.; Chapman, M.H.; McKeon, T.A. Fatty acid and carotenoid composition of Gac (*Momordica cochinchinensis* Spreng.) fruit. *J. Agric. Food Chem.* **2004**, *52*, 274–279. [CrossRef] [PubMed]
33. Le, A.V.; Roach, P.D.; Nguyen, M.H.; Parks, S.E. Optimisation of process parameters for supercritical carbon dioxide extraction of oil from Gac seed kernel powder. *Adv. J. Food Sci. Technol.* **2017**, *13*, 170–177. [CrossRef]
34. Müller, L.; Fröhlich, K.; Böhm, V. Comparative antioxidant activities of carotenoids measured by ferric reducing antioxidant power (FRAP), ABTS bleaching assay (αTEAC), DPPH assay and peroxyl radical scavenging assay. *Food Chem.* **2011**, *129*, 139–148. [CrossRef]
35. Aguilar-Garcia, C.; Gavino, G.; Baragano-Mosqueda, M.; Hevia, P.; Gavino, V.C. Correlation of tocopherol, tocotrienol, γ-oryzanol and total polyphenol content in rice bran with different antioxidant capacity assays. *Food Chem.* **2007**, *102*, 1228–1232. [CrossRef]

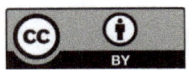

© 2018 by the authors. Licensee MDPI, Basel, Switzerland. This article is an open access article distributed under the terms and conditions of the Creative Commons Attribution (CC BY) license (http://creativecommons.org/licenses/by/4.0/).

MDPI
St. Alban-Anlage 66
4052 Basel
Switzerland
Tel. +41 61 683 77 34
Fax +41 61 302 89 18
www.mdpi.com

Medicines Editorial Office
E-mail: medicines@mdpi.com
www.mdpi.com/journal/medicines

www.ingramcontent.com/pod-product-compliance
Lightning Source LLC
LaVergne TN
LVHW070647100526
838202LV00013B/904